MW01120777

The Hevert Collection

DIETETICS
of NATUROPATHIC MEDICINE

In Their Own Words

Dear Dr. Snow
you are an inspiration to us all!.

[signature] 2015.

The Hevert Collection

DIETETICS
of NATUROPATHIC
MEDICINE

In Their Own Words

Edited by SUSSANNA CZERANKO, ND, BBE
Foreword by BETTY RADELET, ND

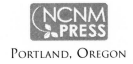

PORTLAND, OREGON

Managing Editor: Sandra Snyder, Ph.D.
Production: Fourth Lloyd Productions, LLC.
Design: Richard Stodart

Cover photo: Louisa Lust

© 2014 by NCNM Press
All rights reserved. No part of this book may be reproduced or transmitted
in any form or by any means, electronic or mechanical, including photocopying,
recording, or by any information storage and retrieval system, without the prior
written permission of the publisher, except where permitted by law.

Published by NCNM Press
National College of Natural Medicine
049 SW Porter Street
Portland, Oregon 97201, USA
www.ncnm.edu

NCNM Press gratefully acknowledges the generous and prescient financial
support of HEVERT USA which has made possible the creation and
distribution of the *In Their Own Words* historical series.
The HEVERT COLLECTION comprises twelve historical compilations which
preserve for the healing professions significant and representational works
from contributors to the historical Benedict Lust journals.

Printed in the United States of America

ISBN: 978-0-9771435-4-2
0-9771435-4-6

The early Naturopaths who built the basis of our nutritional knowledge and its clinical application left a precious trail to follow. *Dietetics of Naturopathic Medicine* is especially dedicated to these pioneers of our profession and to present and future Naturopaths who know that healthy food means healthy people.

TABLE OF CONTENTS

FOREWORD

Congratulations! You're reading this book! It will change your life!

It may even save your life or the life of someone you love. It can't get better than that! Carry on, you're in for a treat!

Though I've been a Naturopathic Physician for 45 years, I've already made some changes that I'm expecting to make my life better, and perhaps extend it.

Dr. Czeranko, N.D. has done an outstanding work of gleaning from our forebears valued and important concepts in relation to dietetics.

What worked in 1913 also works a century later!

The human body is still the same—same needs, same reactions, same results.

Sebastian Kneipp said: "Most of the diseases and cases of ill-health so prevalent in our times may be traced to our incorrect habits of living, and to our accustomed unhealthful diet."

You'll learn how and when to fast, how to treat a fever, take care of a cold, the flu and more.

Your stomach cannot talk! But it lets you know when you've made some wrong choices.

We all eat too much, too fast and unwisely.

What is Fletcherizing?

Watch for adulteration, so prevalent and deadly.

Are you over-weight?

Are you familiar with *unfired* foods?

Who are the Apyrtrophers?

Who is this book for? *You*, of course.

What benefit to *You*? As much as you'll apply it.

Where from here? One step at a time. Keep plodding.

Why is it important? Our daily food is continually necessary, and our choices ever before us. We need to be knowledgeable and have determination to persist, so our latter years are truly *golden* and free from the common exigencies of old age.

How can you accomplish this? Read, and reread this book, digest it and make it yours, physically, mentally, experimentally, actually.

It will be worth every minute.

BON VOYAGE!

Betty Radelet, N.D.
NCNM Class of 1968

A POEM
by Dr. Betty Radelet

Send a smile to your Liver
And kind thoughts to your Spleen
Three cheers to your Kidneys
That keep your Blood so clean

    Speak peace to your Lungs
    Double honor to your Heart
    With its many miles of vessels
    Air and food to every part.

A grand salute to your Brain
The Director Supreme
Of Pancreas, Adrenals
Keeps them working like a dream.

    Many bows to your Stomach
    Keep it happy and content
    'Twill make your life worthwhile
    Ev'ry day and ev'ry moment.

A merry grin for your Bladder
Its best friend is H_2O
Together rid the toxins
From your head down to your toe.

    Save a laugh for your bowels
    Be sure to move them daily
    A necessary job
    Removing all debris.

Your body is a blessing.
God's royal gift to you.
So praise and thank Him daily
For all it can, and does do.

PREFACE

Dietetics of Naturopathic Medicine is the third of the twelve book Hevert Collection series, *In Their Own Words*. This volume highlights many important articles found in the journals published by Benedict Lust from 1900 to 1923 that have become foundational to current dietetic principles. Lust published continuously for fifty years until his death. His commitment to spread the word about health in America did not falter for a second. Diet became unquestionably the most important focus of the early Naturopaths as they grappled with disease and lifestyle habits. It is not surprising to those who know about naturopathic medicine, but important to note nevertheless, that diet was first recognized by the Naturopaths as the key determinant of health and disease. The dialogue on dietetics left behind many more articles than could be squeezed into *Dietetics of Naturopathic Medicine*. Articles on the subject of food and diet dominate the pages of *The Naturopath and Herald of Health*. Mining the rich content of these early works may surprise the contemporary reader in that many of our current ideas of a healthy diet originated over a century ago. As we ponder the shocking state of food production, distribution and preparation today, and it sinks in that our food supply now includes over 10,000 food additives, our complacency regarding food becomes alarming. Yet, even before our era of agri-business and GMOs, when the early Naturopaths first encountered the relatively few additives and preservatives finding their way into the food chain, they collectively mounted an outcry and galvanized their efforts to educate and guide their patients back to health through food.

Vegetarianism (known by our forebears as 'abstinence from flesh foods') was the healthy diet embraced and advocated by the early Naturopaths. It did not take long for the early profession to establish dietary rules to guide their patients in the selection and preparation of wholesome foods which they viewed as vegetarian-based. Nor did it take them long to get creative and formulate different paths to vegetarianism. Today's new rage of raw food and vegan diets is neither unique nor new. In fact, a vegetarian diet of raw food was first promoted by Eugene Christian over a century ago. He paid dearly for his dietary beliefs with outrageous fines and even an arrest in 1907 (thankfully retracted the following year).

By 1913 a regular monthly column appeared featuring George Drews and his dietary regime called Apyrotrophy (from Greek root words meaning unfired food). There are many similarities in the mission of the early Apyrotrophs and today's Permaculturists. Both recognized and cherished the relationship between the environment and the biodiversity of food. Today, we are familiar once again with the taglines of sustainability, land stewardship and the promotion of healthy environmental practices. The naturopaths you will meet in these pages promoted such ideas and approaches to food more than ten decades ago.

Henry Lindlahr advocated a moderate version of vegetarianism which he instituted in his Nature Cure therapies. His wife, Anna, wrote often on the merits of vegetarianism as did Louise Lust who offered guidance in menu planning for those unfamiliar with the vegetarian way of life. Another crystal clear message came from Arnold Ehret who endorsed the mucusless diet comprised of a vegetarian diet of fruits and nuts. His book is still in print to this day and was one of the first books in my dietetics library many decades ago.

Dr. Betty Radelet, the oldest woman Naturopath living in North America today, is a testament to the supremacy of the vegetarian diet. Dr. Betty is in her 94th year and has abided by a strict vegetarian diet since she became a Naturopath in 1968. She has adopted a strictly vegan raw food diet providing her vitality that the rest of us only hope for as we approach the tenth decade of life. When visiting with Dr. Betty to share stories and visions, it is customary to drink tea which she brews. This has been her custom with visitors for over half a century. The tea is delicious. I would like to share her recipe with you.

DR. BETTY RADELET'S TEA

6-7 cloves
Ginger the size of a knuckle sliced thinly
1 stick of cinnamon
2 cups of water

Add all the ingredients into a small pot and simmer for 15 minutes. Strain and add 1 to 2 tablespoons (according to taste) to a cup of hot water and enjoy. Store the remainder in the refrigerator and use daily.

What struck me during my work on *Dietetics of Naturopathic Medicine* were the conviction, clarity and resolve that the early Naturopaths had for health through diet. They were zealous and determined to help their fellows in achieving healthy life habits for themselves and for future generations. Many of the articles in this collection were chosen because they were the first to appear in print on the subject and help us understand the longevity of food as a health determinant. These articles have messages that are as pertinent today as when they were written a hundred years ago. Although disease patterns have changed, one looming causative factor of disease formation has not budged at all, and that is over eating. Today, obesity is chronic, literally bursting at the seams, threatening the welfare of future generations. This book will offer guidance, tools and inspiration for the naturopathic doctor eager to find a prominent place for dietetics in a naturopathic practice.

So many people have their finger prints all over these pages. Without their hard work, this book would still be chugging along somewhere a thousand pages back. I am deeply grateful for the support of my colleague, Dr. Rick Severson, a gifted, dedicated librarian, educator and archivist. His ears listened to my tales when I confronted obstacles along this journey. Dr. Severson would unclutter the path. He knows to convert a barrier into an opportunity, how to locate missing issues which were long felt to be lost (especially issues from 1906 and 1907). We got them, and thus the Benedict Lust journals at NCNM are now one spectacular, coherent and complete, unique collection. He never doubted this project for a nanosecond. His encouragement and guidance make him the rock star of naturopathic medical education library directors. I have been blessed to have had a colleague who is so supportive of this work.

Inside the glossy book cover are hundreds of typed pages which were patiently transcribed by many wonderful students at NCNM. In fact, there are over 1000 articles typed from the Benedict Lust journals in preparation for this and forthcoming books in this series. There are many more articles still in queue as this series emerges. I want to acknowledge every one of those special NCNM students who typed or proof read articles while simultaneously navigating intense course loads and juggling their personal lives. Huge heaps of intense gratitude to *Abendigo Reebs, Adam Dombrowski, Alla Nicolulius, Allison Brumley, Anemone Fresh, Angela Carlson, Avishan Saberian, Delia Sewell, Delores Stephens, Derrick Schull, Elizabeth Wade, Erin Conlon, January Bourassa, Joshua Corn, Katelyn Mudry, Katherine Venegas, Kirsten Carle, Lisa Fortes-Schramm, Lucy-Kate Reeve, Meagan Watts, Megan Hammel, Michelle Brown-Echerd, Natalie Paravicini, Node Smith, Olif Wojciechowski, Rachel Caplan, Renae Rogers, Stephanie Woods, Tina Dreisbach,* and all those whom I am inadvertently missing here. I so much enjoyed working with each and every student who sacrificed scarce, precious study and leisure time for the hard work of meticulous research and transcription. As you launch yourselves into the Naturopathic profession, never forget how special and important your work has been. You have chosen a path of sacred work. You will be loved and cherished by your patients because you listen and truly care. Remember Nature!

I am especially indebted to the tireless work of *Dr. Karis Tressel* who was my diva of anti-chaos and who brought sublime organization and order to the colossal stacks of paper and minutia. Without Karis' exquisite, patient and detailed sense of clarity, I would be gray haired and frazzled. I am deeply grateful for her profound love of Nature Cure and her loving tenacity with this project.

I am very grateful for the unwavering, behind the scenes support of the Board of NCNM, Dr. Sandra Snyder, Susan Hunter, Nora Sande and Jerry Bores who understood from the beginning the importance of this project. Many thanks to Alison Derico for her timely, invaluable assistance during the end stages of reframing and finishing the draft of this manuscript.

I applaud Fourth Lloyd Productions, Nancy and Richard Stodart, my designers and coaches extraordinaire who guided me with alacrity every step of the way. Thank you both for the exquisite care that you took in every minute detail!

This book would be an historical curiosity and irrelevant to the contemporary health landscape, were it not for the thousands of Naturopaths working in their communities keeping the philosophy of our medicine alive. You took the path of nature in the health professions. Your patients know that your work and dedication are a testament that Naturopathic Medicine is as critical now as a century ago when our extraordinary naturopathic pioneers chose to walk a different path.

Lastly, I want to thank my husband, David Schleich, who typically saw the ending from the beginning and much sooner than I could. Writing takes a lot of energy and I am deeply grateful that David shares my love of history and listens to my stories with awe and deep appreciation. He always helps me find my way back to the present when I need to return from my beloved books in the NCNM archive.

You may be reading some sentences written by these early naturopaths that are a mile long, or embellished with words no longer in the current lexicon. Fear not; this is on purpose. These articles have been carefully transcribed and edited to ensure that you are taken back into time and experiencing the actual idioms, vocabulary, syntax and all. So, settle back in a comfortable chair with some of Dr. Betty's tea and enjoy these articles chosen from our pioneering elders *in their own words*.

Blessings,
Sussanna Czeranko, ND, BBE
Portland, Oregon, January 7, 2014

Introduction

The only safe guide in eating is hunger, "not appetite"; this is nature's sign that more food is needed, and that the organism is in condition to take care of it.
—Henry Lindlahr, 1908, 304

If three meals are eaten, the heartiest meal should be taken at midday. The breakfast should be substantial, the evening meal very light, especially avoiding pastry, fats, rich sauces, and hearty foods.
—John Harvey Kellogg, 1908, 321

When the organs of digestion are continually overworked, they weaken and are unable to convert the over-supply of food into the proper constituents for healthy blood and lymph; waste matter accumulates, creating noxious gases and systematic poisons.
—Benedict Lust, 1910, 611

About 90% of all human disease originates in the stomach, caused by errors in eating.
—Eugene Christian, 1912, 6

The most natural factor of every healing process, the instinctive self-help, is to stop eating, whether from accident or chronic disease. Animals do this intuitively.
—Arnold Ehret, 1919, 145

Cooking, when not properly done, destroys the vital or life principle of the food.
—Louise Lust, 1921, 323

If the early Naturopaths had a consistent and pervasive message, it was that diet is the foundation of lifelong health. From this strong conviction, the pursuit of the definitive diet was from the earliest days of the profession a central quest. Today, many others have at times confused and overwhelmed their audiences with new diets, cookbooks and celebrity cooks, the sheer volume and diversity of which information, fads, guidelines and warnings the early Naturopaths and the modern Naturopathic doctor must work hard to help their patients navigate. In such a landscape one diet book can counter another: whole grains or not; paleo or not; vegan or somewhere in between; food pyramids; calorie counters, and cleverly written labels.

What we learn from the early literature, however, is that the naturopathic doctors of the early 1900s were focused from the outset on assembling a reliable, unified dietary message. To be sure, it varied in point of view, but nevertheless illustrated the perennial obsession then and now with diet. For example, vegetarian diets were widely promoted, but so too were the diet regimens of the Apyrotrophers, whose raw food recommendations look remarkably familiar even today. As the years went by and a wider array of options surfaced and spread, we discover in the old literature the focus on dietetics among our early Naturopaths. Their writing about food filled to the brim the pages of *The Naturopath and Herald of Health*.

Diet choice was incrementally complicated in the new twentieth century by the growing economic success which the scaling of agri-business brought, by the growing economic pressures of profit-sensitive shelf-life, and by the high environmental cost of continent-wide distribution funnels supplying wholesale and retail markets. These food products were aimed at consumers increasingly alienated from their food sources. Year round selection, seductive taste, texture and choice augmented consumption and skewed quality. Naturopathic doctors in our own era know that today's food, despite ubiquitous availability and variety, is not the food of our forebears. Naturopathic doctors from a century ago knew that vigilance about food was increasingly important. Contemporary Naturopathic doctors have the same concern.

Among other factors today is that there are over 10,000 food additives in the modern food supply. Food labels often have unpronounceable, unfamiliar, confusingly quantified ingredients. Globally marketed, processed food products, coupled with environmental degradation affecting their production, have generated huge problems within the food systems of both the developed and the undeveloped worlds. Populations all over the planet face chronic epidemics of obesity, allergies, diabetes, hypertension, cancer, and auto-immune disorders among other chronic diseases, many of which the early and the modern Naturopathic doctor attribute to poor dietary habits.

It is not surprising, then, that "Dietetics" constituted the main therapeutic focus of many early Naturopathic Doctors. At the same time, however, the record shows that their dietary counsel was frequently vilified by the allopathic establishment who considered such health guidance as a danger to the public and, at the same time, who considered the naturopaths a threat to their hegemony. Indeed, the literature of the period documents how many early Naturopaths experienced punitive fines and jail terms for their work, including dietetics. In some of the articles in *Origins of Naturopathic Medicine*, the first volume of this series, we encountered records of this kind of vindictive onslaught by the allopathic medical associations of the period, directed against Naturopaths who prescribed vegetarian diets and provided other dietary counsel and therapeutic alternatives to pharmaceuticals and invasive surgeries.

Despite such a political climate, the journals published by Benedict Lust reveal a rich record of dietary advice and research. He and his contemporaries examined every aspect of eating, nourishment and nutrition. Their numerous articles on diet reflect a mission to help their patients choose, prepare and eat nutritiously across a lifetime, from infancy to vital old age. For decades, the influential Lust journal articles addressed many diet questions. Indeed, contributors to these remarkable journals insisted that "most of the diseases and cases of ill-health so prevalent in our times [1900] may be traced to our incorrect habits of living and to our accustomed unhealthful diet." (Lust, 1900, 14)

Our survey of this highly relevant literature begins with the very first article published by Benedict Lust on diet. In it, he extolled the work of Father Sebastian Kneipp. Lust reported in this early piece that Kneipp returned "to a simple, plain, appropriate diet calling attention to the most natural and nourishing foods at our command and the proper way of preparing and using them." (Lust, 1900, 14) He was indebted to Father Kneipp for his own rebound from death and wrote with respect, and admiration about Kneipp's legacy and about his methods of healing. By then Lust had established in New York City one of the first health food stores offering Kneipp herbs and stone milled Kneipp bread, both of which were extensively advertised in his journal. In this first article, Lust gives instruction on the preparation of the genuine, unfermented Kneipp Health Bread and on Kneipp's Strengthening Soup. Kneipp Health Bread was touted as "the best and most nourishing bread made to-day; a boon for dyspeptics and sufferers from constipation." (Lust, 1900, 14)

Another doctor indebted to Father Kneipp was Friedrich Bilz who by the late 19th century had already established a very large sanitarium in Germany and had authored an impressive two-volume encyclopedia of natural healing. Bilz considered "food or diet [as] the most important question in nursing the sick" (Bilz, 1900, 118) and recommended food that did not place a burden on the stomach. Digestion was important, but so too was the subsequent absorption of nutrients. He reminds us, "We do not live upon what we eat and digest ... but solely and entirely upon what is actually assimilated by the body." (Bilz, 1900, 118) At the same time, it is perhaps surprising to learn that over eating was perceived as a problem a century ago too, considering the low incidence of obesity at the time. Bilz observed that "many illnesses arise in consequence of general overfeeding." (Bilz, 1900, 118)

We discover in this literature that a common admonition repeated by these early Naturopaths to patients was that they avoid gorging and over-eating. Lust explains, "People who are in the habit of gorging themselves every day should better fast one day in each week, thus they would give their overworked digestive organs a little rest and many diseases, beginning with stomach-troubles would be prevented." (Lust, 1901, 27) In this regard, digestive issues such as constipation were attributed to "wrong modes of living, overfeeding when not hungry, hot and rich food, pepper, mustard, coffee or too much meat. ... Just the same as the body needs daily nourishment, it also needs daily evacuation." (Lust, 1901, 28)

Lust weighed in often and vigorously on the subject of how to balance eating with illness, and elaborates with details of non-stimulating diets. We can see across the hundreds of articles appearing in his journals the beginnings of a consolidation of the elements of an early dietetic science. He states, "For instance, in many cases the body is overloaded with albumen, fat, etc., and there is deficiency of carbohydrates, salts, and water; in other cases the cause of illness being perhaps exactly the reverse." (Lust, 1904, 173) Careful observation of the patient and his or her diet "must be remedied by a suitable combination of foods." (Lust, 1904, 173)

Drinking excess fluids as a detriment to health was also caused by over eating. Excessive eating was associated with over working the digestive organs resulting in the incomplete metabolism of food left in the body "creating noxious gases and systemic poisonings." (Lust, 1910, 611) Lust continues, these waste matters "contaminate the vital fluid, causing corruption and obstruction in organs and tissues." (Lust, 1910, 611)

The vegetarian diet was at the forefront of the naturopathic movement and a key tool in the treatment of such eating disorders. The so-called "non-stimulating diet" recommended for those suffering with ailments consisted mainly of vegetarian food, especially gruels and soups, which were prescribed depending upon the desired effect. For example, "rice gruel is often useful in cases of diarrhoea. ...An oaten [gruel] has proved itself to be the most certain restorative, and is even efficacious in cases where all other so-called tonics leave us in the lurch; I know no better remedy for building up a broken down constitution." (Lust, 1904, 173-174)

Throughout Lust's journals in addition to well known fare such as gruels and soups, we continuously discover new foods and products to combat sickness. For example, we find an article written on the topic of olive oil as a remedy, reflecting on the somewhat adventurous efforts of the early Naturopaths in their search for health food selections. As presented in *Dietetics of Naturopathic Medicine*, they recommended a vast array of foods was recommended by the early Naturopaths for incorporation into a healthy diet, accompanied by various applications or forms of use. Today, for example, olive oil has become an ubiquitous kitchen staple, yet in 1900 it was used both topically and internally as an excellent remedy for numerous conditions such as laryngitis and hoarseness, dyspepsia, gastric ulcers and diphtheria. (Lust, 1900, 36) As a topical ointment, olive oil was rubbed on the body to relieve inflammation, pain, and fever. To resolve phlegm, Lust explained, "one teaspoon in the morning and in the afternoon will effect a cure." (Lust, 1900, 36)

The coconut as a food was also well known to the Naturopath a century ago. Other nuts such as almonds, walnuts and pine kernels were prepared to make delicious creams and ambrosia. The allure of vegetarianism and novel food items a century ago inspired many recipes. For example, in his article, *Cocoa Bread*, Ammann offers a recipe for a raw bread made from fresh grated 'cocoanut' and rolled oats. Cocoa reminds us of chocolate but the word actually refers to the humble coconut. The recipe did not call for any liquid; rather, what was very important was to press the bread using heavy weights or even a wine press. "This dry mixture, wrapped up in a cotton cloth, is put into a flat form … smoothed out so as to be of the same thickness all over, sandwiched in between two boards and then left under a rather intense pressure for from 3 to 10 hours." (Ammann, 1918, 176) The "cocoa bread is good only when fresh, and therefore, the supply for the day should be made either on the night before or early in the morning." (Ammann, 1918, 176)

The topic of vegetarian diets, inclusive of such new foods to the North American palate, was addressed from the start as the Naturopathic profession emerged, embracing nutrition as the key element of health. For example, in one of the earlier issues of *The Kneipp Water-Cure Monthly,* Lust introduced the benefits of consuming nuts as an excellent substitute for animal protein. Nuts as a food and relished by many, was relatively inexpensive and easily digested. Before long, the Naturopaths seized the opportunity to use nuts in numerous ways. Lust wrote this article on nuts to promote a new food that today we see in every kitchen: nut butters. In 1900, nut butters were being manufactured widely, but the Naturopaths cautioned their patients that "on account of the temperature at which they are produced, a change takes place in the oil, rendering the fat more or less indigestible to certain individuals." (Lust, 1900, 141) From the very beginning, our Naturopathic pioneers educated their patients and each other not only about a wide variety of nutrient sources, but also about appropriate preparation and use.

In this regard, another nut product to capture the attention of the early Naturopathic vegetarian was recommended: "Nut Marmalate and nutlet [are] foods put up in sealed cans, and have a growing popularity. These foods are excellent sliced, or can be made up into stews with potatoes or various other vegetables." (Lust, 1900, 141) These new prepared products were considered superior to raw nuts because they were "more digestible than raw nuts." (Lust, 1900, 141)

Nuts mixed with malt, made to be tasty as a snack, were another option, but Lust and his contemporaries cautioned against such snacks if they were adulterated with less healthy ingredients. Lust explains, when speaking of such snacks, that there were healthy choices available. He writes, "Nuts are combined with predigested starch in the form of malt sugar." (Lust, 1900, 142) Taking one healthy ingredient combined with less desirable ones has been a ploy of the food industry to convince us of the healthy properties of snack foods. Lust saw these malted nut snacks as a healthier choice, "almost pure nutrition, and the starch part being already digested and the nut food thoroughly cooked, they are an excellent food for cases of weak digestion." (Lust, 1900, 142)

Another food that received much attention was bread. Bread was considered a major staple of the diet. Farming practices were still relatively natural, akin to contemporary organic production. Today, however, most conventional farming practices incorporate genetic modifications to crops, involve heavy pesticide and artificial fertilizer use, and are accompanied by the over processing of foods. This cascade of economically motivated activity has generated a significant stigma against wheat and gluten, which are responsible for many adverse reactions by those who eat GMO grains. Naturopathic Doctors have been warning their patients about hybridized and genetically modified grain products for decades and only recently have some latecomer bio-medicine professionals begun weighing in on this severe food supply and consumption problem. These concerns appear in our early literature often.

In the 19th century, for example, flour manufacturing practices underwent a transformation that lead to the introduction of very fine white flour which assured more reliable production, storage and shelf life advantages. These developments triggered widely reported alarm among the early Naturopaths. They recognized immediately the cumulatively disastrous consequences of removing some of the most nutritious elements during the milling process. As a case in point, Henry Lahn recounts the history of the roller mill system. He writes: "The roller mill system (1878) made possible the production of the refined white flour consumed in such enormous quantities by a misguided public today." (Lahn, 1921, 67) The advantages of such milling practices paid huge dividends to suppliers and processors, an economic phenomenon also seen today. "The fact that the fine white flour has much greater keeping qualities than the darker whole grain flour, thus allowing greater amounts to be milled and stored, had an important bearing on this increased production." (Lahn, 1921, 67) Lahn includes more historical insights into milling practices around the world in his article, *Grits Versus Bread*.

The milling practices of a century ago involved not only wheat. Lahn reports, "50 to 75% of the organic salts in the kernel, were not only confined to the wheat grains, but also to barley, rice and other cereals which were peeled and polished to 'improve' the appearance." (Lahn, 1921, 69) To counter these practices, he offers excellent suggestions and recipes for the preparation of grits both for unfired [raw] and cooked grits.

Buettgenbach recounts, "The flour produced by the small mills a quarter of a century ago, retained much more of the nutritive properties of the wheat, than that milled by our so-called improved and patented mills of to-day." (Buettgenbach, 1900, 228)   Buettgenbach cites a story of a dog fed on "bread baked from the finest and whitest flour, mixed with water. After thirty days the dog would not eat this food any more, and ten days later he died—while another dog ... was fed with graham-flour" (Buettgenbach, 1900, 229) and lived enjoying good health. In the human community, white flour was often the culprit for "ailments such as indigestion, constipation, stomach and bowel troubles." (Buettgenbach, 1900, 229) Gluten Graham bread was touted as a simple food that was "very easily digested and very nourishing." (Lust, 1905, 316) Graham flour retained all its nutrients in the process of milling.

As illustrated by Buettgenbach's work, the food message of the early Naturopaths was always for wholesome foods and against highly processed products, such as those emerging from a transforming grains industry. When it came to a grain staple, such as rice for example, the Naturopaths favored unpolished rice which was "ten times as rich in organic salts as the polished rice of commerce." (Carqué, 1906, 36) The criticism of the rice manufacturing process by the Naturopaths was not about its presentation as a product; rather, it was grounded in nutrition concerns. As Carqué writes, "Fashion demands rice having a fine gloss, just for appearance's sake. ... The rice is put through the polishing process which removes some of the most nutritious parts of the rice grains, especially fat and some very important organic salts, as those of iron, magnesium, and silicon." (Carqué, 1906, 35) Carqué adds, "The parts removed by the polishing process are nearly twice as valuable for food as polished rice." (Carqué, 1906, 35)

The Naturopaths of that era had many such suggestions related to nutrition. Take onions, for example, yet another of many foods to assist digestion that the profession pointed to. In fact, they felt that onions were a favorite, a champion among foods. As Lust explains, onions may not have been for everyone's palate, but they were "easily digested [and] ensured the better digestion of other food, and increased the work of the organs designed to cleanse the body." (Lust, 1902, 468) Onions had other valuable properties too, they announced, such as being a "diuretic, dia-phoretic, carminative, and soporific." (Lust, 1902, 468) Lust declared, "Stick to onions if you wish to avoid the doctor sticking to you." (Lust, 1902, 468)

The early Naturopaths recognized individuality of diets and the uniqueness of each person's constitution. They collaborated with their patients to tailor dietary regimes, customized to individuals, and struc-tured to address where the patient was, in terms of health or disease. In the case of fever, as Lust points out, the Naturopath's interaction with the patient is quite specific to that individual, and "best ascertained by measuring his pulse and bodily warmth, for instance more than 100°F or more than 90 to 100 beats of the pulse, or whether he breathes more than 20 times in a minute." (Lust, 1901, 27) The diet for the fever or influenza patient recommended that "cooling beverages or light soups should be given ... for instance soup from boiled sour apples or natural lemonade, or even pure water—but only when there is desire." (Lust, 1901, 27-28) Soups such as Kneipp's Strengthening Soup [recipe found 1900, p. 14] or Whole-wheat-meal soup were efficacious for fevers and hemorrhoids.

No matter what the dietetic concern, Naturopaths had thoughtful, well researched, practical responses. Even water consumption did not escape their attention. In her article, *Should We Drink?* Sophie Leppel addresses the safety of water consumption. Recalling that clean water and good sewage facilities may not have always been available in urban environments in that era, Leppel's comments are especially poignant. She suggests the use of fruits and vegetables that were high in water content as a safe alternative to potentially bad water. She gives the example, "raw peeled cucumbers, eaten like apples, contain abundant juice and they cool without making thin." (Leppel, 1903, 88) Leppel discouraged water in the diet unless the source was assuredly pure and the quantities modest.

Another related, popular diet was Johan Schroth's "dry Schroth diet". "The theory on which Schroth worked was that when little or no liquid is taken the morbid humours in the body ... [are] gradually loosened and thrown off." (Gray, 1904, 184) Described as a regeneration treatment, the Schroth diet was considered excellent "for the removal of toxins and poisons of all kinds from the body." (Gray, 1904, 184)

In another early article, Sophie Leppel introduces a different way of looking at diet choice. The conventional diet, she explains, was comprised of bread, meat and potatoes. So, writing about vegetables was fairly novel. Leppel points out some of the benefits of including lemons, tomatoes, and juicy fruits into the diet. "Lemon-juice possesses curative properties beyond those of any other fruit or vegetable in common use." (Leppel, 1903, 88) Leppel advised that, rightly applied, lemon-juice dissolves hardened substances in the body such as tumours, fibroids, chalky deposits in the joints of the hand, feet, etc., and it powerfully assists digestion." (Leppel, 1903, 88) Leppel wrote about juices and other topics on several occasions in *The Naturopath*, adding to the growing repertoire of content on the subject of dietetics. She classified nuts and fruits by their property to improve brain function and energy, for example. The significance of this particular Leppel article is in how it depicts her preparation of nuts. For instance, Leppel soaked almonds before pounding them into a paste. Today, we have blenders and kitchen machines that have simplified this process. Nevertheless, in an era preceding such kitchen processors, Leppel creates and shares several interesting recipes using dried fruits and nuts for brain workers.

Another who studied the effects of foods on the brain was Dortch Campbell. Campbell dismisses those who "ridicule the idea that there is such a thing as 'brain food'. " (Campbell, 1913, 727) He continues, "We are all aware of the ancient superstition of the value of fish for brain nourishment." (Campbell, 1913, 727) Today, the use of EPA oils to enhance cognitive functions is an established fact and indicative of his prescient work. At the same time, he did not exactly agree with Sophie Leppel's views on stringent choices of fruits and nuts as the only exclusive brain foods. The list of foods that he considered useful for brain enhancement was more extensive and included: "lean meats, fish, milk, eggs, cheese, beans, peas, lentils, nuts and ... certain kinds of fruits." (Campbell, 1913, 727) He qualifies each of these foods in terms of quality and digestibility which diminishes his list to "the very best brain foods—pecans, filberts, walnuts, almonds, butternuts, pine nuts, etc." (Campbell, 1913, 728)

Another person who had much to contribute to the field of dietetics and endorsed whole grains was Scholta, who listed the benefits of some of the common foods of the era. For example, "oatmeal ... is an excellent nourishing food; it is the meat of the vegetable kingdom for the vegetarian."(Scholta, 1904, 139) Roasted oatmeal was especially useful for the promotion of bowel movements. Scholta, though, did not approve of cocoa especially since it was constipating. He agreed with Father Kneipp's assessment and warned against its use. "Cocoa swells in the intestines and forms a kind of paste, which produces constipation." (Scholta, 1904, 139)

While nuts were manufactured into various products, another food, milk, was examined for its protein content and its inclusion in the diet of children and adults. Lust created a table of nutritional values for cow, goat and human milk. In a footnote in this particular article, he reveals the importance of the first milk [colostrum] produced by a mother for her infant as the most important milk. He states, "The watery milk is specially adapted by a wise provision of nature to the digestive capacity of the child during the first days of its life." (Lust, 1900, 180)

The question is raised in this early literature about whether pasteurization was necessary to rid the milk of bacteria. With emphatic resolve, Lust opts for unpasteurized milk. "The best and right way is, of course, to drink it as nature provides it, fresh; and experience has shown that fresh milk is more readily drunk, better tolerated and more easily digested than milk which has been boiled." (Lust, 1900, 180) After exposure to high temperatures, milk will coagulate into lumps in the stomach and cause discomfort. (Lust, 1900, 180)

The early Naturopaths considered milk to be both good and bad, and there were many articles written about its consumption. For the most part, milk was considered a universal healing remedy for kidney and heart diseases, as well as for stomach abscesses, scrofula, anemia and nervousness. (Scholta, 1904, 140) However, caution needed to be exercised, the early Naturopaths warned. They cautioned against overfeeding babies with milk. Cooked or pasteurized milk was condemned, but "thick sour milk and kefyr milk [were considered] excellent beverages for the sick." (Scholta, 1904, 140) In one variation which appears in the literature, Henry Lahmann, promoted the use of "vegetable milk" for the development of children. In his article, *Dr. Lahmann's Vegetable Milk,* we can get a glimpse of an early movement toward dairy-free beverages, pioneered by Naturopathic doctors. Alas, there is no definitive record of the ingredients in vegetable milk, but it was referenced often, as in the work of Dr. Lahmann, as a way of avoiding the dangers of sterilized milk (and promoting his own product for use). He noted that the use of pasteurized milk accompanied a rise in "chronic bowel troubles ... caused by sterilization ... and new illnesses, like Barlow's (a combination of rickets and scrofula)." (Lahmann, 1909, 20)

In any case, milk a hundred years ago came from hormone free and drug free cows. Something called the "Milk Cure" was adopted by many of the early Naturopaths. However, Lindlahr was not one of these. He considered the milk cure as a fad and only appropriate for newborns. Lindlahr cautions, "A strict milk diet has a tendency to cause distension of the stomach, fermentation, biliousness and constipation, especially when the bowels are sluggish and the stomach weak and relaxed." (Lindlahr, 1910, 261) Naturopathic positions on milk consumption today move along a continuum which includes abstention by vegans to Weston Price followers who promote the health virtues of milk.

In an article written by Alice Reinhold, ND, the subject of milk alternatives is explored. She describes the health of children when raised on a pure vegetarian diet. As a Naturopath, she prescribed 'milk of the grain' to children when sick. The recipe for "hard wheat, yellow cornmeal, oatmeal or barley" (Reinhold, 1923, 31) milk provided an alternative to cow milk. The objection to cow milk was that the cows were vaccinated and considered unhealthy and artificial food.

Living in Portland, Oregon, Reinhold gives an account of where children could have benefited from the milk of grain. She reveals, "Just recently there was an epidemic of 'septic sore throat' among children in the suburbs of Portland, Ore., and twelve of the babies and small children died as the result." (Reinhold, 1923, 31) As vegetarian enthusiast, she affirms, "Wise, educated vegetarians take their food fresh from nature's hand and are not troubled with diseases." (Reinhold, 1923, 31)

Overall, diet as a preventative measure against disease was very clear to the early Naturopaths. "Diet is one of the most important questions for the sick as well as the healthy, as it is no doubt easier to prevent illness by a sensible way of living than to cure a disease that has once taken hold of us." (Lust, 1903, 226) Lust emphasized, "Diet is the essential factor in trying to keep this principle, [sensible way of living] as a great number of diseases originate only from poor and unwholesome food." (Lust, 1903, 226) And, Lust cautioned often, a good diet begins with Breakfast. He writes, "We should accustom ourselves from early childhood to eat sufficient and wholesome food in the morning." (Lust, 1903, 226) Coffee, though, as the only sustenance in the first meal was discouraged by Lust. He continues, "It is a very unwise custom of so many people to drink only coffee at breakfast." (Lust, 1903, 226) Instead, Lust suggested beverages at breakfast to include "Kneipp's malt coffee or one of the popular nourishing vegetable salt cocoas, Banana Coffee" (Lust, 1903, 227) and herbal teas.

Many Naturopaths advised that the correct way to begin the day was to eat flour soups. "Those having a good appetite may take some bread, or one or two soft boiled eggs, with their flour soup every morning." (Lust, 1903, 226) Flour soup used rye or whole wheat bread that "was well cooked with milk, water or butter." (Lust, 1903, 226) Naturopaths emphasized the inclusion of bran which made a heavier bread. "Country people eat mostly coarse dark bread, prepared from coarse rye flour (flour with bran) and of their own make, and to a great extent they are indebted for their good health, strength and endurance to this bread." (Lust, 1903, 227) He often wrote about the merits of dark coarse bread with such suggestions as, "It may be added that the coarser the bread the easier digested; the finer it is the more indigestible." (Lust, 1903, 227)

The dietary choices of what and what not to eat were most often presented quite clearly in the journal articles we encounter in the Lust journals. For example, Lust writes, "Condiments, spices, stimulants, pickles, iced-drinks, rich sauces and gravies, lard, glucose, white four, all such panderings to appetite rather than satisfying of hunger, Naturopathy rejects and condemns." (Lust, 1903, 247) In a 1903 article, *Health Incarnate,* Lust even proposes a list of dietary guidelines. He begins by citing the importance of mastication: "If no thirst be present at the beginning of the meal, its appearance before the close is infallible proof of deficient mastication." (Lust, 1903, 247) Lust criticized the chaotic eating habits of Americans at that time. In other guidelines, he laments, "The three meal plan is for most Americans an utter abomination; that from five to eight hours should intervene between meals; that the heavy meal—if there be such—must follow, not precede the day's work; that it should include with post-prandial rest, a full hour and a half." Eating in Lust's mind was never to be predicated on a clock, but rather on the body's sensations of hunger. Lust continues, "The mealtime should be controlled, not by custom, or hospitality, or family feeling, but by hunger, by the condition of the gastric juices, by the digestion of the previous meal, by the character of the work to follow, by the mental attitude, by the age, the occupation, the temperament ... in short the YOU is the arbiter of Naturopathic eating." (Lust, 1903, 247)

Opinions about eating a hearty breakfast or about completely abstaining from consuming breakfast were both presented in these early Naturopathic writings. Lust can be found to endorse substantial breakfast in one publication and in another to promote the book of Dr. Dewey's diet of *The No Breakfast Plan,* a popular diet of the time, which proposed the contrary. Thirteen points are presented to clarify the healthy eating habits of Dewey's "quit breakfast for good and all." The first suggestion is "never eat until hungry." (Lust, 1903, 248) Another familiar suggestion, "Masticate every morsel to the liquefied state of involuntary swallowing." (Lust, 1903, 248)

Mastication was the torch song of many including Horace Fletcher, a wealthy retired merchant of Venice, Italy who published a diet book that in 1905 took the world by storm, *The A B Z of Our Own Nutrition.* (Lust, 1905, 53) A review of Fletcher's book appeared in *The Naturopath and Herald of Health* written by Lust himself. The premise of Fletcher's book was that the primary health problems in modern societies were caused by overeating and unwise food choices. Fletcher proposed that if proper attention was given to mastication, obesity and health problems could diminish. The term 'Fletcherizing' become popular to describe the practice of thorough "chew[ing] food four or five times as long as usual." (Lust, 1905, 55)   Lust embraced the theories of Fletcher and his dietary reform was presented in several articles published about the practice of 'Fletcherizing'. This emphasis on chewing food well appeared frequently. "Prefer rather dry and firm foods to pappy ones," Lust wrote (Lust, 1908, 148). He adds, "The former are more easily digested as they have to be properly chewed; chew everything very carefully." (Lust 1908, 148) And above all, "eat only when hungry." (Lust, 1908, 149) Enriching this taxonomy of advice about how to consume food were many articles building on the journal's frequent introduction of information about the varieties of food to include in a healthy diet, such as fruit.

Carqué was interested in presenting a scientific perspective of fruit in the diet. In California "Likefresh" Fruit, Their Nutritive and Hygienic Value, Carqué endorsed the consumption of fresh and dried fruits. Carqué points out, "Statistics show that of the total amount of money spent for food in the United States, only 5% is expended for fruit, while flesh foods, dairy products and cereals predominate in the average dietary." (Carqué, 1912, 730) Many early Naturopaths, however, were quite concerned that fruit in the diet was increasingly being replaced by the consumption of refined sugars. Carqué was not only espousing fruit consumption, but also cautioning against sugar. This article is particularly significant because it is one of the earliest papers on the dangers of refined sugar and the use of sulfur in the production of dried fruits. Our perspective on sugar consumption is similarly impacted today by volume concerns, but also by substitute sweetener choices. A century ago artificial sweeteners were not widely available, but refined sugar use was expanding rapidly. Its consumption was alarming even then, but the warnings of our pioneering colleagues appear to have gone largely unheeded since today we are consuming more than our own weight in sugar annually. Carqué had been shocked at the modest, but growing data about sugar consumption of his own day: "Statistics show that the average American consumes half of his own weight, or over 82 pounds of sugar every year." (Carqué, 1912, 731)

Not only did Carqué voice his opinion about sugar consumption and the dangers of refined sugar, he also called attention to the value of breastfeeding and the inadvisability of over feeding of children, particularly if such practices involved sugar consumption. "Infants, as well as children, should not be given refined sugar in any form," he declared. (Carqué, 1911, 790) His counsel needs to be heeded today, with the epidemic of tooth decay and the proliferation of dentistry. He continues,

> The use of artificial sweets in connection with white flour products is one
> of the most pernicious customs of the day, causing defective development
> of the skeleton of the infantile body and in later years a morbid softening

of the bones, making dentistry one of the most lucrative professions of the
this country. (Carqué, 1911,790)

Carqué raises the dangers of refined sugar; however, a substitute is
also often discussed in the literature. Sebastian Kneipp reveals some of the
properties of a natural sweetener, honey. Kneipp cautions that "young
people should by no means take much honey, it being too strong for them;
on the contrary, old people were helped on their legs again by it." (Kneipp,
1900, 58)   Kneipp offers several recipes for a honey ointment, a gargle
and mead. Honey's uses as a topical for skin sores and ulcers and internally as a tea were effective in both applications for "dissolving purifying,
nourishing and strengthening" (Kneipp, 1900, 58) the whole body.

Martha Opland's article, *For Mothers and Children,* illustrates the
ingenuity that the early Naturopaths had in substituting sugar with other
healthy foods for children. Opland offers suggestions to the mother to can
her preserves without the use of sugar. She also offers alternatives to canning with drying fruit practices. Another suggestion that Opland makes
is how to sweeten sour fruit dishes. She suggests, "Take one fourth pound
of seedless raisin, (or more) wash well, then run through food chopper,
add the juice from a quart of dried or canned fruit, mix well, then pour
over fruit, mix in carefully with a fork and let stand a few hours or over
night." (Opland, 1920, 449)

While refined sugar was injurious for the body, fruit was nature's
answer for a healthy energy source. Shipping and the production of food
have made great strides today, so it is understandable to hear these early
Naturopaths' objections to the desiccation of fruit with the use of sulfur. Sulfuring was done "to conceal decayed portion of the fruit [and] to
prevent fermentation and decay during the drying of the fruit." (Carqué,
1912, 733) The Naturopaths contended that sulfuring was deleterious
and overworked the kidneys and impoverished the blood "in respect of
the number of red and white corpuscles." (Carqué, 1912,733) Carqué
offers an alternative to the sulfuration process with the use of a dehydra-
tor called the Likefresh.

While white sugar consumption attracted the wrath of the Naturopaths, so too did the widespread use of white, polished rice. Rice as
a staple was also joined with other exotic foods such as the taro root.
Valued for its nutritious elements, it was a good food "for children, invalids, and persons of a delicate digestion." (Lust, 1905, 332) Taro-ena,
in fact, was an early version of a fast food product which was promoted
as a nutritious pre-cooked baby food supplement and a flour substitute.
"Taro-ena, combined with milk, cream or water, will be found a complete
and unsurpassed food, pure, sweet, wholesome and nutritious, and one

that will be easy to digest and assimilate." (Lust, 1905, 333) The easy digestible nature of Taro-ena prompted the Naturopaths to use this for many different conditions. The diversity of food choices at the turn of the 20th century, as illustrated by the use of Taro root, shows us that the early Naturopaths were very curious to scout out wholesome foods from all corners of the world. Such foods were prized and chosen for the naturopathic diet.

The adulteration of processed foods over a century ago, though, cannot compare with Monsanto and the unlabeled additive quagmire of today. In a 1906 article, though, Samuel Bloch was already voicing concern about such food additives. He was outraged that "there is not one article of diet that is not adulterated." (Bloch, 1906, 167) Bloch compiled a list of food staples such as bread, butter, flour, pepper, maple sugar, etc., and included the adulterating compounds found in them. For example, he reported that bread also contained "alum, sulphite of copper, and potatoes." (Bloch, 1906, 167) Another item that we are quite familiar with is pepper which, in those days, could be contaminated with "sandalwood, red sawdust, sand, rice, bean shells, coconut shells, and ground olive stones." (Bloch, 1906, 167) These food additives found by Bloch may not compare with the numbers and types in the food supply today, but Naturopathic alarm was the same.

In this connection, Cora Ives, another conscientious objector of processed foods, points out some of the disgusting chemicals used in selling food. She states, "The butcher tells us that he can't sell his meat unless it is bright red and fresh-looking, and as he must satisfy the demands of his customers, he puts on a preservative, made of the most powerful acids" (Ives, 1906, 230) such as formaldehyde, sulfuric acid, hydrochloric acid, boracic acid. (Ives, 1906, 230) The use of preservatives meant bigger margins and returns in the food production and distribution industries. She poses a very apt question that is as relevant today as a century ago, "Is it not time we stopped to consider our daily food and what enters our stomachs?" (Ives, 1906, 230)

Food additives and preservatives found in processed foods, however, were less likely to be found in fruits a century ago. For this and other nutrition-specific reasons, there was a movement in the Naturopathic circles to adopt a fruitarian diet that included all forms of fruit and nuts. "For perfect health and strength and the 'staying' power boasted of by meat eaters, nothing can beat a fruitarian diet," Hara wrote in 1906. (Hara, 1906, 223) To prove his point, Hara recounts in his article a race of 125 miles from Dresden to Berlin by 32 competitors in 1906. "The first six to arrive in Berlin were fruitarians and vegetarians." (Hara, 1906, 223) This same Hara, who adopted the No Breakfast Plan of Dr. Dewey, spaced his meals at 12:30 pm and 6:30 pm. His meals consisted of 12 to 16 ounces of dried foods such as a variety of nuts and dried fruit plus two to three pounds of any fresh fruit in season. (Hara, 1906, 224) Hara insists, "You will find your magnetic and vital power doubled—nay trebled—by the simple pure food" of a fruitarian diet. (Hara, 1906, 225)

The extreme diet of fruitarians was at one end of the vegetarian spectrum and at the other were green salads and vegetables, as markers of healthy eating. For the vegetarian or health conscious eater in 1900s, vegetables were noted for their therapeutic properties and used as medicine. For example, spinach and dandelions aided the kidneys and celery was tonifying for nerves and inducing sleep. As Clark put it at the time, "Onions, leeks, and garlic increase the blood circulation, promote digestion, and increase the flow of saliva and gastric juices." (Clark, 1906, 254)

Lust in another article on diet addresses the issue of obesity and weight management. Causes of persistent obesity at the time are reminiscent of contemporary factors, such as those which Lust listed in his guidelines, including over eating, sedentary lifestyle and choosing the wrong kinds of foods. Lust advised, "The safest cure [for obesity] is to live on twenty five cents a day and do physical work for your living, for I have not yet seen a corpulent wood-cutter or a fat letter-carrier. These people have to work hard for their living." (Lust, 1908, 38)

The meat diet was one factor in obesity, even though meat consumption a century ago was low in comparison to current figures. In 1909, the average total daily meat consumption was approximately 150 grams compared to current daily consumption of about 350 gms. (Barclay, 2012) To counter this trend in meat consumption and to mitigate its effects, nutrition leaders such as Kellogg and Lust advocated a vegetarian diet. Lust also encouraged drinking "as little as possible during the meal; if thirsty, lemon water; light black malt coffee, dry bilberry, currant or moselle wines (one glass a day)." (Lust, 1908, 38)

In his article, *Diet for Corpulent People,* Lust outlines a daily diet designed to help reduce weight. To help people get accustomed to the new diet of vegetarianism, 16 suggestions were provided which are still relevant today. Besides gradually reducing meat consumption, the readers were advised to "eat rather less than you were formerly used to [and] ... [not to] fall into the common error of too great one-sidedness which impels one to live only from potatoes, white bread and cabbage." (Lust, 1908, 148) Spices, alcohol, and farinaceous foods, such as white bread and pastries, were forbidden on the Naturopathic vegetarian diet. Instead, fresh lemon juice and whole grains were the preferred substitutes. At the same time, some foods, such as peanuts, most particularly because of the way in which they were prepared for consumption, attracted the attention and caution of Naturopaths of the time. Whereas today peanuts have been banned from the school lunch room and have been shown to be responsible for life-threatening anaphylaxis, in Lust's day the concern focused on their digestibility. In a very short article, Lust explains why peanuts are hard to digest. He explains, "The digestibility of the peanut butter depends upon how it is made." (Lust, 1908, 355) In roasting peanuts, the oils of the peanut are released, "which is burned upon the surface, and the peanut is really fried and becomes indigestible." (Lust, 1908, 355) For the proper way of heating peanuts, he advises temperatures of 240° F for roasting peanuts without burning.

The world of healthy food was further enhanced in this period by the work of Professor Metchnikoff who analyzed properties of meat and reasoned that "chronic disorders are due to poisons absorbed from the intestines." (Kellogg, 1908, 269) The poisons that Metchnikoff found were actually anaerobic germs found in meat. Kellogg continues, "The poisons formed by these germs are extremely virulent, and when absorbed into the body gradually break down the liver, kidneys and other defensive organs, and so give rise to a large number of very common and very serious diseases." (Kellogg, 1908, 269)

In response to the challenge of neutralizing pathological micro-organisms, Metchnikoff researched and popularized the properties of yogurt. His work paved the way for healthy microbes to have a place at the table. As Kellogg reports, "Metchnikoff's experiments show that the new lactic ferment has such great vitality that it is not only able to live but to flourish in the colon ... and to kill off the anaerobes." (Kellogg, 1908, 269) In the early 20th century, work to concentrate and encapsulate the ferment from milk was attempted in laboratories. Kellogg was very excited about these prospects that "each capsule contains ten million or more units." (Kellogg, 1908, 270) He adds that "one or two of these capsules taken after each meal ... [would] drive out the invading anaerobes, stop the formation of poisons and give the body an opportunity to clear itself from the accumulated toxins, and thus establish conditions which render recovery possible." (Kellogg, 1908, 270) We now know this ferment that Kellogg is referring to and what Metchnikoff uncovered as "yogurt".

Like the Naturopaths of his era, Kellogg was an avid believer in healthy eating, highlighted in the next article, *The Simple Life in a Nutshell*. He captures in 50 points everything one would need to know to live a healthy life. His comprehensive suggestions, or rules as he refers to them, offer a template to live well. Kellogg did not leave one aspect untended. His first "dietectics rule" was, "eat only natural foods. The natural dietary included fruits, nuts, cooked grains, legumes and vegetables." (Kellogg, 1908, 319) Kellogg leaned towards a vegetarian type diet and many of the other rules reflect his disdain for animal protein. For instance, "Avoid meats of all sorts. ... They are all likely to contain deadly parasites of various kinds and always contain noxious germs, meat bacteria or 'anaerobes', which infect the intestines, inoculate the body with disease, and cause putrefaction and other poison forming and various morbid processes. " (Kellogg, 1908, 319)

Kellogg supported food combining, and recommended against the consumption of sugar, salt, condiments, and poisonous foods such as tea, coffee, chocolate and cocoa which he viewed as poisons. (Kellogg, 1908, 320) He reiterated the Fletcherizing doctrine of "chew every morsel until reduced to liquid in the mouth." (Kellogg, 1908, 320) Within his 50 rules, almost half pertained to eating and the others dealt with exercise, dress, hygiene, sleep and mental hygiene. (Kellogg, 1908, 322)

Howard Tunison also established a list, although shorter. His sixteen guidelines were meant to help people eat within the laws of nature. The guidelines are deliberate and valuable, and like Kellogg's, of enduring value. He assures us that "rules pertaining to diet have been gradually learned by painstaking observers during years of careful study." (Tunison, 1918, 652) Tunison repeats many of the ones offered by Kellogg but also includes, "do not wash down your food, or soak it in any drink before you eat ... never eat while feeling ill ... avoid late suppers; never eat just before going to bed." (Tunison, 1918, 652)

If the rules of Kellogg and Tunison did not dissuade the novice from healthy eating, the number of books on the subject of diet must have for sure been baffling at the very least. In 1909, Louise Lust reveals, "strange to say that there are upwards of 1700 works extant on the subject of diet and cook books. And yet dyspepsia prevails." (Lust, 1909, 98) Our preoccupation with new diets and cookbooks has changed little. Louise Lust added her voice to that dialogue about healthy eating. She recognized that a balance between acid and alkaline foods was important, especially in a vegetarian diet. She writes, "We are learning slowly that the proper combination between acid and alkaline food shall answer this purpose; their reaction on each other, when realized and rightly understood, may give incalculable help in all our considerations with regard to food." (Lust, 1909, 98) The kinds of foods adopted by her were simple. She continues, "One conclusion seems plain—that the grains, the pulses, peas, beans, lentils, fresh vegetables, salads and fruits are the best foods for non-meat eaters." (Lust, 1909, 98)

The diet during sickness was also addressed by Louise Lust. She insists, "Much of the suffering endured by sick persons is simply the result of erroneous diet." (Lust, 1909, 99) "The more inflammation and fever exist, the more fruit and cooling drinks should be given and the less nitrogenous and starch matter." (Lust, 1909, 98) The vegetarian diet became almost the official diet of the early Naturopaths. Many articles were written that subscribed to this doctrine. Failure to follow the vegetarian diet was often attributed to poor food combinations.

The Lust journals returned often to the subject of grains, most particularly flour. A food that the Naturopaths toward the end of the first decade of the twentieth century knew had come to dominate the appetites in America was flour, and in particular 'durum flour'. Charles Cristadodo recounts the history of Durum flour transplanted to America from Russia. "Less than ten years ago, the US Department of Agriculture sent Prof. M. A. Carleton to Russia to investigate the durum wheats grown there." (Cristadodo, 1909, 308) In less than ten years, "the crop amounted to 60,000,000 bushels worth $40,000,000 to $50,000,000." (Cristadodo, 1909, 308)

Analyzed by the US Agricultural Department, durum wheat proved to be superior in color, moistness, and texture when compared to the local wheat of Minnesota. As well, "Durum wheat yielded 16 pounds more dough to the barrel than did the Minnesota spring wheat flour." (Cristadodo, 1909, 308) This article illustrates the ease with which local species have been supplanted, right from the beginning of the twentieth century, in the interests of economic scaling.

Wheat variety changes, though, did not trigger the Naturopaths as much as did changes in the milling process in the early 20th century. The shift in milling methodolgy caused an uproar among them. In Lindlahr's and others' view, grains were increasingly depleted of "positive mineral salts ... stored in the hulls and the dark outer layers." (Lindlahr, 1910, 259) The demand for white flour and rice meant the removal of bran and the outer parts of grains. Lindlahr pointed out that there was no mystery as to why "American vegetarians living largely upon devitalized leguminous and grain products, with a liberal allowance of peanuts and olive oil, often fare worse than people living on the mixed meat diet." (Lindlahr, 1910, 259)

Notwithstanding his contributions to the discussion about milled wheat, probably Lindlahr's most important contribution to dietetics were the scientific platforms and frameworks he brought to his views. In this regard, Lindlahr was influenced by one of his mentors, Dr. H. Lahmann, who became an authority on the chemical composition of food and popularized a theory of nutritive salts. Lindlahr shared Lahmann's ideal diet as "a rational vegetarian diet properly combined, consisting of dairy products, the positive vegetables, and the medium positive fruits with just enough of starchy and protein foods to supply the needs of the body for tissue building and fuel material, will be found to be an ideal diet for human beings fully sufficient to keep them in health and strength under the most trying circumstances." (Lindlahr, 1910, 260)

His rationale for choosing a vegetarian diet was simple. Meat consumption, he contended, "doubles the work of our organs of elimination and overloads the system with animal waste matter and poisons." (Lindlahr, 1908, 302) In understanding how to replace meat from the diet, his contemporary, Edwin Wilson, assembled tables of various foodstuffs with protein. Included were vegetarian prepared products available that simulated or replaced meat protein in the diet. Nuts and legumes offered an excellent source of protein. On the subject of nuts, Wilson notes, "[Nuts are] undoubtedly Man's natural meat. Rich in Protein, Fat, Mineral Salts, and a small amount of Starch they are indeed an ideal type of food, and one that at the present time is not properly appreciated." (Wilson, 1909, 569) Nuts were used to create vegetarian products. He describes them, "If properly cooked, they closely resemble roast or boiled meat. They have the appearance of meat, they smell like meat, and they taste somewhat like meat." (Wilson, 1909, 569)

Although dietetics characterized by such considerations as Wilson's was for most Naturopaths the core modality of their practice, a more comprehensive, scientific understanding of dietetics was tackled by Henry Lindlahr in a series of articles that he contributed to *The Naturopath and Herald of Health* during this period. He had assembled a list of macronutrients compiled from "the five greatest German authorities on food chemistry, viz., Doctor's Lahmann, Koening, Schuessler, Hensel and Bunge." (Lindlahr, 1910, 103) Lindlahr's objective was to "form an indispensable basis for the rational and scientific study of food chemistry." (Lindlahr, 1910, 103) In this article, *The Magnetic Properties of Food*, Lindlahr compiles valuable information on the mineral salts found in food: Iron, Sodium, Calcium, Magnesium and Potassium.

The association of these mineral salts to health and disease was examined in some detail by Lindlahr. He notes, "Iron in the form of Hæmoglobin is all important as a carrier of oxygen from the lungs into the various parts of the body. Combustion is impossible without oxygen, and digestion is simply a slow process of combustion." (Lindlahr, 1910, 103) To illustrate his comprehension of digestion and the physiology of the micro-factors involved, Lindlahr explains the roles of sodium and carbon dioxide in the digestive process. Continuing, "If sodium is lacking in the blood, CO_2 accumulates and gradually asphyxiates the process of combustion on which depend digestion, reduction of waste and heat production." (Lindlahr, 1910, 104)

Food chemistry was also shared by Henry Lindlahr who placed a lot of attention on diet in his treatment protocols. His and his colleagues' need to understand the body and the chemistry in Naturopathy led to their creating theories to support what little science had to offer to the study of nutrition, then in its infancy. Lindlahr developed a natural system of curing disease under the banner of Nature Cure and with it he fashioned supportive dietary principles. He addressed the question of salt in the diet, as a case in point. Recognizing that table salt consisted of sodium and chloride, Lindlahr deduced that "The neutralization and elimination of food poisons depend largely upon sodium." (Lindlahr, 1912, 218) He proposed that if vegetarian foods such as vegetables and fruits "are very rich in organic sodium as well as in all other 'organic salts'," (Lindlahr, 1912, 218) then additional salt in diet of a vegetarian was unnecessary.

In this particular article by Lindlahr and his reference to inorganic salts, we are learning about vitamins and minerals before this body of knowledge migrated into common knowledge. He comments, "As soon as scurvy patients are put on a fruit and vegetable diet, the destruction of tissues, the bleeding resulting from it and other symptoms promptly abate." (Lindlahr, 1912, 219) We now know that scurvy is a vitamin C deficiency and that fruits and vegetables contain this needed vitamin. The line separating minerals and vitamins was quite thin. Lindlahr recognized mineral deficiencies and understood that humans and animals living on soil depleted by mineral starvation would be prone to salt cravings. He described examples of bees and butterflies attracted to salt and not sugar. (Lindlahr, 1912, 220) Among the First Nations people, "the Chibokwe women burn a marsh grass into a potash powder as a [salt] substitute". (Lindlahr, 1912, 220) The First Nation's people have a long history of acquiring their mineral needs from the mineral salts in the ash of the burned and pulverized marsh grass and other botanical plants.

Incidentally, Lindlahr also had definite opinions of the deleterious effects of milk, a food discussed earlier in other articles in the Lust journals. As well, he had a clear understanding of water consumption. He did not share his colleague's practice of drinking copious amounts of water to flush out their systems. He did not agree that the human body was like a sewer needing flushing. He felt that "the cleansing of the human organism depends upon the concentration of vital fluids and secretions, not on their dilution with large quantities of water." (Lindlahr, 1910, 261) He reasoned, "Blood, lymph, saliva, gastric juice, bile, pancreatic juice and all other fluids and secretions of the body are chemical solutions and chemical solutions do not become stronger by dilution with water." (Lindlahr, 1910, 261)

Another who added his voice in the water consumption discussion was J. H. Neff. In the opening line in his short yet concise article, *Drink at Meals,* the message is loud and clear, "Never, no, never drink a drop of any liquid at meals." (Neff, 1911, 381) Neff was adamant that drinking while eating was one of the worst practices that one could do. He continues, "It only prevents digestion and causes ill-health." (Neff, 1911, 381) Neff reminds us that digestion begins in the mouth, and food needed to be "thoroughly saturated with nature's liquid, the only liquid needed—the saliva, which forms the first part of digestion." (Neff, 1911, 381) He reasoned that drinking with meals substituted the need for saliva. Saliva was the first part of the digestive process and enabled gastric juices in the stomach to complete the work. Dilution of these digestive helpers would only cause "stomach troubles and other evils." (Neff, 1911, 381)

Making a difference and having an enduring impact on the health of adults was another important objective. In their view, one of the most significant ways of influencing an adult's health was to start in childhood. Thus, infant care was not taken lightly by the early Naturopaths. Otto Carqué, for example, was an outspoken, articulate Naturopath specializing in dietetics and infant care. "The period of early childhood is decisive for the rest of our life and the amount of vitality to resist injurious influences, aside from heredity, largely depends on the quality of nourishment we receive in the first year of our existence." (Carqué, 1911, 788) The diet of infants was a grave concern in the early 20th century because of high infant mortality statistics. Carqué recounts the infant mortality in NYC in 1907, "About 150 babies out of every thousand born died before they reached the first year of age, from causes which were largely preventable." (Carqué, 1911, 788)

As far as Carqué was concerned, the best food for infants was uncontested: mother's milk. Carqué felt that it was unthinkable for any mother to not nurse her baby. He states, "Any mother who does not nurse her child because it is not convenient, because she does not wish to be tied down to her child during the first few months, is not fit to be a mother." (Carqué, 1911, 788) Breast fed babies were healthier and more robust in comparison to the "bottle-fed babies [who are] much smaller." (Carqué, 1911, 788) In this connection, Carqué presents some interesting information regarding the cow milk that bottle fed babies drank. Carqué is very clear: "The digestion and growth of a calf are quite different from those of an infant." (Carqué, 1911, 788) However, cow milk in itself was not the only problem; rather, the concern was with what was done to the milk. This was the age of pasteurization and Carqué observed the consequences of its consumption. He reports, "Careful experiments with feeding babies on pasteurized milk ... [demonstrate that in] the vast majority of cases, produces rickets and scurvy." (Carqué, 1911, 789) The introduction of sterilized or pasteurized milk led Naturopaths to be distrustful of its consumption.

Another outspoken dietetics expert among the Naturopaths was Eugene Christian. He states, "About 90% of all human disease originates in the stomach, caused by errors in eating." (Christian, 1912, 6) He adds so appropriately as all his colleagues had, "All disease is merely an expression of violated natural law." (Christian, 1912, 6) The question of health rested, then, on correct eating habits. Christian was keen on reducing human disease and suffering with science of nutrition. Blad reports, "Eugene Christian, for 20 years in modest seclusion, has faithfully devoted his life to the mission of discovering the chemistry of the human body, the chemistry of food and method of uniting these two branches of science." (Blad, 1914, 6005) Christian was a principle architect of the statement that "man is physically what he eats" and this still rings true today. Christian declares, "What we take into our stomachs either nourishes and gives us strength and health or poisons and produces disease." (Christian, 1912, 6) He "has shown that when food is properly selected and administered, and eaten according to one's age, occupation and time of the year, it will, in the great majority of cases, produce a perfectly normal result; that is, all the organs of digestion and assimilation as well as those of elimination will work in harmony and automatically." (Blad, 1914, 605)

Christian felt science had much to offer in the advancement of food science. He says, "Knowing the chemistry of the body and the chemistry of our food, we could very easily learn the laws of chemical harmony and ... know how to select food that would remove causes of indigestion, constipation, rheumatism, gout, Bright's disease, obesity and nearly all abnormal conditions we call disease." (Christian, 1912, 7) Christian had his eyes on the future of nutrition science. A contemporary response to his request might well be our preoccupation with nutraceuticals.

The current rage of raw food and living food may seem new to us, but was certainly not for our Naturopathic forebears. From the very inception of the naturopathic movement, raw food was esteemed as the model of health. In 1902 Lust proclaimed, "Not only is it possible to eat all kinds of fruit, vegetables, corn, and all leguminous plants in their raw state, but even it is possible to make them palatable to the most fastidious palates." (Lust, 1902, 107) Cooked foods were considered inferior to raw foods. Cooked foods could be eaten in greater quantities than raw foods which was a strain on the stomach. "The principle failing of all cooked dishes is that they may still be nourishment without having any life-giving ingredients; they do not any more contain the vital, electric, or magnetic tension power." (Lust, 1902, 108) Cooked or boiled foods lack the vitality of raw foods. Lust considered cooked foods as dead, their vitality killed during the heating process.

Louise Lust advocated raw food diets and valued "slow mastication which aids digestion." (Lust, 1921, 323) She acknowledged that there was much prejudice and misunderstanding about raw foods. "The dyspeptic fears raw food and must have everything doubly cooked and made into a mushy mess before he will eat it." (Lust, 1921, 323) Cooking and especially over cooking "destroys the vital or life principle of the food." (Lust, 1921, 323) She proposes, "The change from cooked to raw foods should be made gradually in order to permit the stomach and intestines to accustom themselves to it." (Lust, 1921, 323)

Mrs. Anna Lindlahr, on the other hand, proposed that vegetables could be cooked as long as care was taken to not overcook them. She counsels, "Cook the vegetables no more than is necessary." (Lindlahr, 1910, 107) She continues, "Avoid frying and boiling foods violently. As a rule, it is better cook vegetables slowly and conserve the life force or life energy of the living plant, which is lost in proportion to the heat applied in cooking." (Lindlahr, 1910, 107) Mrs. Lindlahr and her husband, Henry Lindlahr, were staunch vegetarians in their own dietary preferences and in their writings. Mrs. Lindlahr advocated "butter or some pure vegetable fats" (Lindlahr, 1910, 107) in cooking and to "cook vegetables in their own juices; that is, steam or cook them in just enough water to make a sauce to serve with the vegetable" (Lindlahr, 1910, 108) to preserve their organic mineral salts.

Mrs. Lindlahr shared her husband's articulate communication skills and wrote often on dietary matters that included the down to earth details of food preparation. She recognized that processed sugar and starch were unfit to sustain life. She states, "Animals fed on chemically pure white starch, albumen, sugar, gluten, etc., will die sooner than if they receive no food at all." (Lindlahr, 1910, 239) In describing the importance of sun energy, she notes, "The molecules of plant and fruit have become charged with the warmth and the electro-magnetic currents of the great life-giver [the sun]. These forces are liberated again when the molecules disintegrate under the action of digestive ferments, thus furnishing heat and energy for the building up and sustenance of animal and human bodies." (Lindlahr, 1910, 239)

Lindlahr includes her menu for a meal served at the Lindlahr's sanitarium with all of its recipes. Every recipe was vegetarian and delicious. The menu included barley sausage with gravy, water cress and onion relishes, mayonnaise made from scratch, mashed turnips, sago pudding and grape sauce. (Lindlahr, 1910, 240) Louise Lust also contributed many of her menus providing guidelines on healthy eating. Louise Lust and Anna Lindlahr both shared vegetarian interests. Lust wrote an interesting article, *Menus for Purification* giving suggestion on how to prepare for spring season of purification. She recommended eliminating salt, oils and nuts, dairy, and breadstuffs during this period. (Lust, 1918, 278)

In 1913, the raw food movement was galvanized under the name of Apyrotrophy, meaning "unfired" foods. Sherry declares the new terminology thus: "The *new vegetarian* wants his food with all its nutritive value to the system, that is to say, he wants it uncooked, or unfired, and for that he calls himself an Unfired Fooder, or, in Greek, an Apyrotropher." (Sherry, 1913, 50) Lust had created a monthly column for Apyrotrophy which lasted several years in *The Naturopath and Herald of Health*. This trend in eating was popularized by George J. Drews, (*Unfired Food and Tropho-Therapy*, 1910), who wrote a monthly column.

Another 'unfired fooder' was Helen Sherry, Associate Editor, who shared Drews' fervent dedication to this new way of eating. Sherry writes,

> Thousands of men and women who are deeply convinced that a diet of unfired foods is the only one which is absolutely correct, health-giving and founded on scientific research of the most painstaking and authentic character, it now behooves them to effect such a union of forces as will materially increase their numbers and help promulgate the dietary doctrines dear to them. (Sherry, 1913, 50)

Sherry presents several arguments on why apyrotrophy is worth pursuing, namely for health. She contends, "The too frequent tale of men and women is that premature illness and death …[are] brought about by malnutrition." (Sherry, 1913, 51) Adopting a healthy diet of raw food was the answer that the Apyrotrophs offered.

The Apyrotrophs did not stop in the kitchen, but also included in their dietary plan the importance of having a garden to provide fresh food for the table. Like the current permaculture movement, the Apyrotrophs advocated "rais[ing] vegetables in your little back yard, turn[ing] your kitchen into a 'trophery,' eat[ing] your garden stuff unfired, and laugh[ing] at the doctors and the food trusts." (Sherry, 1913, 123)

The garden plot of "twelve foot square will produce all the green vegetables that two people can eat in eight months of the year." (Sherry, 1913, 123) In a diagram of a model city garden measuring 20' by 6', instructions on how to ensure food for the table are given. Some of the varieties of greens included nasturtiums, broad leaved and curled endive, swiss chard, curled and upland cress, whitloof chicory, various lettuces, parsley, sorrel and rampion. (Sherry, 1913, 125)

Many of the plants grown in the trophery have been supplanted today by conventional vegetables grown in distant and often exotic locations, transported and then made available for purchase in our local grocery store. The foods that the Apyrotrophs grew in their small gardens to provide fresh produce their families may seem exotic, largely because our current food supply is constantly shrinking in variety, reminding us that biodiversity is not what it used to be. Curled dock, thistles and dahlias were among the usual and delectable choices for the Apyrotrophs cuisine. Curled dock was "like spinach in all the essential organic salts for toning the blood and for aiding the kidneys and other glands in eliminating from the blood and tissues accumulated impurities, wastes and irritants." (Drews, 1913, 266) The Apyrotrophs planted dock into their gardens that could "be forced to furnish tender leaves during summer and fall when prevented from running to seed." (Drews, 1913, 266)

Thistles of various varieties with their unique flavors found their place in the Apyrotroph's garden too. Drews comments, "One who has never seen nor tasted the root of the Golden Thistle could never rationally expect to find such a delicious root under such cruelly thorny leaves." (Drews, 1914, 832) The pith of the Golden Thistle root [Scolymus Hispanicus] has the flavor of "sweet milk and in this respect the root is sweeter than the pith of the bull-thistle." (Drews, 1914, 832) The foods chosen were for flavor and also for therapeutic effects. As Drews explains, "To those whose alimentary canal is not in a perfectly healthy state, this root has a mild laxative property; but with others it has proven no other property than that of toning the blood." (Drews, 1914, 832)

Dahlia tubers were prized for their crisp texture and warm spicy flavor. Drews offers instruction on how to prepare these roots: "The tubers may be peeled and cut into sections and served like radishes, or they may be chopped and combined with other vegetables and nuts to form salads." (Drews, 1915, 69) Dahlia tubers were used in the making of the synede or salad. A recipe for one Dahlia synede included "chopped celery, chopped cabbage, shredded dahlia tuber and flaked peanuts, dressed with a little honey." (Drews, 1915, 69-70) Drews offers more recipes using the dahlia tuber in the supawn and posset. The supawn is a form of paté and the posset is a tonic drink.

He adds, "The Cruciferae or cross-bearing vegetables and flowers are a family of plants which have four petals arranged like the arms of a cross. This family of plants presents itself in greater variety of form than any other family known." (Drews, 1913, 201) Drews lists the members of this large family: "the cresses, the mustards, the cabbages, the kales, the radishes, the turnips, the kohlrabis, the cauliflowers and many ornamental plants of which, later, both the leaves and especially the flowers may be used as food." (Drews, 1913, 201)

The diversity found in the Cruciferae was impressive and especially the prolific choice that Apyrotrophers had in selecting plants for their table. Drews enumerates the kinds of turnips one could have. He states, "There are also about 64 varieties of turnips." He continues,

"More than 70 varieties of smooth-leaved cabbages and 17 varieties of crimped cabbages are cultivated." (Drews, 1913, 203) Within the

Cruciferae family are edible flowers. "The flowers and leaves of sweet alyssum, candytuft and sweet rocket, cultivated only for ornaments, are perfectly wholesome, but they are, rather, too pungent for most people." (Drews, 1913, 204)

The Apyrotrophs saw the potential for food in many plants found in a garden whether a flower or vegetable garden. They identified and culti-vated many unusual plants, such as the Dasheen. As Drews explains, "the Dasheen is a tuber or corm of a variety of the caladium esculentum, com-monly known as elephant's ear." (Drews, 1915, 399) The dasheen was bland but well suited for a synede of various plants. Drews illustrates the variety of tastes that Apyrotrophs enjoyed, "Nasturtium leaves or flow-ers, garden cress, white mustard leaves, sorrel, French dock, curled dock, dandelions or chicory." (Drews, 1915, 399)

The variety of greens grown in a garden was complemented equally with the variety from the sea. Sea lettuce and dulse were considered "a luxury by some of the wealthier classes who have acquired a taste for it." (Drews, 1915, 714) Dulse was "rich in organic iodine which has none of the harmful after-effects that are known to follow the use of the unorganized and concentrated iodine prescribed by the M. Ds." (Drews, 1915, 714) The Apyrotrophs recommended rinsing dulse to remove the salt and was added "with greens and nuts in the form of a synede (salad)." (Drews, 1915, 714)

We think of raw fooders as salad eaters who probably would not include milk as part of their diet. Milk was included by the Apyrotrophs but only raw milk. Drews explains, "Apyrtrophers do not use much milk because the foods they select are mostly so rich that milk becomes super-fluous, but when they do use milk they want it unfired like all their other foods, i. e., natural as it comes from a clean and healthy cow." (Drews, 1916, 119) Sterilized and pasteurized milk was thought of as "warm dead milk [which] is just the stuff that the tubercle bacilli like to feed on." (Drews, 1916, 119)

As referenced in earlier articles, the early Naturopaths were quite opposed to pasteurization of milk especially "fed exclusively to infants, will produce rickets, constipation and finally, consumption." (Drews, 1916, 120) Milk pasteurized or sterilized caused putrification and milk albumin to coagulate making digestion difficult. (Drews, 1916, 119) Drews elaborates on the differences between the natural process of lactic fermentation and putrefaction of sterilized milk. He warns, "Beware of milk that has been pasteurized and sterilized. It cannot sour, it can only putrefy." (Drews, 1916, 120)

Eating raw and vegan minimized morbid matter introduced into the body. For those who did not eat well or who had exposure to poor dietary habits, fasting was a way of restoring health by removing the accumulated waste products. Fasting was considered one of the best methods of eliminating poisons or morbid matter from the body. The early Naturopaths embraced the fast and throughout the years of *The Naturopath and Herald of Health,* numerous articles appeared extolling the virtues of the fast. Moershell defines the fast as "abstention from all food, liquid or solid, water only permissible." (Moershell, 1915, 104) The basis of disease for the early Naturopaths involved the concept of morbid matter, the accumulation of toxins and waste matter. Fasting enabled the elimination of morbid matter allowing the body to return to homeostasis and health.

William Freeman Havard wrote extensively on fasting, describing the principles involved, "The digestive organs and anabolic function of the liver are given a complete rest, leaving the liver to the more thorough performance of its katabolic function while the eliminating organs—kidneys and sweat glands—are allowed full play to carry off the effete matter which has acted as an encumbrance to normal physiologic action." (Havard, 1920, 277) Havard outlined in his article, *Fasting,* a clear set of guidelines and rules on how to conduct a curative fast that was effective and successful. Havard's first rule: "Put aside all fear of starvation." (Havard, 1920, 280) Havard warned, "Fasting is not advised unless the patient thoroughly understands his condition, or unless he is under the care of a competent physician." (Havard, 1920, 277-278)

Moershell rationalized, "since the greater amount of excretory materials is deposited by the mucus cells, special effort should be made to clear these surfaces." (Moershell, 1915, 104) Moershell advised that hot water be drunk to clear the mucus and as well to ensure that the liver and bowels be cleared with enemas. (Moershell, 1915, 104) To those who were novices, he warned "against the long fasts, fasting until the return of natural hunger or what is sometimes termed 'fasting to the finish'." (Moershell, 1915, 105) The significance of the coated tongue, foul breath and other fasting symptoms are explained in Moershell's article. Moershell explains how to break the fast when the fast comes to completion. He states, "I have my patients take about three or four tablespoons of grape juice and one tablespoon of water every three hours for the first day." (Moershell, 1911, 592) Moershell slowly introduced foods which he describes in detail.

Another author on the fasting cure was Arnold Ehret who wrote several books on rational fasting and the mucusless diet. He concurred with Moershell on fasting, that it was an excellent means of restoring health and advocated individualized treatment. In the time of illness, fasting and drinking water were often quite capable of generating a cure. Ehret concludes, "In the most severe cases, nature heals by refusing to eat; hence the logical conclusion that a sick person cannot eat too little." (Ehret, 1917, 257) Ehret's observes, "The most natural factor of every healing process, the instinctive self-help, is to stop eating, whether from accident or chronic disease. Animals do this intuitively." (Ehret, 1919, 145) The quantity of food intake did catch the attention of the early Naturopaths. Ehret speaks on this subject, "Although the minimum requirement of food for the sick, as well as the healthy, is not yet fully established, every follower of Naturopathy knows that all maladies are caused, more or less, not by too little nourishment, but by overfeeding." (Ehret, 1917, 257)

Undigested food in the body leads to the formation of mucus. Ehret developed principles to help others to eliminate and "successively withdraw all contaminating mucus-forming food, which consists of meat, eggs, milk and its products, bread, potatoes, and all carbohydrates." (Ehret, 1917, 259) Ehret advocated a return to a natural diet based upon fruits and vegetables. He theorizes, "I employ vegetable and lettuce salads as purifying mucus–cleansers to augment the aperient, cleansing effect of fruit, with due regard to choice and combination." (Ehret, 1917, 259)

Ehret's mucusless diet brought salvation to a population who gorged and over ate the wrong kinds of foods. Over eating, especially foods that were poor nutritional choices, could lead, in his opinion, to actual starvation. Axel Emil Gibson points out that over eating had other implications. He states, "Starvation from food is only one of the dangers that arise from indulgence in ill-balanced food mixtures—poisoning, auto-intoxication, is another." (Gibson, 1915, 99) He estimated that "the world's diseases [are] 90% due to errors in diet." (Gibson, 1915, 99) The continuing eating of devitalized and processed foods eventually results in the inability to assimilate any nutrients that leads to starvation.

As the prevalence of food sensitivities and allergies escalated, Gibson continued describing what he witnessed, and what we as a society continue to perpetuate. He continues, "sooner or later, however, the effect of our dietetic transgressions will come into evidence. In place of rising from the table with a feeling of buoyancy, energy and optimism, we experience dullness and dizziness ... accompanied by sour stomach and general discomfort." (Gibson, 1915, 100)

When numbers and values are presented, a different kind of awareness develops. In the article, *The Cause of Disease*, Eales addresses the problem of over eating. Previously, we learned that our meat consumption has more than doubled in the past century. A century ago, the numbers, were already staggering. Eales reports, "If computed in terms of animals [this] would mean that a man at seventy had eaten 30 oxen, 200 sheep,

100 calves, 200 lambs, 50 hogs, 1,200 fowl, 300 turkeys, 24,000 eggs, [etc.]" (Eales, 1919, 276) The Naturopaths felt excess eating was a huge problem. Eales states the obvious question, "With the expenditure of the vital energy necessary to digest and assimilate such vast and unnecessary quantities of food, is it any wonder that degeneration of the vital organs should take place and disease manifest itself?" (Eales, 1919, 276)

In the next few articles, William Havard, a Naturopath from Chicago, presents his theories of diet. Havard was articulate and strived to establish a solid and unified foundation for the Naturopathic curative diet. In his first article, he proposes definitions which may seem simple to us today but at the time of writing were novel and innovative. Havard recognized that the diet for the sick and well were different. He saw that many of the food scientists were only concerned with food that was edible. He continues, "Some [food scientists] make little or no distinction between sick and well people, but try to bend everyone to their ideas of a 'balanced diet'." (Havard, 1920, 505)

Havard identified three main categories of diet: diet of growth, diet of maturity and diet of cure. Throughout *The Naturopath,* authors addressed the first two dietary regimes; i.e. raising healthy children and maintaining healthy adults with nutrition. The curative diet emphasized the importance of proper quantity and quality of food to maintain the state of health. However, the early Naturopaths recognized that the requirements during health and disease differed. Havard explains, "In disease the body requires principally organic salts to effect the elimination of accumulated wastes before proper metabolism can be re-established." (Havard, 1920, 506) He identified and defines the steps in eliminating waste material from the body. The morbid matter or waste material resulting from abnormal quality of food or the digestion of quantities in excess of the body's need resulted in disease and called for fasting.

Havard continues on the need for fasting. He writes, "Cure or healing is a process which begins with the elimination of old accumulations of waste products and disease refuse, and one of the most valuable procedures to effect complete elimination is rational fasting." (Havard, 1920, 508) The liver's role in preparing waste or endogenous toxins to be eliminated from the body was well understood by the early Naturopaths.

The curative diet as recommended by Havard was the rational fast. In his following article published in 1921, Havard provides rules during the fast as well as case studies. He addresses topics such as water consumption, exercise, bathing, duration and breaking the fast. Breaking the fast was "the most important period of fasting, because on it depends whether or not the benefits secured will be lasting." (Havard, 1921, 29) He provides a case as an example of an incorrect way of breaking a fast.

A young man fasted for 27 days for chronic constipation and indigestion. "On the 28th day he ate a meal of beef steak, potatoes, bread and butter and coffee." (Havard, 1921, 29) He continues with the negative consequences of such practices with several more cases.

The rules of fasting apply today as when written a century ago. Havard's suggestions included, "Be properly prepared for the fasting ordeal by thoroughly cleansing the alimentary tract with a raw vegetable diet and nightly enemas for three days preceding the fast." (Havard, 1921, 30) He includes guidelines for exercise and rest and assures us to "put aside all fear of starvation." (Havard, 1921, 30)

After the fast, he provides more suggestions to stay well such as, "don't bolt your food. Chew it thoroughly in order to gain the greatest benefit." (Havard, 1921, 31) He adds, "Don't mix fruits and vegetables at the same meal, particularly while on a curative diet." (Havard, 1921, 31) He advises against the use of vinegar and recommends "Lemon juice should be substituted for vinegar, in salad dressings and sauces." (Havard, 1921, 31) He also viewed refined foods as inedible. "White flour, white sugar, canned goods, pickled products, have forfeited their right to be classed as foods. They belong in the list of chemicals." (Havard, 1921, 31) His adoption of vegetarianism resulted in his condemnation of meat in the diet. "Flesh of animals cannot rightfully be considered fit food for humans." (Havard, 1921, 32)

Instead of meat or processed food, Havard chose for a healthy diet acid fruits such as lemons, and a raw vegetable diet. In a follow up article, Havard presents menus for specific conditions, such as digestive ulcers, consumption, rheumatism and fevers. He illustrates examples of health producing foods for those who had conducted a fast and wanted to live healthier. One example that Havard gives us is adding lemon juice for "rheumatic conditions or other liver disorders together with a moderate mixed diet." (Havard, 1921, 89) Another example is garlic and onions. "Garlic is an excellent purifier of both the intestines and blood, as well as a wonderful nerve tonic." (Havard, 1921, 90)

Havard also presents the milk diet which was very popular. Perhaps, less than ideal today, milk was considered then "a building food [that] affords all the nutritive elements that the body requires" (Havard, 1921, 92). Havard determined that "after a fast, after an acute illness or after a period of a strictly eliminating diet, the milk diet is the safest." (Havard, 1921, 92) Havard continues, "Experience has proven that the unpasteurized milk from Holstein Cows is best suited for human consumption." (Havard, 1921, 92)

While Havard extolled the virtues of milk, Louise Lust advised "it is better to keep away from milk in any shape or form while there is any tendency to indigestion." (Lust, 1921, 324)   She instead qualifies milk consumption.   She writes, "sour milk or buttermilk [which] exert a less injurious action upon digestion than fresh milk but the merits of sour milk and its germs are much exaggerated." (Lust, 1921, 323-324)

Ross, who continues this discussion on meat consumption, states, "All varieties of 'meat' or flesh are greatly productive of uric acid in the process of digestion." (Ross, 1922, 117)   He adds in this category of foods that produce acid, "white-sugar, pastries, bread, and cereals of every sort and potatoes as well, are perhaps the chief causes of stomach-fermentation of the wrong sort." (Ross, 1922, 117)   People who complained of acidity or 'acid stomach' often avoided acidic foods.

Ross clarifies that fruits such as citrus fruits and other sour fruits are not necessarily acid foods.   He writes, "The 'acids' in these foods are not only good and beneficial for all who eat them, but chemically they even cease to be acids, but instead turn alkaline almost as soon as they enter the stomach." (Ross, 1922, 117)

The question of cooked versus raw was persistent and voiced by many of the contributors to the Lust journals.   Gibson answered this question quite cleverly, suggesting, "In cases of constitutionally high-strung and over-wrought subjects—with their nervous system constantly quivering under interior irritation, the cooked fruit would be more agreeable, while to the easy-going well-poised, phlegmatic nature the raw fruit is preferable." (Gibson, 1922, 371)

Food combining theories were beginning to take place within the Naturopathic dietary scope long before William Hay popularized his diet in the 1920s.   Gibson counseled against eating meats with fruit because they were digested at different rates.   He states, "The mistake in combining fruit with meat is readily seen when realizing the former ... only requires 70 minutes for its digestion, while meat, grains and vegetables need a period varying from three to six hours before its ready to leave the stomach." (Gibson, 1922, 371)   The debate about mixing or combining of starch and fruit was also presented by Gibson.   "The main argument against combing fruit with starches is based on the danger of fermentation and alcoholization, which, unless the digestive system of the individual is powerful, is practically unavoidable." (Gibson, 1922, 372)   The theories of food combining were complemented with eating locally.   Gibson suggests, "The rule holds good that fruits should be enjoyed in their fresh uncooked state wherever they are found growing." (Gibson, 1922, 372)

Kennedy concluded that there were three essential rules to obtain proper nutrition, as applicable today as when they were made.   First, the diet must consist of "pure, digestible foods, free from poisons or injurious substances." (Kennedy, 1923, 385) Secondly, Kennedy stressed, "eating at regular intervals and of proper combinations." (Kennedy, 1923, 385) The third counsel was to ensure that when we eat we are not consumed with worry or vexing thoughts nor engaged in "strenuous mental or physical work immediately after meals." (Kennedy, 1923, 386)

Diet, then, was as fundamental to naturopathic medicine a century ago as it is now.   Foundational to lifelong health, a healthy "dietetics" was a central strategy for our early Naturopathic doctors. Their clinical expertise, the cumulative wealth of their research and investigations, and their deep commitment to helping people become and stay well are legacies which persist to this very day.

Sussanna Czeranko, ND, BBE

Kneipp Health Food
Benedict Lust

Olive Oil As A Remedy
Benedict Lust

Honey
Mgr. Sebastian Kneipp

Diet For Patients And Convalescents
Friedrich Eduard Bilz

Nut Foods
Benedict Lust

Milk
Benedict Lust

Biscuits, Light Bread, Or Whole Wheat Bread?
F.J. Buettgenbach

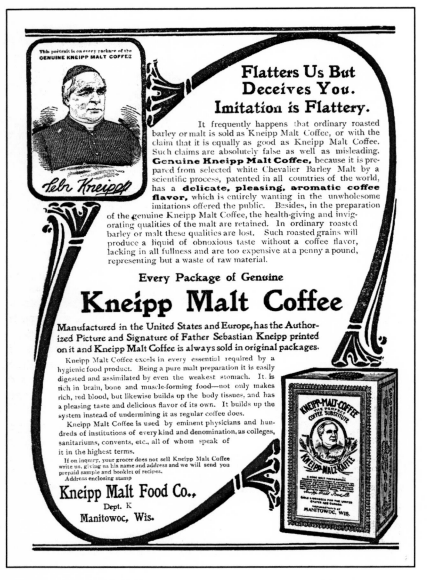

This portrait is on every package of the
GENUINE KNEIPP MALT COFFEE

Sebr Kneipp

Flatters Us But Deceives You.
Imitation is Flattery.

It frequently happens that ordinary roasted barley or malt is sold as Kneipp Malt Coffee, or with the claim that it is equally as good as Kneipp Malt Coffee. Such claims are absolutely false as well as misleading. **Genuine Kneipp Malt Coffee**, because it is prepared from selected white Chevalier Barley Malt by a scientific process, patented in all countries of the world, has a **delicate, pleasing, aromatic coffee flavor,** which is entirely wanting in the unwholesome imitations offered the public. Besides, in the preparation of the genuine Kneipp Malt Coffee, the health-giving and invigorating qualities of the malt are retained. In ordinary roasted barley or malt these qualities are lost. Such roasted grains will produce a liquid of obnoxious taste without a coffee flavor, lacking in all fullness and are too expensive at a penny a pound, representing but a waste of raw material.

Every Package of Genuine

Kneipp Malt Coffee

Manufactured in the United States and Europe, has the Authorized Picture and Signature of Father Sebastian Kneipp printed on it and Kneipp Malt Coffee is always sold in original packages.

Kneipp Malt Coffee excels in every essential required by a hygienic food product. Being a pure malt preparation it is easily digested and assimilated by even the weakest stomach. It is rich in brain, bone and muscle-forming food—not only makes rich, red blood, but likewise builds up the body tissues, and has a pleasing taste and delicious flavor of its own. It builds up the system instead of undermining it as regular coffee does.

Kneipp Malt Coffee is used by eminent physicians and hundreds of institutions of every kind and denomination, as colleges, sanitariums, convents, etc., all of whom speak of it in the highest terms.

If on inquiry, your grocer does not sell Kneipp Malt Coffee write us, giving us his name and address and we will send you prepaid sample and booklet of recipes. Address enclosing stamp

Kneipp Malt Food Co.,
Dept. K
Manitowoc, Wis.

A popular coffee substitute, Kneipp Malt Coffee was sold in Benedict Lust's Health Food store in NYC.

KNEIPP HEALTH FOOD

by Benedict Lust

The Kneipp Water Cure Monthly, I(1),14. (1900)

Nobody will deny the fact that most of the diseases and cases of ill-health so prevalent in our times may be traced to our incorrect habits of living and to our accustomed unhealthful diet. It is time for us to consider this matter seriously. Our highly developed civilization makes increasing demands on our faculties and energies, and we ought to be careful to keep the body in such a condition as to enable us to meet all our duties with ease and confidence. Otherwise our strength is sure to fail and we will be left behind by our competitors in the struggle for life.

We ought to overcome inherited weakness or debilitating influences of our occupation and surroundings, or we will sooner or later succumb to adverse conditions.

We ought to make our health and our diet a study, rejecting stimulants, condiments and all kinds of food or drinks that are not natural, nourishing and harmless.

In this we may be well guided by the advice of authorities, who have experimented and studied in this direction. To Mgr. Kneipp principally is the merit due of showing us the necessity of returning to a simple, plain, appropriate diet calling attention to the most natural and nourishing foods at our command and the proper way of preparing and using the same.

Kneipp's Health and Strength Foods are well-known preparations and are cheap as well as good. Thus they will be found invaluable for the healthy and the sick, and of a price suited to every purse. They are not patent medicines sold at an enormous profit, but sold for a few cents and within the reach of all.

All the following preparations have been made according to Mgr. Kneipp's personal directions and have been examined and approved by eminent practitioners, being the most easily digested, blood and muscle producing foods made. They should be used in every family where health and healthful food-products are appreciated.

THE GENUINE, UNFERMENTED KNEIPP HEALTH BREAD

Made of whole wheat and rye, should be free from any artificial leaven or yeast. It is the best and most nourishing bread made to-day; a boon for dyspeptics and sufferers from constipation; the real staff of life for children and adults.

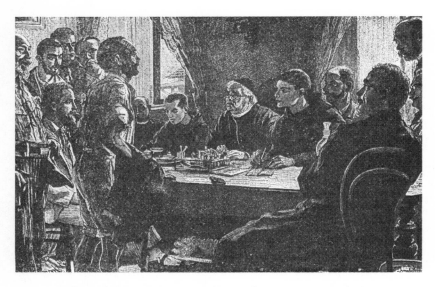

Father Sebastian Kneipp consulting with patients in Wörishofen.

HOW TO BAKE KNEIPP'S WHOLE WHEAT BREAD.

In *My Watercure* the following recipe for baking bread from such flour is given:

> Of this flour take 2, 4, 6 or 8 lbs. (according to the number of persons for whom the bread is going to be made), put it in a kneading pan, and make it into dough with hot water. Put the dough in a rather warm place, where it should remain during the night. Neither leaven, nor salt, nor any other spice may be mixed with it. The next day little loaves, or rolls, are formed out of the dough, and baked in an oven heated as for ordinary bread; they are left in the heat for an hour and a quarter to an hour and a half. As soon as the bread is taken from the oven, it is thrust into boiling water for 3 or 4 seconds, then put at once into the oven again for a short time to dry.

In a community of Franciscan Sisters the Kneipp Bread is prepared as follows:

> The flour is mixed with warm water and a little compressed yeast. After 4 or 5 hours this dough must be well kneaded. Then let it rise from 2 to 3 hours, then form it into loaves and put these into bread pans. Let the loaves again raise for ½ or ¾ of an hour, and then put these in a well heated oven for 1 ½ hours. The larger the loaves are the longer it takes to bake them.

STRENGTHENING SOUP

This strength giving Soup Meal is the best thing for weak and sickly children, because it is easily digested, very nutritious, and a cure for anaemia. It is also used with great benefit in kidney and stomach troubles, etc.

How to prepare it: This Soup is made in three different ways:

1) A small loaf of Kneipp Bread is cut into strips and toasted in a pan, then pulverized. Then put two or three tablespoonful for each plate of soup into boiling beef or mutton broth, let boil for twenty minutes, add egg and serve; soup greens and potatoes boiled with the meat will give an extra fine flavor to this soup.

2) Very nourishing soup is prepared by boiling the meal in milk with a little butter or an egg.

3) It may be boiled in water and seasoned to suit to taste.

Mgr. Kneipp says: "I am convinced that a great many sick people might be made well and happy if the value of this soup was understood and turned to advantage. It should be used in every household."

This soup meal can also be bought at Kneipp-stores and Kneipp-bakeries.

Good Health

depends as much upon your discrimination in the selection of foodstuffs as anything else.

OLIVE OIL is a wholesome food and builder of health when its production and preparation for market is protected all the way from the pressing of the native fruit to bottling and canning of the pure oil.

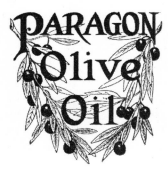

PARAGON Olive Oil

is a perfect product produced under the most modern sanitary conditions—it is pure and wholesome.

Packed in 5 Gallon, 1 Gallon, Quart, Pint and one-half Pint Tins. Your Jobber can supply you. Order from him now!

Paragon Olive Oil is used by the best Naturopaths and the Natural Life and Nature Cure People everywhere. Endorsed by physician, connoisseur, cook, housewife and those who know!

Magnus, Mabee & Reynard, Inc.

257 Pearl St., New York City

Established 1895

One of many olive oil ads found in *The Naturopath and Herald of Health*.

Olive Oil As A Remedy

by Benedict Lust

The Kneipp Water Cure Monthly, I(3), 36. (1900)

Since years codliver-oil is used as a remedy to strengthen weak children, while according to Kneipp this oil possesses very little value as a strength-giver. Kneipp was of the opinion that codliver-oil should only be used to soften heavy boots, but for no other purpose. On the other side he considered olive-oil an excellent remedy for many ailments, for instance:

For obstructions with phlegm.

For laryngitis and hoarseness.

For dyspepsia.

For ulcers in the stomach.

For fever-heat.

For diphtheria.

For obstructions with phlegm in the organs of respiration and laryngitis from 10 to 12 drops of olive-oil taken with a piece of sugar three times a day will work wonders. In cases of laryngitis it is advisable to rub the inflamed parts of the larynx with olive-oil. For ulcers in the stomach one should use 30 drops of olive-oil three times a day. For fever-heat a teaspoonful in the forenoon and in the afternoon will do. For diphtheria olive-oil is a very good remedy. One teaspoonful in the morning and in the afternoon will effect a cure by dissolving the phlegm.

For weak-breasted young people olive-oil cannot by recommended too highly. It is only used externally in such cases. Two or three times a week the breast of such patient is rubbed well with olive-oil. People who have to talk much, as priests, teachers, etc., etc., will find that rubbing olive-oil will give relief of pains in the breast which are a result of their work.

In cases of nervosity rubbing of the back with olive-oil will render good services.

Linseed-oil has pretty near the same effect as olive-oil but does not taste as well. Linseed-oil is a very good remedy for burns; it will stop the pain and heal the wound.

HONEY

by Mgr. Sebastian Kneipp

The Kneipp Water Cure Monthly, I(4), 58. (1900)

HONEY

From Producer to Consumer

Honey is a purely vegetable product—a natural food, delicious strength giving and health giving.
The craving of the human system for sweets is perfectly natural and Honey is a perfectly *natural* sweet to supply this need.

I am a *specialist* in Honey selling directly to the consumer. My Honey is ripe, rich, thick, delicious, and *I fully warrant it's purity under all Pure Food Laws*.

Place Honey on the table every meal. Use it partly in place of nut butters or creamery butter. Costs only half as much and will take its place in part. Give it to children in place of candy.

I sell two colors and flavors—light and dark. The dark is preferable for flavoring.

Prices;—10 lb. pail $1.30 by express. 4 (10lb) pails $5.00 by freight. *Freight charges much less than express.*

Sample by mail and copy of "Honey as a Health Food". 10c.
ALBERT G. HANN, Pittstown, New Jersey

Ad for "Honey as a Health Food".

The former generation maintained that young people should by no means take much honey, it being too strong for them; on the contrary, old people were 'helped on their legs again' by it.

I have made manifold use of honey, and have always found its effects excellent. It operates in a dissolving, purifying and strengthening manner.

It has long been used as an admixture with tea for catarrh and obstructions of phlegm.

Country people know well how to apply honey ointment for exterior sores or ulcers. I strongly advise those who are not skillful enough to treat such sores with water, to make use of this simple, harmless and effective remedy rather than of any other smearing stuff. The preparation is most simple. Take equal portions of honey and white flour, and stir them well together by means of a little water. Proper honey ointment should be solid, not liquid. Honey is also a good interior remedy for different lesser complaints. Smaller ulcers in the stomach are quickly contracted, broken and healed by it. I would not advise honey to be taken by itself, but I strongly recommend it taken mixed with a suitable tea. Without admixture this superior extract operates too strongly; before it has passed the throat, it has make it already quite 'rough'.

If on account of catarrh, or any other similar complaint, swallowing becomes difficult, let a teaspoonful of honey be boiled in a cup of water; by so doing, every singer will obtain the best and sweetest gargle.

Even if a drop happens to go down, there is no need to be afraid of injuring the stomach, or of poisoning.

The purifying and strengthening honey-water for the eyes is well known. Boil a teaspoonful of honey in a cup of water for five minutes, and it is ready for dipping in the linen for the eyes.

I know of an old gentleman above sixty years of age, who prepares his daily table-wine. He puts a tablespoonful of pure honey into boiling water and lets it boil for a while, and the drink is ready. It is said to be wholesome, strengthening and relishing. "I owe my health and my vigorousness in my old age," said he, "to this honey-wine." May be! This much I know from my own experience (I have prepared a great deal of honey-wine, seen a great deal of it drunk, and sometimes drank a glass of it myself): it is dissolving, purifying, nourishing and strengthening; and it is good not only for the weak sex, but for the strong sex too.   It always reminds me of the honey-mead of the ancient Germans.

PREPARATION FOR HONEY-WINE

(Very recommendable for the healthy and the sick.)

The ancient Germans had little or no wine. The brown beer was not known to them, because there was no such thing. Their food was very simple, and yet nevertheless they were a powerful race; they attained a great age and enjoyed an extraordinary health. They attributed this great age and extraordinary health to the 'mead' (honey-wine). It is a great pity that this good drink is so little known, and that its place is now occupied by the everywhere-known brown beer, which is often so much spoiled by art that it can no longer be considered a wholesome drink. In the larger works on the breeding of bees recipes are generally given for making honey-wine. But the complaint is often heard, that one has tried to follow these recipes, but has never arrived at a good result.

I generally prepared it as follows: I have from 60 to 65 quarts of soft water put in a very clean copper vessel. When this has become rather warm about 6 quarts of honey are stirred in it, and then it is left to boil quite gently for an hour and a half. From time to time the scum is removed from the top. When the time for boiling has expired, the honey water is emptied out into tin or earthen vessels, and when it has cooled (to a temperature a little higher than that of water heated by the sun), it is put in a thoroughly clean cask. The bung is put on, but not fastened. If the cellar is rather warm the fermentation begins after five to fifteen days. After about fourteen days fermentation this new fermented honey wine is drawn off into another cask. The dregs of course are left behind. In the second cask, the fermentation comes quite calm, so that nothing more is heard in the cask, then the bung-hole is closed. After three or four weeks, it will be clear and fit for drinking. It is then drawn off into bottles, and these are well corked and put into sand, it will effervesce in a few days rather strongly. This beverage is very cooling, and is therefore liked by those ill with fever. When sick people cannot drink either beer or wine, such honey-wine is a cordial for them. But it is also a good drink for the healthy; it ought, however, to be drunk in small quantities only, otherwise it cause disgust.

DIET FOR PATIENTS AND CONVALESCENTS

by F. E. Bilz

The Kneipp Water Cure Monthly, I(7),118-119.

It is a great mistake to suppose that patients and convalescents can benefit from a so-called strengthening diet, by which term is generally meant meat, wine, eggs, extract of meat, beef-tea and the like. On the contrary, by taking such food recovery is only retarded and relapse is often called, because a weakened organism can only digest the very lightest of food. A disordered or weak stomach or one suffering from the effects of an illness lately thrown off should only have rice boiled in water together with stewed plums, apples, etc., (later on a little browned butter), as well as thin soup made of ground groats, meal and coarsely ground wheat (patients with disordered stomach should not take too much whole-meal bread or coarsely ground wheat soup); moreover, fruit raw or stewed and later on milk, etc., may be given, and then by degrees, pass on to a non-stimulating diet. By proceeding in this way recovery and gaining of strength will be ensured without the danger of a relapse.

Many diseases, such as those in which the stomach is not irritated, are cured most quickly if for some time only whole-meal bread and fruit are given.

People of weak digestion may try addition of a few drops of lemon juice to their food, as this promotes digestion; fresh pure soft spring water only should be given to drink. It may, however, be mixed with a little fruit juice and sugar.

As the food of man is, so is his blood, as his blood is so is his energy, and his energy, so is his health.

Non-stimulating food, free from disease germs, forms pure, healthy blood free from germs of disease, and the same is true of pure or impure air.

As both in the question of food and medicine great errors prevail amongst the people to the prejudice of the patients, we here also call attention to the "Opinions of Medical men on the Taking of Medicine" with a view to convert the injurious inclination for drugs, which is so prevalent among the people, into abhorrence, and destroy their misplaced faith in medicine.

It is not always sufficient to prescribe a non-stimulating and easily digestible diet for all patients, but it must be suited to the particular patient and his ailment and tested from time to time as to its good or contrary effect, a procedure which is, unfortunately, only too rarely attended to even by Natural Healers.

Food or diet is the most important question in nursing the sick.

The art of determining a suitable diet consists chiefly in selecting such food as the stomach can digest perfectly and without too much exertion, and in such a manner that the nourishment which the body has received in too small or too great a degree, e.g., fat, starch, albumen, etc., or perhaps water, for lack of which the disease may also have been caused, may be supplied in proper quantity.

Moreover, in observing the nourishment of the body, and particularly of a sick body, the rules regarding the utilization of food must be more carefully followed by the attending doctor than has been the case hitherto.

We do not live upon what we eat and digest, i.e., upon what is merely acted upon by our digestive organs, but solely and entirely upon what is actually assimilated by the body. Everything else passes off as waste material, not only without benefiting, but often causing serious injury to it.

Further it should be remembered that what is unnecessarily inflicted upon the body in the form of nourishment, in the time of illness, feeds the disease rather than the body; the so-called nourishing and stimulating food must be withheld, in order to cut off what matures the disease. Abstention of food permits the organism to do its healing work most effectually, because if left alone and not burdened anew by superfluous ballast, it is in a position to expel the morbid matter, in which the illness has its origin, and to heal itself with what it extracts from non-stimulating, easily digestible food.

Taking too much food is overfeeding, by which we mean not always merely taking too large a quantity of food, but by overloading the body with food which contains too small a percentage of that particular kind of nourishment, i.e., albumen, fat, etc., which the patient particularly requires.

It is, therefore, necessary to consider and compare the relative value of foods as well as the condition and state of the body and its activity.

The following elements are the chief component parts of the human body:—Oxygen, hydrogen, nitrogen, carbon, sulphur, phosphorus, iron, sodium, potassium, etc.

The principle nutritious matter required by the human system are:
  I. Albumen.

  II. Fat.

  III. Carbon Hydrates (as starch, sugar, dextrine, etc.), which are chiefly found in cereals and their products (flour, bread), potatoes, vegetables, plants, etc.

  IV. Water (this simple nutriment), consisting merely of oxygen and hydrogen, is in spite of its simplicity of the greatest importance for the human body; the body of an elderly person consists of 75%, that of a younger one still more, even as much as 90% of water. Consequently our food should contain water in the same ratio, except in certain illnesses in which a dry diet should be observed.

V.   Mineral Salts.

These five principles species of nutriment must be supplied and be present in the body in a certain proportion if man is to be healthy and remain so.

If, however, too much or too little of one or more of these be taken, disorders in assimilation, i.e., illness results.

Diseases thus caused can only be healed by removing the primary causes just as in other illness, i.e., by increasing or decreasing, as the case may be, the proportion of the various kinds of nutriments.

It has been ascertained by recent investigations that the highly important nutriment called albumen only builds up the body but cannot supply it with heat or strength, and that is done by fat and carbon-hydrates, a fact which must be most carefully considered in prescribing a form of diet.

Many illnesses arise in consequence of general overfeeding.

Further, the temperature of the food taken, which may vary according to the patient, should be considered.

In many cases cool nourishment is advisable, in others food should not be above 90° F.

Dr. Sturm says, "Proper diet is the basis on which the art of healing should rest. This is the very foundation without which no attempt at healing can be justified. For as the organs are built up of nutriment, it is only from this that the possibility of living exists in our body."

Many diseases are never cured for want of a proper diet. The incurability of many diseases may be attributed to the imperfect study of other influences on the body.

If a patient be given the food which his ailment requires, he will in the majority of cases recover.

In concluding this article I must still call attention to the fact that sufficient perseverance is indispensable both in taking food suitable to the organism as well as in careful attention to the modes of application adapted to the disease in question.

Unfortunately the contrary is experienced too often, viz: that a patient, who has suffered for years from a deep-seated ailment and has changed his medical adviser a number of times, has taken the waters of some famous springs or has resorted to quacks and patent medicines of all kinds and finally has recourse to the Natural Method of Healing. (As a rule the experiment is not made until there is no other hope and the patient is not practically beyond recovery.) If in a few days or weeks the patient does not notice a very considerable improvement (slight improvements are scarcely acknowledged), he says there is nothing in it and gives it up.

Such patients are certainly not the kind we would like. He will only find sure and certain cure, if such be possible, who with firm faith and confidence and stern will recognizes the Natural Method of Healing as the only true method and, adopting it, continues it for a sufficient length of time.

This perfect confidence in the Natural Method of Healing is only to be acquired by experience; he who has no experience not only does not place it higher but frequently lower than any other method, and that is, considering the prevailing opinion with regard to this new method, hardly to be wondered at. Still whoever has had sufficient experience will agree with me that as truly as only one sun exists for our earth, so truly does only one method exist for the sick and ailing, and that is the Natural Method of Healing and its various branches.

Non-stimulating food, free from disease germs, forms pure, healthy blood free from germs of disease, and the same is true of pure or impure air.

We do not live upon what we eat and digest, i.e., upon what is merely acted upon by our digestive organs, but solely and entirely upon what is actually assimilated by the body. Everything else passes off as waste material, not only without benefiting, but often causing serious injury to it.

NUT FOODS

by Benedict Lust

The Kneipp Water Cure Monthly, I(8), 141-142. (1900)

By those who desire to leave of animal foods, such as eggs, milk and flesh meats, there has been a long-felt want for some food which will supply an abundance of nitrogenous matter in easily digestible form. While the grains contain a proper proportion of nitrogen, fruits and vegetables are deficient on this point. The legumes (peas, beans and lentils) contain an excess of nitrogen, and could be used to advantage with the starchy vegetables, such as potatoes, etc., but they are somewhat difficult on digestion, especially so for people of sedentary habits, and hence any foods which would supply nitrogen in an easily digestible form are of great value to the vegetarian. Such foods we have in nuts; but it is often the case that nuts eaten in the raw state, and perhaps not well masticated, are not well borne by the stomach. For this reason a series of foods have been prepared, after much experimentation and outlay, which have the following characteristics:

ADVANTAGES OF NUT FOODS

1. They furnish nitrogen in an excellent form.
2. They supply an abundance of oil, partially emulsified, so that it is more readily handled by the digestive system.
3. They contain a comparatively small amount of starch, and hence are an excellent food in cases of starch indigestion.
4. They are relished by most people.
5. They are cheap, as compared with meat and other animal products. A pound of nut food contains much more nitrogenous matter than a pound of meat, besides a lot of carbonaceous material. One can readily see that persons eating flesh would do well to take up the nut foods from an economic standpoint.
6. They contain none of the poisonous substances which are so common in meat, and are not so likely to become decomposed as meat.
7. They furnish a large amount of nutrition in small compass, and hence are excellent for travelers. They can be conveniently carried without danger of contaminating other articles of food, or damaging clothing. They are always ready for use, being thoroughly cooked. As the sealed goods are sterilized in the process of manufacture, they will keep fresh indefinitely.
8. They are more digestible than raw nuts.

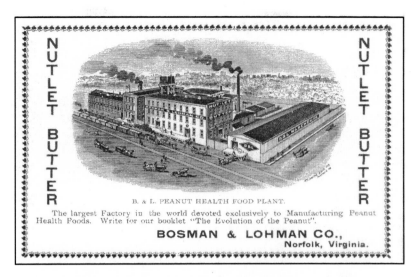

NUTLET BUTTER   NUTLET BUTTER

B. & L. PEANUT HEALTH FOOD PLANT.

The largest Factory in the world devoted exclusively to Manufacturing Peanut Health Foods. Write for our booklet "The Evolution of the Peanut".

BOSMAN & LOHMAN CO.,
Norfolk, Virginia.

The introduction of nut butters as health food began in the early 20th century.

The first of these foods put on the market was nut butter, and it has had such a remarkable success that it is now manufactured all over the country, in a small way, by families and by small manufacturers. It is proving a boon to many people, but on account of the temperature at which it is produced, a change takes place in the oil, rendering the fat more or less indigestible to certain individuals; so in a certain portion of cases it is found to disagree. Notwithstanding this, it is probably used, on account of its cheapness, to a greater extent than any of the other nut foods.

Nut Marmalate and nutlet are foods put up in sealed cans, and have a growing popularity. These foods are excellent sliced, or can be made up into stews with potatoes or various other vegetables. In fact, there are many ways in which, by the aid of these foods, appetizing and healthful dishes can be prepared. The manufacturers furnish recipes on application.

There is another series of foods, in which nuts are combined with pre-digested starch in the form of malt sugar. These foods, bromose, malted nuts, etc., are very delicate and toothsome, and occasionally we find a case where patients who can eat nothing else thrive on these. They are wonderful foods to lay on fat with. These foods may be said to be almost pure nutrition, and the starch part being already digested and the nut food thoroughly cooked, they are an excellent food for cases of weak digestion. They should take the place of the oil which has been obtained by drying out rotten cod livers, in the treatment of wasting diseases; and where they are so used they will be found to have a very beneficial effect.

MILK

by Benedict Lust

The Kneipp Water Cure Monthly, I(10), 180. (1900)

From the fact that milk is, or ought to be, the exclusive article of nourishment of children as well as of all mammalia, during the first months of their existence, we see that it contains all the materials necessary for the formation and growth of the body.*) Milk is, therefore, one of the best articles of nourishment that we possess.

We give a table showing the constituent parts of the kinds of milk most commonly used.

	Water	Fat	Casein and Albumen	Sugar of Milk	Residue
Cow's milk	87.7	3.5	3.7	4.4	0.7
Goat's milk	86.9	4.0	3.9	4.4	0.8
Mother's milk	87.9	3.3	2.6	5.7	0.5

Milk should, therefore, not only form the exclusive article of diet for infants, but should be an important constituent of our nourishment in later life. It should, therefore, be added to the food, or drunk between meals, in all cases, in which it is desired to increase a patient's strength, or to improve the condition of the blood and the humors by means of a somewhat more nourishing diet, as in convalescence after exhausting diseases, such as scarlet fever, diphtheria, typhus, etc.; also after painful deliveries, or in scrofulous, rickety, and consumptive subjects.

We now come to the question: "Ought milk to be drunk fresh or boiled?" The best and right way is, of course, to drink it as nature pro-

---

* Milk is produced in the lacteal glands. The secretion of milk commences at the birth of the offspring, and continues during the whole period of suckling, nine to twelve months or even longer. The secretion of milk ceases with the occurrence of a fresh pregnancy. The milk secreted immediately after birth is thin in quality and contains comparatively few solid constituent parts. It is often withdrawn and thrown away before the child is put to the breast under the mistaken idea that it is of little value, whereas the watery milk is specially adapted by a wise provision of nature to the digestive capacity of the child during the first days of its life.

vides it, fresh; and experience has shown that fresh milk is more readily drunk, better tolerated and more easily digested than milk which has been boiled. The practice of boiling milk owes its origin mainly to an exaggerated dread of bacilli. It is supposed, of course, that any bacilli in the milk will be destroyed and rendered harmless by the process of boiling. As if all men, in spite of every precaution, did not constantly breathe air laden with myriads of bacilli, in the streets and in public places, theatres, concert rooms, public houses, etc., without any harm resulting to their health, except in cases where the system has been weakened by other causes and the soil has been, as it were, prepared for the reception of the germs of infection.

The exaggerated dread of bacilli is, therefore, uncalled for in the case of milk. Any danger likely to arise from the presence of a few isolated bacilli in milk is more than compensated for by the greater palatability and digestibility of fresh milk.

Many people say they are unable to take milk because it produces a feeling of discomfort in the stomach. But this only happens when people, whose stomachs are naturally weak, suddenly take to drinking milk in large quantities, e.g., a tumblerful at a time. Under the action of the acids in the stomach, the albumen in the milk is coagulated into a lump, only the upper part of which can be acted upon by gastric juice. The presence of this mass in the stomach for some length of time gives rise to a feeling of pressure and pain in that organ. We, therefore, recommend to those suffering from weakness of the stomach, to drink milk, a mouthful at a time, and to eat a little bread at the same time. By this means the milk is more evenly distributed and prevented from coagulating into lumps; it is then more easily digested and causes no discomfort. In this manner, this excellent article of food can be digested by the weakest stomach. For infants and small children, by whom milk taken alone is not well borne, and in whom it is apt to cause discomfort, the milk should be mixed with a little groats or water-gruel, for the same object.

Thick and curdled milk can also be recommended. It is more easily digestible than fresh milk, because the first stages of digestion, the coagulation of the albumen, is already accomplished. Moreover, it has a favorable effect on the activity of the bowels in those who complain of a tendency to constipation after drinking fresh milk.

It is, at all events, desirable that the drinking of milk should come more into vogue in towns, and that people should cease to regard milk as an article of food only fit for infants. In many families it would be better for mental and bodily health, as well as for the pocket, if milk were substituted for pernicious alcoholic beverages.

BISCUITS, LIGHT BREAD, OR WHOLE WHEAT BREAD?

by F. J. Buettgenbach, Minerva, Oregon

The Kneipp Water Cure Monthly, I(12), 228-229. (1900)

About 2700, B.C., the introduction of wheat for food-purposes for mankind is recorded in Chinese history; after that we often find this grain mentioned in the old testament, and the ancient history, where we are told about bread made out of wheat and many other kinds of grain; Oatbread, barley or rye bread. Furthermore, we find in ancient history descriptions of how they cleaned these grains, ground them into flour, mixed them, baked them into bread, and that they enjoyed a long and healthy life because they ate in their bread all the elements that constitute the basis of all vital and strength-giving foods.

History tells us how the ancients, as also all the various races, up to the present century, ground these grains.

They first put them into a mill, and after they were ground into a flour, they used the whole of this product for bread, not minding the looks of it. They ate the whole of the wheat kernel, which contains, as is shown in modern chemistry, all the elements found in the human body:—Oxygen, hydrogen, nitrogen, phosphorus, carbon, calcium, sodium, potassium, magnesium, sulphur, chlorine, florine, silicon and iron. All which in right proportion help to rebuild the mental and physical forces and replace the daily waste.

The outer portions of the "Wheat," including the seed, contain "Protein" and mineral particles that constitute 12 of the 14 elements of the whole kernel. These are commonly known under the name of "Gluten."— "Gluten contains the 12 elements necessary for the sustainment of life."

Gluten contains phosphorate, or nutritive salts, without which no kind of food gives us any nourishment. "Gluten makes muscle, bone and teeth-enamel."—"Gluten makes the blood red, and new nerve and brain tissues."—"Gluten contains highly effective digestive agents, which would take the place of peptone and malt extracts."—"Gluten contains an oil equal to the best olive oil." When making "white flour," all the gluten is lost and therefore "biscuits" or light bread made with this flour, are almost "good for nothing."

The flour produced by the small mills a quarter of a century ago, retained much more of the nutritive properties of the wheat, than that milled by our so-called improved and patented mills of to-day. Since the opening out of the great wheat districts of the West, inventive genius has been taxed to its utmost to produce machinery which would make the whitest flour.

But by this procedure, only three of the above essential elements are retained in right proportion—"oxygen," "hydrogen" and "carbon."

And the wheat-flour is thus robbed of its most nutritive elements: Those which make bone, muscle and brain—in reality, the life-giving attributes of the grain.

Biscuit or bread made from this "robbed" flour might be compared to the "ballast of a vessel."

A trial of the comparative value of each flour was made in Bavaria (Germany).

They fed a dog with bread baked from the finest and whitest flour, mixed with water. After thirty days the dog would not eat his food any more, and ten days later he died—while another dog of the same age and proportion, which was fed with graham-flour-bread mixed with water, still enjoyed good health after these forty days, and if thus fed continuously, would only die of old age.

For the last half century the white flour drove away the golden, yellow-looking nutritious flour, only to please the eye, and the natural sweetness has been taken out of the flour to be replaced by artificial sweetness, which destroys the teeth, as well as the stomach. By these two factors the whole system of a person may soon be worn out, and this only on account of habit or custom, because people don't think about it or don't know any better.

Now, if you want to enjoy a healthy and happy life, live reasonably, eat reasonably, and in the first instance, don't spoil your constitution—for only in a healthy body can there be a healthy soul. Go back to the good and wholesome food which your grandparents used to eat. A good many people in the old country, but unfortunately, only a few people in this country eat nowadays, instead of light bread and biscuits made out of "white flour," the bread made out of graham flour which contains the whole of the wheat-kernel, just as the Creator gave it to mankind, only mixed with either milk or water and nicely baked. Don't put in any salt, for nature has already put it into the wheat. Don't put in any of those thousand different baking powders, which are mostly adulterated with either soda, alum, etc.; remember that your stomach is not a wash-tub, but that it and your bowels will get hurt by eating those mineral baking powders.

Furthermore, it is not necessary to use any other kind of yeast for bread, for whole wheat bread is easily digestible even if cold. To eat and drink hot food is dangerous for teeth, stomach and the whole constitution, and is very often the cause of severe sickness. If you will eat whole wheat-bread instead of the white-flour-bread, you will find out pretty soon how your bodily vigor and good health will increase, and your ailments as indigestion, constipation, stomach and bowel troubles will all cease, and you will have a good stool without the use of drugs, tablets, etc. But if you still persist in using the white flour, and won't listen to reason, you will find out your mistake: After the ball is over, i.e., when it is too late. Don't get deceived by the sayings of some of the rich people who say they like hot and white bread; well—they may like it, but they eat only the crust of the bread or half of a biscuit, leaving the rest on the table, but take sufficient nourishment from some of the seventeen other dishes on their table.

When making "white flour," all the gluten is lost and therefore "biscuits" or light bread made with this flour, are almost "good for nothing."

If you will eat whole wheat-bread instead of the white-flour-bread, you will find out pretty soon how your bodily vigor and good health will increase, and your ailments as indigestion, constipation, stomach and bowel troubles will all cease, and you will have a good stool without the use of drugs, tablets, etc.

DIET TREATMENT
BENEDICT LUST

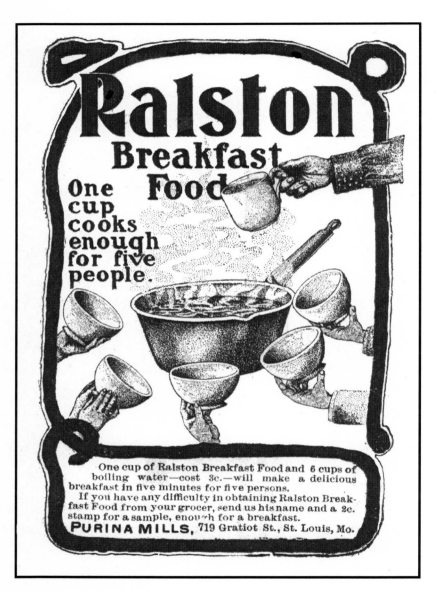

The origins of fast food at breakfast.

Diet Treatment

by Benedict Lust

The Kneipp Water Cure Monthly, II(1), 27-28. (1901)

A Series Of Articles By The Editor

What I designate hereafter as "Diet-treatment" does not only mean the enumeration of the different kinds of nourishment but also includes general directions as far as the limited space permits it.

After an observation of a number of years I have come to the conclusion, that a proper diet does not only enable the body to keep in good health, but in certain cases will even recuperate the health of the individual in question.

It must be remembered however, that as in some cases the body has been vitiated by a wrong treatment of many years, it should not be expected that after a fortnight or perhaps a four weeks treatment, a complete cure (which could indeed be called a wonder-cure) could already be effected. This would perhaps need several years, until new blood and especially better juices have filled the body.

Therefore in the following diseases I simply want to indicate principally the appropriate diet for invalids or reconvalescents. That for each sickness it would be impossible to define a proper diet, is of course self-evident, for in each case of sickness the diet must be appropriate to the constitution of the individual in question, and well may the patient bless himself who has a physician treating him, who understands fully the importance of a natural diet.

If a physician orders for the patient a diet consisting of bouillon, chopped meat, wine etc., he acts directly against the laws of nature, for in most cases the patient has almost an aversion against such nourishment, and rather longs for fruits or similar articles. It is really ridiculous (to say the least) when physicians say to the patient: You must eat plenty of meat, wine etc., so that you may regain your strength, as if the bedridden patient had to perform any hard manual labor! In most cases it is the digestion that is impaired and the stomach cannot be coerced; at most digestion might be stimulated by light bread-soups or a spoonful of lemonade made from fresh lemons.

As soon as health returns, then also the healthy appetite returns with it; and with a healthy appetite, the strength of the patient also returns; especially if the patient has plenty of fresh air.

Many people are frightened if, when they feel slightly out of sorts, they have no appetite, and they cannot fill themselves with food, as they

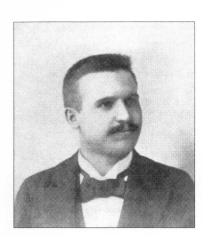

Benedict Lust.

are accustomed to. They, however, should not interfere with their digestive organs and when hunger returns again, they should stimulate it with easily digestible soups.

People who are in the habit of gorging themselves every day should better fast one day in each week, thus they would give their overworked digestive organs a little rest and many diseases, beginning with stomach-troubles would be prevented. Overfilling the stomach and too rich diet are certainly more liable to cause disease then a little hunger.

It must be remembered to allow the patients always a little variety in their nourishment.

DIET FOR FEVER PATIENTS

Whether the patient has fever is best ascertained by measuring his pulse and bodily warmth, for instance more than 100° Fahrenheit or more than 90 to 100 beats of the pulse, or whether he breathes more than 20 times in a minute.

Fever-patients as a rule have generally no hunger but only thirst. Only cooling beverages or light soups should be given them, for instance soup from boiled sour apples, or natural lemonade, or even pure water—but only when there is a desire for some.

Is the patient delirious, and the fever very high the nursing person should observe carefully the patient's heat, and from time to time give him a cooling drink with a spoon.

Sweet beverages are not advisable, as they only occasion more thirst; but there may be given either sour milk, oat-meal soup, Kneipp's Strengthening soup, Whole-wheat-meal soup etc., to the patient, if they prove palatable to him.

If the patient is suffering from excessive heat, he should be given a cold pack, and this should be renewed as soon as warm again; or be placed into a cold bath, which is beneficent to the patient and lessens the fever.

If suffering from Cold, a bed-steam-bath may be applied.

Should he also be constipated, which is generally the case, enemas should be applied, and also retained, because they cool, but no medicines be given. There should always be plenty of pure fresh air in the room, therefore keep the windows open.

Diet In Case Of Influenza

Cause: Formerly this disease was called Grippe and was cured in a short time by fasting and sweating. But after humanity has advanced more and more and become more modern and thus deviated from the laws of nature, this illness, as well as many others, appears in a much more violent form, because the blood has been generally weakened and also vitiated. Influenza has therefore grown into a malignant disease.

Symptoms: Days and even weeks before, loss of appetite, tiredness, headache, heat or frost, etc., etc.

Treatment: Never force the stomach to take food, rather suffer a little hunger, but you may as often drink natural lemonade as you like. A good march of from 2—3 hours in the open air, but so that you start to sweat, often kills the disease in the bud. After the long march, take an entire ablution, and protect the body from catching cold.

Should you, however, be compelled to lie in bed, apply 1—2 bed-steam-baths or trunk pack, or leg pack, and if also suffering from headache, cold-water compresses on the forehead should be applied.

Give the patient natural lemonade or broth from boiled sour apples, as many times as he desires them. Other diet is the same as in fever. Always be particular to have plenty of pure fresh air in the room.

If when passing water there is also passed blood or albumen with it, the diet ought only to consist of light, slimy soups (if there is appetite), natural lemonade and soup of boiled sour apples etc. If this treatment is strictly carried through, and the plain diet adhered to for several weeks, the disease will leave no ill after-effects, especially if plenty of exercise in the open air is resorted to.

Medicines, especially Antipyrin and Quinine, only suppress the morbid symptoms, but never cure radically.

Diet In Diseases Of The Rectum (Piles)

Cause: Piles or coagulation of the portal veins in the rectum, are mostly caused by sedentary habits, too little exercise in the fresh air, from working too much at home, from the excessive use of beer, strong coffee, hot and spicy foods, too much meat, leading a dissipated life, also from sorrow, anger, or overwork.

Symptoms: In the portal veins there flows the thickest blood, and these blood vessels all reach into the rectum. Should the blood now become vitiated by any or several of above causes, it is only too self evident that these tender little veins in the rectum will become swollen and form hemorrhoidal knots; these knotty formations then cause great pains, and sometimes burst and cause bleeding and other disagreeable symptoms.

Treatment: Should the patient possess enough energy or will-force, and if his work permits it, the disease may be cured or at least much ameliorated by a vegetarian diet, especially if the primary cause is abstained from.

Every morning whole-wheat-meal or Gluten-meal soup with fruit should be taken, this will at once regulate the stool. In the fore- and afternoon a few sips of fresh water, also natural lemonade.

For dinner vegetables with very little, or better still, no meat. Evenings sour milk with stewed fruit and bread and butter, pot cheese etc. Here are also to be recommended Kneipp's Strengthening and Kern soups, because they don't cause any flatulency. Kneipp said: "You don't believe how healthy such a Kern soup is." At night an abdominal pack which is taken off after 2–3 hours. In the mornings take a cool ablution of the whole body, drink a few sips of water, and then take a few hours exercise, not forgetting to take deep breaths of fresh air, so that the lower portion of the body is affected, thereby the blood-circulation of the lower regions of the body stimulated, and the constitution is improved in general.

Also gymnastic exercise is to be recommended. During the walk an occasional run should be taken if possible up a small hill, then breakfast will really be enjoyed and beneficial.

If someone wants to make an excuse that "the morning-walk is only tiring him" this is proved not to be true, if one considers how many thousands of workingman walk long distances to their work and back home again in the evenings, besides having to work hard all day.

One should go to bed every evening at 10 P.M., and get up at 5 A.M., then he can have concluded his morning-walk by 6:30 to 7:00 A.M.

In the evenings occasionally Sitzbaths (90° F.) should be taken for about 10–5 minutes. If constipated take an enema and massage the stomach from left to right. When applying the enema, a little almond-oil may be mixed with the fluid to be injected. After evacuation has occurred, take an enema of about a wineglassful water and retain some in rectum. The best remedies are gymnastics, bicycling, splitting wood, mounting hills etc., etc.

DIET TREATMENT FOR CONSTIPATION

Cause: It may be hereditary or be caused by wrong modes of living, overfeeding when not hungry, hot and rich food, pepper, mustard, coffee or too much meat. Sitting too much or leading a dissipated life may also cause it. Secret vices and pollutions also dry up the mucous membranes of the rectum. Further also the repeated non-observance of the regular stool.

Just the same as the body needs daily nourishment, it also needs daily evacuation.

But the most common cause of constipation is the continuous use of purgatives, especially patent medicines.

Treatment: First and foremost abstain from the partaking of all rich, hot and spicy food, and instead eat Whole-wheat-bread or soups, plenty of fruit, and take occasionally a few sips of water, but not too much, otherwise the desired effect will be lost. At a certain time each day take an enema with tepid water. Many people think that constitution will soon get used to this, but this is not so, for as soon as the constitution is all right again, the enemas are unnecessary. Further treatment same as in Piles: packs, massage, plenty fresh air, exercise, deep breathing, gymnastics, mounting hills, etc., etc.

It is really ridiculous (to say the least) when physicians say to the patient: You must eat plenty of meat, wine etc., so that you may regain your strength, as if the bedridden patient had to perform any hard manual labor! In most cases it is the digestion that is impaired and the stomach cannot be coerced; at most digestion might be stimulated by light bread-soups or a spoonful of lemonade made from fresh lemons.

REGENERATION
BENEDICT LUST

IN PRAISE OF THE ONION IN MEDICINE
BENEDICT LUST

One of the Many Reasons

Why YOU should be particular in the matter of using G r a p e juice and insist upon

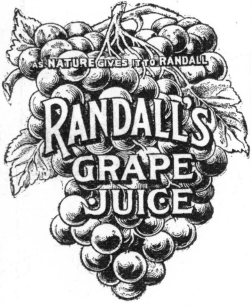

RANDALL'S GRAPE JUICE

Its mild fruit acids promote normal action of the digestive organs followed by a natural m o v e m e n t, which g e n t l y cleanses the system at the same time.

We guarantee our grape juice to be unfermented, strictly pure, containing no alcohol, glucose, preservatives, or artificial colorings.

THE

Randall Grape Juice Co.

Ripley, N. Y.

Unfermented fruit juices were endorsed by early Naturopaths.

REGENERATION

by Benedict Lust

The Naturopath and the Herald of Health, III(3), 107-109. (1902)

What shall we understand to be live food or raw diet? Everything that is offered us by Nature, just as it is, without any alterations. The oftener and the more thorough this alteration is under-taken with any food the greater becomes their deterioration by the hand of man—we call it unboiled, living, natural or raw diet fare.

Not only is it possible to eat all kinds of fruit, vegetables, corn, and all leguminous plants in their raw state, but even it is possible to make them palatable to the most fastidious palates. I know well that the spoilt stomachs and dainty palates of our present mankind will at first only unwillingly adopt these, and demand the customary appetizers. But a strong resolve and consistency will bring in a very short time a blessing to the strong-minded ones, and will procure them daily new pleasures, and they will feel better, lighter in spirits, full of good health, and feel as if regenerated, and will improve both in strength of body and mind.

Adoption of the raw fare.—Just the same, when someone who has remained in a place full of vitiated air, will greet his advent into the fresh, pure air full of joy, and derive much satisfaction from it; this is also the case with the raw fare, and therefore the question, whether to adopt it gradually or at once, is decided in the favor of the latter. All Nature does not produce a single instance of hot nourishment; no animal eats any hot or even warm food, even if very hungry; it will wait till it has cooled off—and anyhow, will prefer unboiled food. To the unspoiled man of nature all boiled dishes are unsavory, also all spirits. When the little daughter of Emin Pascha—Ferida—came to Berlin, she would know nothing of any such dishes, nor of any kind of footwear.

It is also well known that pointers and retrievers, if fed with warm food, get spoiled for the retrieving of animals—and how many men have lost all sense of smell or taste?

I would also like to draw the attention of all the eaters of boiled food to the following: "The earthy particles contained in water (and all water contains some) remain behind after evaporation from boiling; to prevent the food burning more fresh water is added. The body is forced to absorb this unusable matter. Thus we may imagine the formation of the gout, the calcination of the veins, the lessening elasticity of the bones (their easy breakability), the many difficult births, etc., etc.

The purest water is, however, contained in fruits; just sufficient to replace its waste in the body by evaporation, breathing and urination.

In coarse wheat, about a third of its weight is contained therein.

In apples, pears, plums, 75 to 87 per cent; even nuts contain 50 parts of water.

In oranges, cucumbers, and melons water forms over 90 parts of their weight. They are nothing but water, remarks the flesh-eater, sneeringly. But stop! we will reply that even lean beef meat contains 77 parts of water, and we will tell the gourmandizer that oysters contain 80 per cent. of their weight in water.

Even mother's milk contains 85 to 87 parts water. I will not talk here about the detrimental influences to the teeth and mouth; these are all well known, even if not in their entire extent. The many poisoning cases through meat, sausage, or cheese, are only made possible by the smelling and tasting senses having been weakened through the warm diet.

But nothing is told about the disadvantages caused to the other digestive organs, which all get weakened, and lost their strength and useful capacities; wherefore the continuously increasing quantities of food wanted by a boiled-food eater.

For this weakening only one example: it is well known that the stomach will throw up certain things which don't agree with it, if they are eaten cold; but if these are eaten when warmed, they will be retained on account of the warmth weakening the organism thereby.

The art of cooking, says Hufeland, knows how to retain such a good friend in the palate, that all the arguments of the stomach are in vain; and because the palate is tickled by some new pleasant process, the stomach sometimes gets two or three times as much work as it is able to cope with.

What is only a palate tickle, is considered real appetite; thereby man gradually loses the principal props of his health, i.e., the knowledge when he has had enough.

The poor stomach cannot talk; only sometimes it gives vent to its dislikes by some grumbling noises. Sometimes nourishment in concentrated form is given the body by bringing the strength or contents of several pounds of meat, etc., through pressing or boiling, into the space of a soup plate.

Then they believe to have achieved something great, to bring by this method such an extract of nourishment directly into the blood, without having it first masticated by the teeth, and thus saving the stomach its labor.

But Nature's institutions can not be overlooked with impunity. All the juices are overheated by this procedure, and cause a continuous overfilling of all vessels.

Articles which are at once taken up by the stomachial vessels, like meat broths and any other kind of concentrated soups, fluid nourishment, alcohols or sugar in concentrated form; all these cause above symptoms.

Every article of food should go through the regular digestive process; in the mouth it should be entirely masticated; in the stomach worked upon and permeated by the gastric juice, and then only enter the bowels; that is to say, only when it will be assimilated to Nature by the action of the mouth and stomach.

But the principal failing of all cooked dishes (also meatless ones) is that they may still be nourishment without having any life-giving ingredients; they do not any more contain the vital, electric, or magnetic tension power.

The original ways of Nature or of vitality we will never be able to explore; and Albert W. Hollern says very appropriately: "Into the interior of Nature no creative mind will penetrate;" and Hahnemann says: "Even if all elements of the human body are to be met with in Nature, they work in this organic conjunction in such a peculiar, extraordinary way (for which we only have one general name—vitality), that this special vital art of the animals amongst themselves and against the exterior world can be judged in no other measure and explained in no other way."

Not even by any of the known doctrines of mechanics, or statistics, physics or chemistry. . . . According to Goethe: "He who is satisfied with pure experience and acts accordingly, he has enough truth."

In its effects and expressions the natural forces show definitely that they stand in eternal dependence and relation to the earth power, may we call them either electricity or magnetism.

The beneficial influences of light, air, and warmth are recognized everywhere in theory. Every one knows that cellar-plants strive towards the light, and only after having reached it they take color. The strength of the earth and the surrounding atmosphere, however, is something new, or rather something already forgotten. In former times it used to be recognized, although not always called by the right name: instead of the appropriate name "sympathy," they talked about "Kabbala," secret wonderful powers, previous wonderstones, etc.

Something of this strength is felt by everybody, but especially by those suffering from nervousness; if when lying upon the naked ground they feel excited, falsely thinking this to be pernicious, this shall then be caused by the exhalation (!!) of the earth.

If we enter a room we miss something in it; it is not oxygen, because that could not have been used up; or if we were to remain in a hermetically closed compartment, and by help of chemistry were to maintain herein contained air in its complete and correct parts, that is, to replace the used-up oxygen, and to restrain the carbonic acid gas, we should still believe in a very short time that we were going to perish. There is something missing, in spite of all chemistry, which we cannot express, but the loss of which we feel most acutely. The magnetic tension power of the free

Nature, whose vitality is most beneficently noticeable and appreciated in the open air.

This natural strength is to be found in the raw diet, and only in this kind of diet, and is completely killed by boiling, i.e., from a boiled apple, pea, etc., it is impossible to obtain any new fruit, and they also decay the quickest, for they are vegetable corpses, as is also evident by their changed appearance—the power that we use in masticating the fruit, goes over, as we may say, into our bodies.

Not only is it possible to eat all kinds of fruit, vegetables, corn, and all leguminous plants in their raw state, but even it is possible to make them palatable to the most fastidious palates.

. . . the principal failing of all cooked dishes (also meatless ones) is that they may still be nourishment without having any life-giving ingredients; they do not any more contain the vital, electric, or magnetic tension power.

In Praise Of The Onion In Medicine

by Benedict Lust

The Naturopath and Herald of Health, III (XI), 468. (1902)

Few will deny that the palates of some people are not favorably disposed to the pronounced flavor of the onion. Still it must not be forgotten that onions are diuretic, diaphoretic, carminative, and soporific. Diuretic—increasing the action of the kidneys; diaphoretic—increasing the secretive and expulsive work of the cutaneous glands; carminative—toning up the stomach and thus assisting in the digestion of food; soporific—quieting the nerves and inducing sleep. It is thus apparent that onions are more than a wholesome article of the diet, for they are not only easily digested, but ensure the better digestion of other food, and increase the work of the organs designed to cleanse the body of dead matter. The good offices of onions are most needed in hot weather and by nervous people, while all people will find this vegetable nutritious at all seasons. It should be eaten more largely than it is when the debilitating hot weather has so affected the stomach that the appetite is weak and digestion unsatisfactory. People who at that time "can't eat anything," are weak and languid, and at night are restless—slow to sleep and often disturbed in sleep—will find onions just what they need. And who does not know of the efficacy of onion syrup in cases of croup and cold? The mother who knows how to use onions, internally and externally, for croup and all colds affecting the throat and chest, is possessed of information that will be of priceless benefit to her children. Stick to onions if you wish to avoid the doctor sticking to you.

Still it must not be forgotten that onions are diuretic, diaphoretic, carminative, and soporific. Diuretic—increasing the action of the kidneys; diaphoretic—increasing the secretive and expulsive work of the cutaneous glands; carminative—toning up the stomach and thus assisting in the digestion of food; soporific—quieting the nerves and inducing sleep.

A GOOSE'S GASTRONOMY

would be insulted by a lot of the junk that our friends the Health-horrorites swallow for food. We don't know of any law that forbids enjoying what we eat—we do know of an instinct that precipitates dyspepsia the minute we eat a thing because some fellow with spectacles and a squint solemnly analyzed it.

When you're tired consuming chips and sipping dilutions of anaemia, suppose you try some of these real foods:

Whole Wheat Bread, Lust's (without hulls or a leprous look) .... .10

Fruit Crackers (delicious for luncheon, picnics, etc.) .... .10

Kneipp Malt Coffee (tastes something like coffee) .... .15

Banana Coffee (a novelty both food and drink) .... .20

Nutritive Salts Cocoa (a splendid nerve food) .50

Pure Swiss Milk Chocolate (Genuine candy? Yes) .... .25

Apple Tea (sounds interesting) .... .25

Straight-Edge Date-Nuts (oh so good)....... .05

Taroena (any stomach can digest it)........ .30

Cresco Gluten Grit (jollies along complaining kidneys) .... .25

Barley Pancake Flour (for people not too hygienically good) .... .20

Ko-Nut (to fry the pancakes and other things) 3 lbs. .... .75

Unpolished Rice (only kind fit to eat)...... .15

Kneipp's Pea Soup Flour (pure and nourishing as fresh peas) .... .25

Salted Peanuts (you can wash off the salt for conscience sake) pkg.................... .05

Banana Figs and Banana Flour, pkg........ .15

Pure California Honey (to sweeten health-reformers) .... .25

Welch's Grape Juice (good for sick and well) .... .25

and

Hundreds of other delicacies, five cents to five dollars.

☞ **Special Introductory Offer.** Put a dollar bill in an envelope and mail to me at once; then I'll send you by express a lot of sample goods, to the value of $1.25. I know if once you get acquainted you'll want our things right along. Catalogue for a stamp—anyway you can afford that.

THE REAL FOOD STORE

BENEDICT LUST, Proprietor.

124 EAST 59th STREET   **NEW YORK CITY**

Benedict and Louisa Lust operated one of the first health food stores in NYC called 'The Real Food Store'.

1903

CEREO:
The Leader of all Coffee Substitutes
PRIDE OF UTAH

Takes the

place of

Coffee, Tea,

and other

Cereal

drinks.

Money

refunded if

not

satisfactory

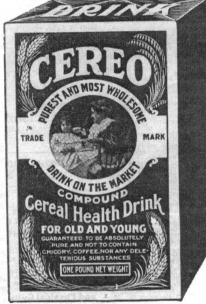

The best

Naturo=

pathic

Cereal

Coffee on

Earth.

Nothing

like it on

the

Market.

Beats

them all.

It is pure, healthful and nourishing. The only cereal drink that is guaranteed absolutely pure and not to contain chicory, coffee nor any deleterious substances.

What Cereo Is

Cereo is a True Food Product or Liquid Food, not a stimulant; therefore builds up the Nervous System in place of deadening. or inciting it.

Cereo is a Regulator, Blood Purifier and Strength Producer as it contains nothing but the Pure nutriment of the grain and fruit.

Cereo is the best food for the young and delicate as it requires neither masticating nor digestion; it being a Pure Liquid Food there is no wood nor pulp to burden the weak organs, but it is in a pure state to be taken up by the blood and build up the weak parts.

Yours Sin-Cereo by
THE CEREO MF'G. CO. LOGAN, UTAH.

Price 25 cents per large package. For sale at all Grocers. Eastern Wholesale and Retail Depot.
PURE FOOD STORE, 465 Lexington Avenue, New York City.

Another coffee substitute.

SHOULD WE DRINK?

by Sophie Leppel

The Naturopath and Herald of Health, IV(4), 87-89. (1903)

Science tells us that less than one quarter of the human frame is composed of solid matter, more than three quarters being water. Many people conclude from this that the laws of health require that they should imbibe a certain quantity of either water, tea, coffee, cocoa, or alcoholic drinks, etc., to supply the needed fluid which is daily excreted by the kidneys, lungs, and skin. Many people drink, not because they feel thirsty, but simply for the reason that they see almost everybody else drink and they assume that it is the right thing to do. We know that all water, especially in large cities, is tainted in a greater or lesser degree with organic impurities and it is probably the most potent of known media for conveying infection. Its unfitness for use is always a matter of degree only. The role of the illustrious who owe their death to water is an appalling one. We need mention only the late lamented Dr. M. L. Holbrook, G. W. Stevens, and the greatest of Russian composers, Tschaikowsky; to these we might add, practically the great majority of the victims of those plagues and epidemic which have not yet ceased to afflict humanity.

Personal experience and professional observation alike convince me that neither water nor any other of the drinks mentioned above is necessary to health provided one can obtain those juicy fruits and juicy vegetables which contain the liquid needed by the system in the purest and therefore the healthiest form. Dr. Evans in his book *How to Prolong Life* demonstrates clearly that the use of water tends to produce disease and premature aging. Many forms of kidney diseases are now attributed to bad water. Distilled water is not available for all and many find it insipid. Many people believe that without some of the ordinary drinks they would become shriveled up, wrinkled, and thin. This is a vain fear if suitable juicy fruits and vegetables are taken in right quantities. For instance, raw peeled cucumbers, eaten like apples, contain abundant juice and they cool without making thin. There is a general belief that cucumbers are indigestible. This is not the case when they are rightly combined with other suitable foods. Lemon-juice is also cooling, but if too much is taken, it impoverishes the blood and makes one thin. Stout red-faced persons may freely indulge in lemon-juice. Lemon-juice possesses curative properties beyond those of any other fruit or vegetable in common use. Rightly applied, lemon-juice dissolves hardened substances in the body such as tumours, fibroids, chalky deposits in the joints of the hand, feet, etc., and it powerfully assists digestion. When lemon-juice, in place of salt, is sprinkled over meat, fish, or vegetables, it makes the food tasty and facilitates the digestion of other nutrients.

★★

The Vitalism Series of Publications.

(THIRD EDITION),   Sent to any address on receipt of the prices named.
In which THE LEPPEL DIETARY SYSTEM is expounded.

1. SUITABLE FOOD AND PHYSICAL IMMORTALITY.
The author explains in this pamphlet how she can, by taking specified combinations of foods, make herself either prematurely old or youthful looking. The vegetarian dietary is given which makes her yellow, irritable, and nervous. Eczema, boils, a blotchy skin, etc., can be as easily produced by her as these disfigurements can be cured. 15 cts.

2. HINTS FOR SELF-DIAGNOSIS.
In "Hints" interesting information is given respecting the cause of the unsightly appearance of most men and women, and the methods are indicated by which diseased and ugly persons can be made healthy and good-looking. 25 cts.

3. VITAL AND NON VITAL FOODS.
Twenty Lists of Classified Foods. Brief but to the point. Lists of foods are given for the aspiring who wish to feel more "fit," or to do their work more efficiently, also lists of food which induce or increase certain complaints. 25 cts.

4. THE DIETETIC WAY OF HEALTH AND BEAUTY.
Deals with such popular fallacies on dietetic habits as "One man's meat is another man's poison," "It is a virtue to live on cheap foods," etc. Different dietetic systems are also discussed. 5 cts.

5. THE TEA QUESTION.
Describes the injurious effects of tea-drinking. 5 cts.

6. THE MISSING LINK IN DIETETICS.
Discusses the importance of taking rightly combined and proportioned foods. Attention is also called to the unhealthy appearance of many vegetarian leaders and Theosophists, and the cause thereof is given. 5 cts.

7. A NUT AND FRUIT DIETARY.
The properties of fruits and nuts in common use are given, with recipes and general rules. 5 cts.

8. WHAT IS THE DIFFERENCE BETWEEN THE DENSMORE AND LEPPEL DIETARY SYSTEMS ?
Interesting Letters and Testimonials. 5 cts.

9. SEXUALITY AND VITALITY.
Affirms that the average man and woman sacrifice their Vital powers on the altar of their animal passions. Cause and cure given. 10 cts.
The above 9 pamphlets for a dollar bill.

FOR THE ABOVE PUBLICATIONS ADDRESS : **Naturopath Publishing Co., 111 East 59th St., New York.**
★★★★★★★★★★★★★★★★★★★★★★★★★★★★★★★★★★★★ ★★★★★★★★★★★★★★★★★★★★★★★★★★★★

Sophie Leppel, an apostle of dietetic reform blamed careless living and over-indulgence in eating and drinking as the primary cause of disease.

Tomatoes of a good quality are excellent for rheumatism and gout. Mineral waters which are so often prescribed for curing these complaints only add to the mass of foreign or unsound elements which the system is unable to expel, their retention being the cause of the trouble. Mineral elements, like table salt, soda, iron, phosphates, etc., cannot be assimilated by the human body and if the system is too weak to expel such foreign substances, they produce ill-looks, disease, and premature death. Although temporary relief may sometimes be found by taking mineral waters, experience proves that ill-health is sure to follow sooner or later when elements are taken into the body which are not suited to its needs. Sufferers from kidney diseases will rapidly improve when abstaining from ordinary drinks of all kinds because thereby less work is thrown upon the kidneys. Acids are not usually relished by this class of people and they should therefore take only a little lemon-juice to assist digestion of other foods. Orange and lemon-juice mixed to suit the taste, without sugar or water, will be found very nourishing and stimulating, for thin and pale-faced persons. Fresh, juicy, uncooked, sub-acid fruits (apples, pears, grapes, berries, oranges, etc.) rejuvenate and beautify and at the same time supply the liquid required by a well-sustained body.

Some kind of nerve and brain food (meat, fish, dairy produce and almonds) should always be combined with fruit and vegetables, to ensure a healthy action of the bowels and to supply the system with sufficient brain or nerve power. Also some starchy food (porridge, bread, rice, sago, chestnuts, etc.,) is needed to keep the muscular system strong. Starch, if combined with other foods and well digested, controls the weight. A stout person should decrease his daily portion of starchy food and the thin person should increase his usual quantity bearing in mind all the time that starch must be combined with a right amount of brain or nerve food, fruits, and vegetables, to avoid mal-assimilation. That starchy foods, if taken in wrong portions, are one of the principle causes of ill-looks and ill-health, is admirably illustrated by Dr. Densmore in his book *How Nature Cures*. Suitable starchy foods nourish the hair, teeth, and nails and make the hair grow thick and strong but meat alone (as far as my experience goes) can restore faded hair to its natural color and lustre.

A diet consisting of brain or nerve food, fresh raw vegetables, fresh, uncooked fruits, and some starchy food, must ultimately supersede all drinks in common use—with those, I mean, who intelligently seek lasting health. I have taken no drinks of the ordinary kind for thirteen years. I have no desire whatever for the usual artificial stimulating drinks such as tea, coffee, chocolate, alcohol, etc., and ordinary water is distasteful to me.

I am convinced that temperance reformers would accomplish much more good if they would take up the food question and learn to advise those addicted to alcoholic drinks to take foods which do not produce thirst, but which contain all the liquid needed for a healthy condition of the body.

Sophie Leppel, Editor, *Diet Versus Drugs*,
26 Clovelly Mansions, Gray's Inn Road, London, England.

Many people believe that without some of the ordinary drinks they would become shriveled up, wrinkled, and thin. This is a vain fear if suitable juicy fruits and vegetables are taken in right quantities.

DIET

by Benedict Lust

The Naturopath and Herald of Health, IV(8), 226-227. (1903)

Diet is one of the most important questions for the sick as well as the healthy, as it is no doubt easier to prevent illness by a sensible way of living than to cure a disease that has once taken hold of us. Therefore, it is and always will be one of the most important principles to teach wise living in order to prevent diseases. Diet is the essential factor in trying to keep this principle, as a great number of diseases originate only from poor and unwholesome food.

It depends so much upon what a man eats, as his body is built up by the food he takes. In any case it is of vast importance that a certain regularity be observed. Irregularity in meals alone causes disturbances in many cases. Three meals a day, in the morning, at mid-day and at night, are the best rule for all to observe; all eating between meals is superfluous. Besides, the center of gravity for all eating and drinking should be put on the first two meals, viz. with the morning and midday meals.

BREAKFAST

We should accustom ourselves from early childhood to eat sufficient and wholesome food in the morning. It is a very unwise custom of so many people to drink only coffee at breakfast; in this way we do not take any nourishing substances, but only a stimulating beverage, as coffee does not contain any nourishment but only excites the nerves and "animates." We become stimulated and animated to work without, however, receiving the substances that give us the strength to work, or to build up our body. Coffee taken in the morning must, therefore gradually become the origin of many diseases. And even if coffee is taken in the morning, be it without bad results for years, the consequences will gradually manifest themselves by nervousness, sleeplessness, etc.

We should therefore accustom ourselves from childhood to take a strong rye or wheat flour soup every morning well cooked with milk, water or butter or oat flour soup. This will keep the body strong and healthy and will never be harmful.

It is of the greatest importance that children should be brought up by these rules, and then we will not hear complaints that one cannot give up coffee and the other thinks flour soups do not agree with him. Those having a good appetite may take some bread, or one or two soft boiled eggs, with their flour soup every morning; and if they absolutely need a beverage they may drink Kneipp's malt-coffee or one of the popular nourishing vegetable salt cocoas, Banana Coffee, Malt Creamlette, Kneipp's Family Nourishing tea, Apple-tea etc.

BREAD

The choice of nourishing bread is of the greatest importance. The custom to make one's own bread has become a thing of the past, much to our disadvantage. We find this custom only in the country, everywhere else bread is bought from bakers, who never trouble about its preparation and whether it is nourishing. Good bread will always be the principle food for most people, and it is very regrettable that the public at large are so indifferent in regard to the bread question.

Among all classes of people perfection of the milling industry is praised in high terms, but nobody considers that the finer the flour the more unwholesome for us. The larger mills have even discarded all apparatus that grind the grain with the bran. Usually the bran is at once separated from the grain and in this way the flour is robbed of its best nourishing qualities, as the bran contains nutritious gluten. The bread we get from the baker does not contain any of this gluten and is therefore very insufficient as a food.

The bran should be retained as is the case with soldiers' ration-bread or graham-bread. The so-called Whole Wheat bread of the Hygienic Bakery, 100 E. 105. St., New York, is also very good bread, as in preparing the flour the really nutritious qualities of the bran are retained, while those parts of the bran which form the outer husk and do not contain gluten and are indigestible, are removed by certain separators. This flour makes excellent bread and is widely known for its superiority.

Those who cannot procure Whole Wheat-bread, Graham-bread, or Steinmetz's strong-bread should try at least to get country-made rye bread, as this is usually stronger and better than the city-made bread. The plainer bread is prepared the better. Turn your back on fancy bread. If possible we should bake our own bread and purchase only the flour.

Country people eat mostly coarse dark bread, prepared from coarse rye flour (flour with bran) and of their own make, and to a great extent they are indebted for their good health, strength and endurance to this bread. But look at the cultured city people; from generation to generation their teeth become poorer and poorer and nowadays false and decayed teeth are very prevalent. The reason for this is that their food is too refined, too much deprived of its nutritious qualities that it does not suffice to build up a strong and healthy body.

It is lucky that country people for lack of means have to support themselves in a simple manner; but this keeps them well and hardy.

It may be added that the coarser the bread the easier digested; the finer it is the more indigestible. The bread made by the baker or confectioner from finest wheat flour is constipating while Whole Wheat-bread, although looking like lead, is easily digested and at the same time acts as a physic.

The limited space does not permit to discuss this highly important bread question as it deserves, but the suggestions given will doubtless appeal to the thinking public.

WAY OF EATING

The opinions about a proper way of living are very different. It is a downright shame to see how every animal without erring finds out that food which is the most beneficial that Nature has given him, while man, who considers himself the head of the creation has a thousand doubts about the simplest questions regarding his way of living.

Professor Dr. Jager is right when he says that in many things man can learn very much from animals. If from this stand-point we look at the controversy whether vegetarianism or mixed vegetarian-carnivorous (meat-eating) diet is the right one, a feeling of great shame must come over us. As these questions, however, are in the focus of the movement for natural treatment it would be a sin of omission should we pass it by without due consideration.

Three meals a day, in the morning, at mid-day and at night, are the best rule for all to observe; all eating between meals is superfluous.

Coffee taken in the morning must, therefore gradually become the origin of many diseases. And even if coffee is taken in the morning, be it without bad results for years, the consequences will gradually manifest themselves by nervousness, sleeplessness, etc.

The opinions about a proper way of living are very different. It is a downright shame to see how every animal without erring finds out that food which is the most beneficial that Nature has given him, while man, who considers himself the head of the creation has a thousand doubts about the simplest questions regarding his way of living.

A NATUROPATHIC SILHOUETTE

by Benedict Lust

The Naturopath and Herald of Health, IV(9), 247-249. (1903)

Condiments, spices, stimulants, pickles, iced-drinks, rich sauces and gravies, lard, glucose, white flour, all such panderings to appetite rather than satisfying of hunger, Naturopathy rejects and condemns.

An infallible test for the wholesomeness of a food is a short fast. Go without eating for a day, and notice the character of the first craving. It will not be for fried oysters, or mince pie, or ice-cream soda. It may not be for the same food your friend might crave—the needs of the two systems may differ. But it will be for a real nutrient.

After all, the important points in Dietotheraphy are Mentality, Mastication, and Post-Prandial Period. The first will be considered later under Mental Therapeutics, the third under Hesukotherapy.

Mastication is the index both of hunger and of digestion. A really hungry man cannot bolt his food—it is a physical impossibility. An acquaintance of the writer broke a three week's fast on the juice of a single orange. He took an hour to finish it, and declared the sixty minutes the most rapturous of his life.

No food is ready for deglutition till the secondary taste has been extracted, complete liquefaction taken place and the swallowing process become involuntary. And if no thirst be present at beginning of meal, its appearance before the close is infallible proof of deficient mastication.

Drinking Water is a point omitted by most Dietists, but peculiarly emphasized by Naturopathy. The human system requires three or four pints of pure liquid daily. Fruit and melons furnish it in most desirable form—distilled and vitalized. Distilled and aerated is the only approximate substitute and is obtained through the modern aerating Stills, such as the Cuprigraph, Sanitary, Ralston, and Puritan. Mechanical impurities are eliminated by such filters as the Berkefeld which is the only one recommended.

But mineral rather than animal matter is coming to be recognized as the defilement of drinking-water. With the exploding of the germ-terror and the knowledge that Senility is simply arterial deposit of earthly matter, attention is directed now to preventing deposit rather than to making corpses of germs.

The average American's drinking supply is undeniably foul, and the less inhibited the better. A still is practically indestructible, comparatively inexpensive, and offers the only approach to fruit-juice yet devised.

Meal-time is a bit of senseless tradition that needs puncturing by the projectile-points of Naturopathy. Strict Nature-Curists plead to abolish it altogether and to forage as the animals do. Naturopathy does not go so far. It does maintain however that the meal-hours of your fathers and your family are not necessarily the meal-hours for you; that the three-meal plan is for most Americans an utter abomination; that from five to eight hours should intervene between meals; that the heavy meal—if there be such—must follow, not precede the day's work; that it should include with post-prandial rest, a full hour and a half; that meal-time should be controlled, not by custom, or hospitality, or family feeling, but by hunger, by the condition of the gastric juices, by the digestion of the previous meal, by the character of the work to follow, by the mental attitude, by the age, the occupation, the temperament, and other neglected personal elements;—in short the YOU is the arbiter of Naturopathic eating.

For instance: this morning your employer gives you a present and a half holiday—you have rice and soft boiled eggs for Luncheon, and the time and temper to eat properly—you spend the afternoon in a gymnasium—and by four o'clock you could digest a hearty Dinner. To-morrow you learn the funeral of a friend is set for the early afternoon—you choke down a plate of salmon and hard boiled eggs—you let your grief poison every digestive juice in your body—and by seven o'clock there is still a heavy mass of half-digested food clogging normal hunger. And yet you religiously and ceremoniously observe the same Dinner-hour to-day, to-morrow, and forever.

Now Naturopathy prescribes four meals for certain cases, one for others; but in general the Two-Meal No-Break-fast Plan is the American's salvation. I have never known a purposeful man or woman to omit Breakfast long enough for a fair trial, and then to lapse back into the matin cakes and coffee. The rational is too plainly and perfectly described in Dr. Dewey's book *The No-Breakfast Plan* to warrant repetition here. But the furred tongue, the "dark-brown taste," the biliousness, the listlessness, the nervousness, the irritableness, the morning headache, the fitful appetite, all the faithful familiars of the American-spirit, these dote on Breakfast. And generally they have sufficiently choked individuality to prevent one's being different in this or any other particular.

The article *The Dissection of a Dead Day*, presents special phases and variations of this most crucial topic. (In January and February Vol. III. 1902.)

In a very inadequate way, the whole matter of Dietotherapy may be summed up in the following.

SUGGESTIONS

1. Never eat until hungry. Laugh at the archaic Dinner-bell. Smile in conscious superiority at the well-meaning but ill-advised friends, who beseech you to "eat and get strong;" delight in the growing conviction that you are your own master.

2. Distinguish carefully between Hunger and Appetite; satisfy the one, conquer the other. To the really hungry man liquor, tobacco, spices, and their kin are absolutely revolting. Dietetic Error is the mother of all Intemperance.

3. Masticate every morsel to the liquefied state of involuntary swallowing. This applies particularly to rice, mashed potato, soup, and foods already diluted. Suction, milk, mastication are truly saliva-precipitants as the most vigorous dentition. The babe chews its milk every grasping of the nipple.

4. Quit Breakfast for good and all. A little grape-juice, or orange-juice, or a warm drink, is not objectionable, but every atom of solid food vitiates just so far your mornings work and noon-digestion.

5. Put your one hearty meal where it will do the most good, at whatever period of the day you have an hour and a half undisturbed. This will probably mean the reconstruction of your culinary arrangements. The beings who yield to conditions and surroundings die at thirty-five, the men who make them live to the age of Gladstone and Bismarck and Verdi and Pope Leo—you can take your choice.

6. Don't be a fool or a Faddist. Chronic experimenters are not safe guides and the cons are more important that the pros of any theory you propose trying. No Diet or Dietery will be of any use whatsoever until you are rationally and emotionally convinced of its beneficence. Moreover no single food is of value whose eating violates natural craving. Eat what you crave, but eat it right.

7. Remember that the real desideratum is not what you eat, but how and when and why. Naturopathy tells you what and how and when, conscious selfhood tells you why.

8. Never drink at meals. If thirsty take a few sips before eating. A single cup of Cocoa or other nutrient-beverage is often advisable, provided it be chewed as food, not gulped as drink.

9. Always sip a pint or so of cool water, pure spring or aerated, distilled or filtered, on arising and retiring; other times simply satisfy thirst. Hot water, salt water, lemon water, oatmeal water and other modifications are preferable in special instances. In the absence of a Still, certain bottled spring waters are to be commended. The normal man who eats right is thirsty a half-hour before eating and two hours after.

10. Gradually accustom yourself to nuts and fruits. In later life you will have to avoid meats, cereals, and other so-called staples which

further the accumulation of arterial deposit. Begin the change now—
Will is a better master than necessity.

11. Get some good work on Dietetics, study it, and don't believe it. There
is no single book yet written that represents or satisfies Naturopathy.
But there are several with glistening grains of Truth. And the important thing is that you become interested.

12. Remember that the stomach is a muscle, and under the dominion of
the brain. When Doctors announce that fasting is fatal, ask them
whether a muscle that is strained, wrenched, fatigued, inflamed,
should be worked or tested. When Predigested-food concocters urge
this or that costly manufacture, ask them if they strengthen the biceps
by investing in slings and cork arms. When Panacea-peddler was
rapturous over this or that Dyspepsia-Cure, ask them if they cure a
sprained ankle with cocaine. When anybody attempts to think or act
or prescribe for you, assert fearlessly the rule of your brain over your
stomach. And you will not go far wrong.

13. Let the lesson of Dietetics take its proper place—insignificant and
inconsequential—in the vast realm of Self-knowledge. It is the greatest single factor in physical welfare, and the least understood. But it
becomes infinitesimal beside the everlasting entities of Soul-unfold-
ment. And when you come to yourself—if you ever do, the food
question will lose itself in the great problem of fulfilling your destiny.

Food and Drink are but the acknowledgment of man's still insistent
dependence on the material. And when you begin to enter the penetration
of Life itself, the toy objects of mere physical existence will appear to you
as to the man who has "put away childish things".

No food is ready for deglutition till the secondary taste has been extracted, complete liquefaction taken place and the swallowing process become involuntary. And if no thirst be present at beginning of meal, its appearance before the close is infallible proof of deficient mastication.

Meal-time should be controlled, not by custom, or hospitality, or family feeling, but by hunger, by the condition of the gastric juices, by the digestion of the previous meal, by the character of the work to follow, by the mental attitude, by the age, the occupation, the temperament, and other neglected personal elements;—in short the YOU is the arbiter of Naturopathic eating.

Distinguish carefully between Hunger and Appetite; satisfy the one, conquer the other.

Remember that the stomach is a muscle, and under the dominion of the brain.

Pure Juice of Wild Fruits

Extensively used as Therapeutic Agents

Nature has endowed Fruits, especially WILD FRUITS, with the most perfect and beneficial stimulative, tonic, and laxative properties.

WAGNER'S
PURE JUICE of WILD FRUITS

Are put up expressly for THERAPEUTIC uses in accord with tried and proved scientific methods—Natural, Unsweetened, Uncooked, Non-alcoholic—guaranteed to be FREE from the addition of any chemicals whatsoever.

A Therapeutic Gift from the Natural Resources of the Wild Forest—

FOR THE WELL—THE SICK—THE INVALID—
THE CONVALESCENT—THE CHILD—THE AGED

WAGNER'S PURE JUICE OF THE WILD CHERRY—an excellent Therapeutic Agent in anæmia, malnutrition, general debility, and the nervous system, especially for women. Also contains mild laxative properties.

WAGNER'S PURE JUICE OF THE WILD BLACKBERRY—Saturated with Organic Iron Oxide. A builder of healthy red blood, indicated in anæmia.

WAGNER'S PURE JUICE OF THE WILD ELDERBERRY—A valuable therapeutic agent to "tone up," regulate, and promote normal functioning of the Female Regenerative Organs.

WAGNER'S PURE JUICE OF THE WILD BLUEBERRY—A mild tonic, indicated in anæmia, nervousness, and general debility, especially where there is a delicately balanced organism, with a sensitive stomach.

Dr. Benedict Lust recognizes and acknowledges the great Food and Therapeutic value of WAGNER'S PURE JUICES OF WILD FRUITS—and uses it extensively in his institutions.

Eastern distributor, wholesale and retail:

DR. B. LUST'S PURE FOOD STORE
110 E. 41st St., New York, N. Y.

Ad for Wagner's Pure Juice of Wild Fruits.

SOME FOODS AS REMEDIES
A. SCHOLTA

THE NATUROPATHIC KITCHEN: NON-STIMULATING DIET, VEGETARIAN OR NATUROPATHIC
BENEDICT LUST

MODERN SYSTEMS OF HEALING: THE SHROTH CURE
JOHN A. R. GRAY

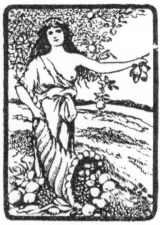

Carqué's California

BLACK MISSION FIGS

Are the Best

SPECIAL OFFER

Ten pounds of this delicious, wholesome Fruit will be sent Express prepaid to all stations of the Wells Fargo and American Express Co. for $1.50. Add 25c. to the other stations.

Carque California **FRUIT LAXATIVE**

A food of excellent remedial quality, composed of carefully selected sun-dried California fruits. Absolutely free from all forms of medication. Package by Mail, 15c.; 3 doz. small packages or 10 large packages, $3.50 Express prepaid.

CARQUE PURE FOOD CO.

Magnolia Ave., Cor 16th St.
Los Angeles, Cal.

Headquarters for Pure California Food Products Unsulphured Dried "Likefresh" Fruits, Nuts, Nut Cream Butter, Olive Oil, Whole Rice, Honey, Fruit-Laxative, etc.
Descriptive Circulars and Price Lists on Request

NEW YORK AGENCY:

B. LUST, PURE FOOD STORE
112 E. 41st St. - - - N. Y. City

Otto Carqué, a leading food expert marketed many products from California's harvests.

Some Foods As Remedies

by A. Scholta, Representative of Naturopathy, Freiburg, Saxony

The Naturopath and Herald of Health, V(6), 139-140. (1904)

All food products can also be remedies if properly prepared. Diet as such is a healing factor.

1. *Oatmeal*

    It is an excellent nourishing food; it is the meat of the vegetable kingdom for the vegetarian. Its specific effect on the intestines is not sufficiently valued. Oatmeal causes a moderate movement of the bowels; this particularly refers to roasted oatmeal. There is nothing better for people suffering from emaciation and diarrhoea. Those subject to constipation will do well to try whether their condition does not become worse by eating oatmeal. Buckwheat-meal can be recommended to them.

2. *Cocoa*

    The cocoa commonly used is over-praised in all medical magazines. I do not agree with this praise of its merits. Kneipp is right if he warns us against it. Exceptions of this are the recently discovered wheat and nutritious salt cocoas, which make blood and do not contain alkalic substances. Cocoa swells in the intestines and forms a kind of paste, which produces constipation. It is often indispensable to those who suffer from chronic diarrhoea or whose mucous membrane of the intestines has been weakened, or, as the physician says, at chronic catarrhs of the intestines and other complaints of the mucous membrane of the intestines; it does not, however, need to be applied in cases of acute diarrhoea. Nervous people and children should take no cocoa whatever, or use it only as a stimulant. The stimulating part of it is the theobromine.

3. *Almond Milk*

    After a feverish attack, or even during fever, it is frequently advised to have an easy digestible, palatable and refreshing beverage. Almond-oil is one of them. If it cannot be bought ready-made, pound sweet almonds fine and mix them with water until they form a thick paste, which afterwards can be diluted and used like milk. A similar effect is attained by the rather very sweet vegetable milk of Lahmann.

4. *Red Whortleberries*

    The juice of red whortleberries diluted with water is a favored thirst-satisfying beverage, and is often used for feverish patients. Like all sourish beverages (apple, fruit and bread-crumb water) it satisfies in the same way that fresh water does, an instinctive requirement of the patient.

Red whortleberry water can especially be recommended for acute articular rheumatism and gout. There is no other beverage that acts so blood-cleansing on the organism as juice of red whortleberries. It is the greatest enemy to uric acid.

People suffering from stomach catarrh and poor digestions should not use sour red whortleberries, not even if they are sweetened. Too many sour things cause a diminution of the red blood-corpuscles; small quantities of natural vegetable and fruit acids promote the formation of blood-corpuscles.

5. *Huckleberries*
An old proverb says: "If huckleberries are scarce there are many diseases," which is very true. Huckleberries to the city folks in summer are the same as the spoonwort is to the Greenlander in spring.

Owing to the tannin they contain huckleberries act constipating on most people, while with others they have the opposite effect. The latter may be explained as an irritation of the glands of the bowels; the former as a contraction of same by the tannin. As a remedy against diarrhoea they have a palliating effect.

They are an excellent cure in cases of acute catarrhs of the mucous membrane of the mouth, the throat and the urethra, if cooked and locally applied. They particularly give relief to defects of the mucous membrane, discharges owing to weakness of the mucous membrane and catarrhs with stoppage of the blood, particularly in the mouth and the larynx. They are indispensable in cases of chronic gonorrhoea, catarrh of the larynx and defects of the mucous membrane of the cheeks.

6. *Milk*
No benefactor of mankind has been so neglected as just milk. All juices of animal tissues and blood contain healing qualities, and the freshly-milked, and to some extent also the uncooked milk, have these qualities. They are lost by cooking.

Milk is a universal healing remedy for kidney and heart diseases. Those who do not know that scarlet fever patients must get milk in order to prevent inflammation of the kidneys should not wonder if, notwithstanding a natural treatment, dropsy and scarlet fever set in. People suffering from abscesses of the stomach will find sweet milk of great benefit if they take much of it and drink it possibly by the spoonfuls. "No scrofula can be cured without milk," says Kunze, although this is a little exaggerated it is a fact that with the poor scrofula, which has usually been caused by excessive use of potatoes, is best cured by milk.   Anaemia is overcome by drinking plenty of milk and not taking other liquids (soups). Anaemia and nervousness require milk, because it contains the proper composition of nourishing qualities.

Milk, however, can have a bad effect if used inexpediently.   If babies are fed too long on milk alone they are apt to get throat trouble. The great quantity of water which is contained in milk wears away the tissues and the tissue-salts are carried off.   The child anaemic, cold and has not the proper support to build up its bones.   Therefore, babies, from their sixth month, should receive more substantial food (such as fruit, grits, oatmeal, bread, soups).

Cooked milk often causes constipation, and also the so-called sterilized milk from old cows often does not agree with people.   The so-called children's milk should not be heated more than ten minutes on eighty degrees Celsius (180 degrees Fahrenheit).   Too fatty milk produces acid in the stomach and constipation.

Thick sour milk and kefir milk are excellent beverages for the sick; the latter is especially adapted for stomach, lung and heart diseases, and to promote appetite and digestion.

7.   *Linen Tea*
"Linseed Tea," as the people call it, is a tea made from linseed.   Boiling water is poured over the well-cleaned linseeds, left for fifteen minutes and then strained, and the tea is made.

Ulcers of the stomach, erosions, painful stomach catarrh, constipation, bladder catarrh, catarrh of the urethra, if at an acute stage, require a linseed decoction. I would not like to miss linen tea in my extensive practice. It protects the lining of the stomach from self-digestion by sour gastric juices, it covers the dry intestines with mucous, promotes a movement of the bowels and can even give relief from chronic diarrhoea, if the latter is caused by lack of mucous in the intestines.

8.   *Calves Feet Soup*
Those who have not tried its effect should give it a trial.   There is nothing better for sufferers from chronic diarrhoea.   It is indispensable in cases of tuberculosis of the intestines, ulcers and cancers of the stomach and the intestines, inflammation of the intestines, and particularly appendicitis.
The calves feet are cooked like other meats, with vegetables, rice, oat-

meal or buckwheat, noodles, etc., and prepared as soup, etc. Wherever it is permissible an egg may be added.

9. *Pumpkin Soup.*
Pumpkin soup and cooking of the pumpkin rind are well-known and harmless kidney cures, and are also applied for dropsy.

10. *Bean Soup*
Bean soup has reputation of driving water out of the system and is used for heart disease.

Cocoa swells in the intestines and forms a kind of paste, which produces constipation.

Almond Milk *after a feverish attack, or even during fever, it is frequently advised to have an easy digestible, palatable and refreshing beverage.*

Cooked milk often causes constipation, and also the so-called sterilized milk from old cows often does not agree with people. The so-called children's milk should not be heated more than ten minutes on eighty degrees Celsius (180 degrees Fahrenheit).

The Naturopathic Kitchen:
Non-Stimulating Diet, Vegetarian Or Naturopathic

by Benedict Lust

The Naturopath and Herald of Health. V(7), 173-175. (1904)

Most diseases originate in a more or less erroneous dietary; therefore, besides using the following non-stimulating foods, the greatest care must be taken to arrange a proper combination of nourishment for each individual patient. For instance, in many cases the body is overloaded with albumen, fat, etc., and there is deficiency of carbon-hydrates, salts, and water; in other cases the cause of illness being perhaps exactly the reverse. In many instances, also, the cause is insufficient digestion of food, but often both of them contribute to the result. Disease frequently consists in one or more organs of the body being too well nourished or not active enough, and the reverse. All this requires most careful consideration, which is one of the doctor's most important functions.

If, for example, an excess of one or more kinds of nutriment, such as albumen, fat, carbon-hydrates, etc., or a deficiency of these is present, often only to be detected after careful observation and consideration on the part of the doctor, the disease must be remedied by a suitable combination of foods.

Should the cause consist of inadequate digestion of food, an increase of the functions of the body or capacity for using up food must be brought about, or rather facilitated. If one or all of the organs be too well nourished, or the reverse, *i.e.*, not active enough, in the first instance the overfeeding must be discontinued, and in the second the deficient activity increased or the reverse.

By non-stimulating diet we understand, firstly, all kinds of bread, particularly whole-meal wheaten bread, then all foods made with milk and eggs, vegetables, porridges and soups, made palatable with milk or butter.

We draw special attention to beverages and soups made with whole-meal, the latter of grated whole-meal bread, fried in a little butter, perhaps made palatable with a little milk or cream; then, above all, curds, buttermilk, sour mild, fruit, stewed berries, which may be partaken of at every meal.

The chief beverage should be pure water, as soft as possible, which may be mixed with the pure juice of fruit, such as raspberry and lemon juice, German unfermented wines, grape juice, Pomona, cider or sugar. Then milk, buttermilk, chocolate, cocoa, Kneipp's family tea, apple tea, etc. Then extracts made from roasted wheat or barley, and decoctions of young strawberry, blackberry and woodruff leaves; further, artificial coffees, substitutes for coffee, malt coffee, banana coffee, malt, creamlet, cocoa, Bilz-Lahmann and Prager's nutritious salt cocoas, etc.

Meat, broths and meat extracts are to be avoided on account of their heating properties, by which febrile diseases especially are aggravated. Should a piece of meat be specially desired, it may be partaken of occasionally in light cases of illness without fever, but the quantity should be small; for instance, a little piece of roast veal, tender beef, young poultry, fish or the like. On the other hand, all smoked or pickled meat, or such as has been overboiled for soups should be avoided by invalids, as well as strongly spiced and salted dishes. In most cases, too, vegetable with husks should be avoided (on account of the indigestibility), as well as alcoholic drinks, such as brandy, strong beer, strong wine, etc., likewise strong coffee and tea.

GRUELS

Persons will do well to provide themselves with a vegetarian cookery book or with vegetarian recipes, in order to obtain a clear idea of what is meant by non-stimulating diet.

These are very thin sorts of porridge. They are particularly suitable for convalescents after acute illness, or in obstinate cases of constipation, etc. Wheat-, maize-, rye- and oatmeals are used in making gruel. About two dessert-spoonfuls of meal must be mixed with cold water, and boiled slowly for fifteen minutes. Rice gruel is often useful in cases of diarrhoea.

ANOTHER SORT OF GRUEL, between porridge and gruel. Flour or oatmeal is usually employed; half a pound of flour and three pints of water is the right proportion. Cook for about twenty minutes. Raisins, currants or dried berries may be added if desired.

WATER SOUPS

FLOUR SOUP.—Stir a tablespoonful of good wheat flour or rye-meal into cold water, beat into half a pint of boiling water, and boil up a few minutes with salt and fresh butter, stirring all the time.

FRUIT SOUPS of every kind can be prepared with any sort of fruit, dry or fresh, or sultana raisins. These must be boiled with plenty of water, the whole then stirred up with rice, barley or oatmeal, or with sago to make the soup thick. Sugar according to taste.

HARICOT-BEAN, PEA, AND LENTIL SOUP.—These vegetables must be boiled thoroughly in soft water. If hard water only be obtainable, boil them up and let them get cold again before using. Rub off the husks (not necessary for persons in strong health) and finish cooking with butter, potatoes and herbs. White bread fried brown in butter, or simply toasted and cut into dice, is very good with bean or pea soup; with lentil soup an addition of dried damsons may be used.

MEAL SOUPS are all made in the same way: three quarts of water with salt brought to a boiling point, then half a pound of meal (wholemeal, flour, oat or barley-meal) stirred into cold water, and boiled up a few times together. If currants, raisins or dried cooked fruit be added, it is more palatable; a little butter must not be forgotten.

PANADA.—The crust of brown bread, pumpernickel or rye bread soaked over night in cold water, then thoroughly boiled with plenty of water and put through a sieve. Add butter, salt and sugar and slices of raw apple; or, instead of the latter, raisins previously boiled (sultanas are best) or damsons; then boil up again. Instead of adding fruit, milk and aniseed may be stirred into the soup when ready. (To three quarts of soup half a pint of milk.)

ROLL SOUP.—Cut a small stale Viennese roll into slices, pour boiling water over it; beat thoroughly and pass through a sieve; add a little salt and fresh butter, and boil again. Or the roll may be sliced into a plate, salt and butter added, boiling water poured over it, and the whole stirred.

POTATOE SOUP.—The potatoes must be washed clean, well covered with water and boiled till done; sweet herbs, green leeks, celery (or dried) herbs) are boiled soft separately in water and then added. Add butter or oil according to taste, and oil all together with whole-meal, flour, oat or barley-meal. Or the potatoes may be pushed through a sieve.

PREPARATION OF OATMEAL.—Oatmeal soup, gruel, porridge and oatmeal water are preparations of oats and water, and may be partaken of lukewarm or cold. Groats and oatmeal, or even the grains of oats, may be used, but the latter must be thoroughly boiled down. This glutinous and digestible food possesses remarkably valuable nutritive properties; it is healing and strengthens the nerves, improves the composition of blood, promotes the various functions of the body, especially the secretions of the kidneys, and is at the same time perfectly harmless. This food renders the greatest service in diseases of the kidneys and bladder, in all kinds of rheumatic affections, in a morbid condition of the humors of the body (cachexia), in nervous and in all kinds of febrile diseases. Professor Becquerel speaks of it as follows in his *Handbook of Hygiene*: "It is far more nourishing than is usually imagined. It is often found that the stomach will retain this when it rejects every other sort of liquid nourishment. It is well known that gruel is frequently used in febrile diseases, especially inflammation of the mucus membrane, as a demulcent remedy promoting the secretion of mucus, and it is only to be regretted that people, when in health, make too little of this excellent article of food. Gruel is probably the best substitute for that wretched coffee, which only wastes the strength and makes people nervous. There is no better morning drink for children." The best method of preparation is as follows:

Wash the groats (for four people a cup or four brimming dessert-spoonfuls) and boil them in plenty of water for from one and a half to two hours, till the soup is glutinous. Then rub it through a fine sieve, add lemon juice, raisins and a little sugar, cook over a slow fire for half an hour, and finally add some butter.

When made of oatmeal, the soup is not so good, but the preparation takes less time.

Three desertspoonfuls of oatmeal (for four people) are thoroughly stirred with a little water, and then poured slowly into three pints of boiling water, in which a little salt and a half of a dessertspoonful of butter have been previously dissolved, stirring all the while. Go on stirring while it boils up, then draw the saucepan on one side, and let the soup simmer for a quarter of an hour at the side of the fire, stirring occasionally. It is not necessary to take oatmeal soup in large quantities.

An oaten dietary has proved itself to be the most certain restorative, and is even efficacious in cases where all other so-called tonics leave us in the lurch; I know no better remedy for building up a broken down constitution. I advise every one suffering from weakness to take porridge and gruel daily, and I know that they will be grateful to me for this advice. Thin and emaciated persons can be "fed up" on this diet in a short time. Anaemic girls, and delicate women suffering from the effects of confinement, who are visibly getting worse while partaking in beefsteak, broth, wine and preparations of eggs, take a turn for the better at once on being fed on porridge and oaten soups. This food also agrees excellently with pale and badly-developed children, particularly during their school-days, when such large demands are made on their youthful constitutions; they become rosy, strong and blooming. In short, oats are unequaled as a restorative, and can therefore be as strongly recommended to invalids as to persons in health.

RICE SOUP.—Stew two or three ounces of well-washed rice till soft with a little water and butter. Beat a little flour, some salt and butter well into a quart of boiling water, and boil until it forms a thin, glutinous soup. Then add the rice.

Most diseases originate in a more or less erroneous dietary; therefore, besides using the following non-stimulating foods, the greatest care must be taken to arrange a proper combination of nourishment for each individual patient.

By non-stimulating diet we understand, firstly, all kinds of bread, particularly whole-meal wheaten bread, then all foods made with milk and eggs, vegetables, porridges and soups, made palatable with milk or butter.

Modern Systems Of Healing: The Shroth Cure

by John A. R. Gray

The Naturopath and Herald of Health, V(8), 184-185. (1904)

The Schroth Cure

The Schroth method of healing is the treatment par excellence for the removal of toxins and poisons of all kinds from the body. It is sometimes called the "regeneration treatment," and it well deserves the name, because after successfully passing through it one has indeed been physically remade. Crowds of diseased men and women, of all classes, who have been ineffectually treated by some of the ablest medical men in Europe, have at last found relief and health through the "Schroth" cure. It is not, of course, equally good for all diseases and this is not claimed for it.

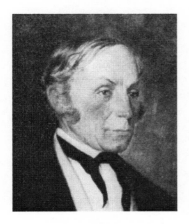

Portrait of Johann Schroth.

Who Was Schroth?

Johann Schroth—born in 1798 and lived till 1856—was a farmer and a jobbing contractor of Lindewiese, in Austria. Like the great majority of laymen who have turned their attention to health study, Schroth was drawn to the subject through personal need of health. In 1817 he was kicked by a horse and his right knee-cap fractured. The medical treatment left a good deal of inflammation in the joint and Schroth became lame. He could no longer bend his knee. Unable to walk by the side of his loaded cart he used to climb up and rest on the top. One day a traveling monk reproved him for riding in this way. Schroth explained his misfortune and the monk advised him to bath his knee frequently in cold water. As this was inconvenient Schroth fastened on a wet bandage instead, renewing it at intervals. And with splendid effect too, for at the end of ten weeks the stiffened leg was as supple as the other. So the foundation of Schroth's health knowledge was laid.

He began to recommend his treatment to others with beneficial results. Thus he went on. As he gained experience he reasoned that what was good for a diseased knee should be good also for internal disease. And on trial he found it so. As his knowledge of healing increased first one part of the body was subjected to his treatment and then another, until at length the entire body was his province.

Through noticing the conduct of wounded animals, and the effect of water-drinking on his horses while at work, he was gradually led to adopt a dry form of diet in the treatment of the sick and diseased. To the present hour this is the salient feature of the Schroth cure. Like Rikli, he used water and other natural means—but as auxiliaries.

SCHROTH'S DRY DIET

Now let us look at this principal factor on which so much depends—the dry diet. The theory on which Schroth worked was, that when little or no liquid is taken the morbid humours in the body are pressed into service, the stomach, and digestive organs generally, are obliged to use up their own secretions so as to dissolve the dry food. The consequence is that poisonous matter in the system is gradually loosened and thrown off. The whole digestive apparatus is granted rest, assimilation is improved and the whole mass of the blood, humours, and body is purified, renewed and invigorated.

There are three parts to the treatment—the preliminary, the main, and the supplementary. The preliminary is a gradual weaning from the usual to a simplified diet, and the supplementary is the gradual return to the usual diet after the principal treatment. I can only outline the main part of the cure. For breakfast and supper the patient has stale rolls and biscuits. For dinner semolina, barley or gruel with stale rolls. A couple of hours after dinner a glass of light wine is taken. Great thirst may be relieved by slowly sipping a little lukewarm water. At night the whole body is packed in a wet sheet. Over this go a couple of blankets and a rug. The wet sheet has the effect of relieving the thirst and equalizing the temperature, as well as carrying away toxins. Of course the treatment must be suited to the strength of the patient. The cure may cover from one to three months according to the nature of the case. It is regarded as complete when the patients tongue is moist and perfectly clean, and the urine no longer contains sediment after standing.

IN CONCLUSION

So much that is interesting remains to be said of Schroth: his wonderfully reliable diagnosis of disease, his unselfish nature and his kindly heart. Schroth was unscrupulously attacked by medical men, not one of whom were fit to unfasten his shoe latchet. But over this we draw a veil.

His worth and ability were recognised in his own time, and as the world frees itself more and more from medical superstition, the higher he will be esteemed. (*Scottish Health Reformer*)

New Theory On Eating
Benedict Lust

About The Value Of A Good Gluten Graham Bread
Benedict Lust

The New Tuber Food
Benedict Lust

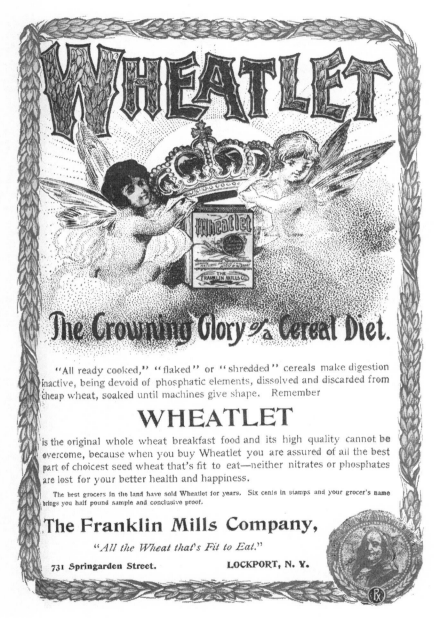

WHEATLET

The Crowning Glory of a Cereal Diet.

"All ready cooked," "flaked" or "shredded" cereals make digestion inactive, being devoid of phosphatic elements, dissolved and discarded from cheap wheat, soaked until machines give shape. Remember

WHEATLET

is the original whole wheat breakfast food and its high quality cannot be overcome, because when you buy Wheatlet you are assured of all the best part of choicest seed wheat that's fit to eat—neither nitrates or phosphates are lost for your better health and happiness.

The best grocers in the land have sold Wheatlet for years. Six cents in stamps and your grocer's name brings you half pound sample and conclusive proof.

The Franklin Mills Company,

"All the Wheat that's Fit to Eat."

731 Springarden Street. LOCKPORT, N. Y.

Before Monsanto and GMO, wheat was a healthy food.

New Theory On Eating

by Benedict Lust

The Naturopath and Herald of Health, VI(2), 53-56. (1905)

We All Eat Too Much, says Horace Fletcher.

Be really hungry, he advises in his work *The A B Z of Our Own Nutrition*. He asks if Man is competent to be Chauffeur of his own body.—An interesting review of the idea of *Fletcherizing Food,* by Dr. Kellogg, of the Battle Creek Sanitarium.

Mr. Henry Bool hands us copies of Horace Fletcher's new books, *The A B Z of Our Own Nutrition*, and *The New Glutton or Epicure,* together with the interesting article published below from the pen of Dr. J.H. Kellogg; and appearing in *Good Health,* and which is a review of the theories of Mr. Fletcher, the discoverer of the benefits of food liquified and rendered tasteless in the mouth before swallowing, and now known as "Fletcherizing."

Mr. Bool has convinced himself that great benefits are to be derived by practicing Fletcher's theories; hence his desire to have the idea promulgated and generally adopted.

Horace Fletcher is a wealthy retired merchant from Venice, Italy, and is a great traveler. He declares in his new book, *The A B Z of Our Own Nutrition*, that Americans eat too much and unwisely. The result, he says, is a loss of energy and an invitation to disease. The majority of those who violate the laws of health by overeating do so, he asserts, through ignorance and not because they are gluttons.

The author has found a way how not to eat too much, according to his own statement, and at the same time eat all the appetite desires and in a way combining a maximum of good taste and a minimum of cost and waste. The monetary saving by economic nutrition, he adds, is of little matter as compared with the saving of the waste of energy and the menace of disease.

In his introduction Mr. Fletcher says: "Nature never intended that we should weaken, depress and distress ourselves in the way that is common to present day living, as is made evident by the prevalence of discomfort and disease relative to our daily food. Nature's plan of evolution does not work that way in general, does not retrograde in the progress of the improvement of plants and dumb animals and certainly does not intend that man, the first assistant of Nature in the cultivation of things and in the domestication of the powerful natural forces, should suffer and become degenerate contrary to the general law."

―――

[Editor's note: Benedict Lust re-published a review that John Harvey Kellogg published in *Good Health*.]

Under the caption, "Some Pertinent Questions," Mr. Fletcher asks:

Considering my body as an engine, would I accept myself as a competent engineer on my own examination and confession?

Were I an iron and steel automobile instead of a flesh and blood automobile, which I really am, could I get a license for myself as a chauffeur to run myself with safety, based upon my knowledge of my own mechanism and the theory and development of my power?

Were I an owner of valuable live stock, would I employ a farm hand or a stableman, even at so low a wage as $15 a month, who knew as little about the proper feeding of my animals as I know about the proper feeding of myself and children?

The "B" of *Our Own Nutrition* deals with the mechanical and chemical physiology of nutrition.

"First, last and all the time be sure you are really hungry and not pampering false appetite," instructs Mr. Fletcher. "If true appetite that will relish plain bread alone is not present, wait for it. Especially beware of the early morning habit craving. Wait for an earned appetite if you have to wait, until noon; then 'chew,' 'masticate,' 'munch,' 'bite' and 'taste' everything you take into your mouth except water, which has no taste. "Sip and taste milk and all liquids that have taste, as the wine tasters do. They never drink wine and yet they get all the enjoyment there is in it and waste none. In a short time sipping and tasting liquids and masticating solid food for 'all they are worth' will become an agreeable and profitable fixed habit. Whether we 'eat to live or live to eat,' why not do as above?"

The following is the article in full of Dr. Kellogg on "Fletcherizing Food," published in *Good Health*, and referred to above.

For some years Mr. Horace Fletcher has been making experiments respecting the increased value of food when thoroughly masticated. He has published the results of these experiments from time to time, and recently has succeeded in interesting the most eminent physiologists and scientists of the world in his observations. Mr. Fletcher is a social reformer, and has taken up the question of dietetics from a purely philanthropic standpoint. From the very foundation Mr. Fletcher is a social reformer, and has written much and profoundly upon the subject of social reform. His writings have indeed shown a penetration of the foundation principles of social reformation equaled by few living writers upon these themes.

In Mr. Fletcher's opinion, dietetic reform is the foundation of all reform. The improvement of man must begin, according to

Mr. Fletcher, with an improvement in body. The slum-region will exist as long as it is cultivated by bad diet, bad dress, bad dwellings, and whatever deteriorates the physical health. Hog wallows would not exist if there were no hogs to wallow, or if hogs could be cured of the disposition to wallow.

Mr. Fletcher made the interesting discovery that everybody eats too much; at least everybody who can get a chance, or whose stomach is still tolerant. According to the results of experiments which Mr. Fletcher has made upon himself and others, the so-called daily ration which has been established by scientific authorities is at least fifty per cent larger than it ought to be, and even this is exceeded by multitudes of hearty eaters. According to Mr. Fletcher's observations, a pound of water-free food is ample for anybody, and if care is taken to masticate the food thoroughly, the amount actually required is considerably less.

Mr. Fletcher's experiments, made under the most careful scientific supervision, have shown that if care is taken to chew the food four or five times as long as usual, the food is utilized to so much better advantage that its sustaining power is wonderfully increased, and hence the amount required is considerably diminished. The amount of energy needed for the digestion of food is very considerable, and varies greatly with different foods. Pawlow has shown, for example, that bread and butter requires five times as much energy for its digestion as an equivalent amount of liquid. This is a most important consideration, not only as regards economy in food, but as regards the greater economy in vital energy. The energy consumed in the digestion of food cannot be utilized in any other way, hence the larger waste of energy which occurs through the neglect to masticate the food properly must detract to a very considerable degree from the vital energy available for useful purposes. Mr. Fletcher has proved this to the satisfaction of the most eminent scientific critics, both in England and in this country, and the saving of energy has been shown to be so very great that such eminent men as Sir Michael Foster, of England, Prof. H. P. Bowditch, and Professor Chittenden, of Yale, have thought it worth while to make a special, personal investigation of the matter, and Professor Chittenden has recently given public expression, in his interesting article in the *Popular Scientific Monthly* to his endorsement of Mr. Fletcher's views.

The military department of the United States government, recognizing the importance of this question in relation to army regiment, has detailed twenty men to give their entire time for several months to an exhausting series of researches, the aim of which will be to subject Mr. Fletcher's claims to the crucial test of exhaustive experimentation. The writer has no doubt that the observations which have already been made by Sir Michael Foster and other eminent scientists will be confirmed by these extended researchers, and that the result will be the revision of views which have heretofore been held by most physiologists respecting the quantity of food required for the maintenance of weight and working power, and also respecting the amount of proteids required for daily consumption. Upon the latter point there has been a wide difference of opinion. Mr. Fletcher's experiments have shown that an ounce and a half of proteids daily is ample for the perfect support of the body even when subjected to arduous physical labor. This is scarcely a third of the amount ordinarily consumed, and will be represented by the amount of proteid material furnished in about six ounces of beefsteak or seven eggs. Proteids constitute the most expensive element of human food supply. Starch and sugar are cheap; fats are more expensive and proteids are most expensive of all.

If Mr. Fletcher's theories are confirmed, and if the public can be educated to the adoption, the result will be an enormous saving. The amount of food material may be reduced at least one third, and the cost may be, to say the least enormously reduced. Suppose, for example, the actual saving in quantity may be estimated at not less than one-half pound per day for each individual, which will amount to a saving for the seventy million people in the United Sates of more than seventeen thousand tons daily. A ton of flour, one of the cheapest of food, is worth at the present time about sixty dollars. Seventy thousand tons of flour would have a value of about $1,020,000. The saving of this enormous sum daily would in a few years pay off the national debt, and be sufficient to provide the comforts of life for every needy person in the country. This is proof that the dietetic reform may be made the foundation for a great and thoroughgoing social reform; may be made to solve economic questions of the most tremendous importance. Mr. Fletcher argues that in this question of the proper mastication of food is to be found a key to the most serious problems relating to human welfare.

Another interesting observation which has been made by Mr. Fletcher is the fact that when the food is properly chewed, there is marked absence of those fermentation and putrefactions which are so often present in the alimentary canal, not only in the stomach, giving rise to flatulence, but also in the small intestine, particularly in the colon, resulting in the formation of poisonous substances which thin the blood and permeate the tissues, interfering with all the vital functions, giving rise to a variety of chronic diseases as well as neuralgia, neurasthenia, insomnia, rheumatism, degeneration of the blood vessels, Bright's disease, hardening of the liver, and other degenerations and ailments too numerous to mention.

The small residue which results when the food is thoroughly masticated is remarkably aseptic. Putrescent processes are almost altogether absent. Fecal matters are comparatively inoffensive, and greatly diminished in amount, and one of the greatest burdens under which the body struggles, through the necessity for eliminating from the skin, the lungs, and other excretory organs the enormous quantities of poisons produced by the decomposition of foodstuffs in the alimentary canal, is lifted, and as the result, the individual experiences a lightness and clearness of intellect, increased vigor, endurance, and resistance of disease, which is almost past belief until one has actually experienced this delightful transformation.

That these views of Mr. Fletcher are not mere fancies has been demonstrated again and again, not only by himself and his immediate friends, but on a large scale at the Battle Creek Sanitarium and Naturopathic Sanitaria all the world over, where, for many years, these ideas have been more or less thoroughly inculcated, and especially within the last two or three years. Any one can easily demonstrate the truth of Mr. Fletcher's contention by experimenting upon himself. The habit of chewing thoroughly is very easily and quickly acquired, and when once the habit is formed, the increased satisfaction experienced in eating, the marked increase of energy, and the sense of well-being which results from this manner of eating, become sufficient incentives to lead to the continuance of the practice. Mr. Fletcher is doing an immense amount of good in his earnest propagation of these wholesome and health-saving ideas. It has been suggested that the thorough method of chewing which he advises, and which differs so widely from the current practice, should be termed "Fletcherizing." The treatment of food by heating at such a temperature as to destroy germs, so as to increase its keeping qualities, is generally known from the discovery of the process as Pasteurizing. "Fletcherizing," or thoroughly chewing the food, increases its digestibility to such a degree that decompositions are prevented, and it thus becomes a sort of physiological method of sterilizing, or ascepticizing the food, and hence the name suggested seems entirely appropriate.

It is reported that "Fletcherizing" is getting to be a very common practice in some portion of New England as well as in Great Britain, where the influence of the royal example has led to the formation of munching parties in various parts of the kingdom. Parents and teachers would do well to give this matter careful consideration. It is but little trouble to train a child to the habit of thoroughly masticating the food and the habit once acquired is likely to be followed through life. The readers of this magazine will hear more of this subject from time to time, as this question is one of which physiologists are bound to recognize as of vital importance, and will unquestionably receive, in years to come, more attention in public school and medical college textbooks than heretofore. Mr. Fletcher is an optimist, and has the most profound faith in the final triumph of truth.

It has been suggested that the thorough method of chewing which he advises, and which differs so widely from the current practice, should be termed "Fletcherizing."

Mr. Fletcher's experiments have shown that an ounce and a half of proteids daily is ample for the perfect support of the body even when subjected to arduous physical labor.

About The Value Of A Good Gluten Graham Bread

by Benedict Lust, N.D.

The Naturopath and Herald of Health. VI(11), 316. (1905)

The nutritive value of a good Gluten Graham Bread is prized and esteemed only by those who make use of the same. A good Gluten Graham Bread is very easily digested and very nourishing, provided you partake of it in moderate quantities, as it is not the quantity but the quality of the food which benefits the bodily system. No sooner are the muscles of the digestive organs strained, then they become lax in their activity and will be unable to withstand any length of time the bulk of food heaped upon them, and the consequence is, their normal state is disturbed by all sorts of stomach disorders. But those who satisfy their appetite with a diminished supply of plain food of the best quality, are not only free from the ailments stated above but also enjoy good health and rare strength and are better able to resist any attack of those dreaded maladies.

To be strong and healthy, or to become such, it is not necessary to indulge in luxurious living and expensive and manifold delicacies and beverages, but to the contrary, the plainest and simplest foods, if properly chosen, attain to the desired end and have the advantage of being reasonable in price and within the reach of the man of moderate means. This is the teaching of wisdom, but which a great many people do not want to comprehend, though so easily understood. Moreover, all the abounding social misery and wretchedness that turns up before our eyes in its many and varied phases, could surely be alleviated by these methods, if not entirely remedied.

To exercise temperance in eating and drinking, and a life of regularity in labor, rest, recreation and bodily care as well as the selection of proper nourishment are the fundamental principles necessary to a happy and contented life. Those who become in time accustomed to eating a half a pound of Gluten Graham Bread daily—the bread not being too fresh, but rather stale—to chew it well, or should the teeth be not fit for the performance, to cook a good soup, and partake of some vegetables with other dishes cooked of Gluten Graham Flour, and occasionally some fruit, will find it a good, desirable and rather inexpensive bill of fare.

We should eat Gluten Graham Bread, because it is of greater value to our health than any other bread. Once you are used to it, you will prefer it to any other baked goods, though it seems discreditable at first. Gluten Graham Bread is a substitute for meat, and as it is in no way an irritable food, it prevents any temptation to take to alcoholic drinks. But it must be a good Gluten Graham Bread as mentioned before.

Gluten Graham Bread is, in short, a splendid substitute for meat, it is easily digested and of a highly nourishing quality.

THE NEW TUBER FOOD

by Benedict Lust

The Naturopath and Herald of Health, VI(11), 331-333. (1905)

Whatever may be claimed as to the superiority of the fruits of the temperate, as compared with those of the tropic zone—to the tropics *must* belong the credit of producing that primate among vegetables, the taro. Like rice, maize and wheat, taro, a tuber known to botanists as the *arum esculentum*, or *colocasis esculenta*, is, or has been, the food-staple for the people of vast geographical areas.

The universal experience of the foreigners who have made the land of the taro their permanent home or their temporary residence, also declares in favor of this tuber as more satisfying and nutritious than any other vegetable. The fondness for taro comes as naturally and requires no more education than for wheaten bread, rice, or potatoes, and the taste, once acquired, no other vegetable seems able to take its place. It is the opinion of the writer, that no one who has had opportunity to judge and has made prolonged trial of both taro and potato at their best, but would give it as the result of his experience that for power to sustain and satisfy, and in a large measure to take the place even of wheaten bread, for long periods of time, the choice, as between taro and potato—or any other vegetable—would lie wholly with taro.

With taro and the addition of a small amount of meat, or fish (as preferred by the Hawaiians), the Anglo-Saxon or Polynesian laborer is able to keep himself in condition for active labor for an indefinite period of time. My experience would not permit me to make the same statement in regard to rice, or Indian corn.

The most important use to which taro can be put, in any place far removed from its place of growth, is that of supplying a bland and nutritious aliment for children, invalids, and persons of a delicate digestion. For adaptation to this threefold purpose nothing can surpass the preparation of taro known as Taro-ena, which is made from taro already cooked. When mixed with milk, it easily lends itself to the preparation of baby-food. Owing to the minuteness and consequent superior digestibility of its starch-cell, Taro-ena is to be recommended for the use of those who find difficulty in digesting other forms of amylaceous food.

Taro-ena, in a greater degree than any other preparation overcomes the physiological objection which holds against the use of any kind of starchy food in infants below the age at which the starch digesting functions have attained their full vigor, from the fact that a considerable percentage of the starch of the taro is converted into dextrin in the process of preparation.

Taro-ena in the hands of any one who has not the least knack and inventiveness, will, either alone or mixed with flour, easily lend itself to

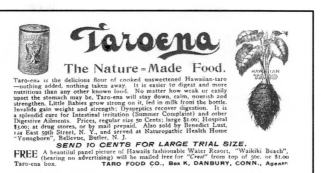

Taroena
The Nature = Made Food.

Taro-ena is the delicious flour of cooked unsweetened Hawaiian-taro —nothing added, nothing taken away. It is easier to digest and more nutritious than any other known food. No matter how weak or easily upset the stomach may be, Taro-ena will stay down, calm, nourish and strengthen. Little Babies grow strong on it, fed in milk from the bottle. Invalids gain weight and strength; Dyspeptics recover digestion. It is a splendid cure for Intestinal irritation (Summer Complaint) and other Digestive Ailments. Prices, regular size 50 Cents; large $1.00; Hospital $3.00; at drug stores, or by mail prepaid. Also sold by Benedict Lust, 124 East 59th Street, N. Y., and served at Naturopathic Health Home "Youngborn", Bellevue, Butler, N. J.

SEND 10 CENTS FOR LARGE TRIAL SIZE.

FREE A beautiful panel picture of Hawaiis fashionable Water Resort, "Waikiki Beach", (bearing no advertising) will be mailed free for "Crest" from top of 50c. or $1.00 Taro-ena box.   **TARO FOOD CO., Box K, DANBURY, CONN., Agents**

the making of delicious cakes, muffins, biscuits, porridges, puddings and baby foods. Mixed with hot or cold water and allowed to stand until fermentation can be perceived, and then eaten with a boiled fish and salt—if coarse, so much the better—the reminder of the Hawaiian national dish will be so strong as to transport one in imagination to the Pacific.

In enumerating the advantages of Taro-ena as a model food for the young mother, we would direct especial attention to its well known flesh-producing properties. The Taro-ena-fed woman invariably presents the appearance of one who is exceptionally well nourished, one whose tissues and tissue-juices (especially her mammary fluid) contain sufficient fats and proteids to enable her to spare some for her child. And it is upon these two essential ingredients of her milk that the latter thrives.

Again, according to the various chemical analyses submitted (Ch. Bulletin, No. 68, U.S. Department of Agriculture, p. 13), Taro-ena furnishes starch and mineral matter in such form that it is readily absorbed into the blood and utilized; the former constituent, of course, being transformed into glycogen or animal sugar. As sugar and the mineral salts are both important elements of breast milk, which aid in the finer coagulation of its casein, it will be seen that a food which furnishes these ingredients in proper amount and proportion, will prove of more than ordinary value to both mother and child.

The wonderful digestibility of Taro-ena is doubtless one of the chief points in its favor as an ideal food for the nursing mother; but just here it is our object to lay special stress upon the advantages we have mentioned— i. e., of prescribing a food in these cases which furnishes in amount, form and proportion, as combined by nature, the exact ingredients (fats, proteids, sugar and mineral salts) essential to a supply of healthy, rich breast milk. We believe that Taro-ena does this as no other food will do.

During this trying period when the baby is most liable to stomach troubles and bowel complaints, Taro-ena will be found of great value and the safest food that can be used. To thoughtful mothers and to those to whom the care of babies and children is given, Taro-ena is offered as one which the most delicate stomach will retain, and which will nourish and build up a weak and exhausted system. Unlike other vegetable and cereal foods it contains little taste or indigestible matter and is therefore readily assimilated into the blood. The mineral salts which it contains are found by chemical analysis to be in the exact proportion demanded by nature for the bone-making elements, and the child thus fed becomes strong, rugged and healthy, with no one-sided development in any respect.

If the baby is weak and frail, peevish and fretful, wakeful and restless at night, if it suffers from colic and stomach disturbances and is backward in growth, Taro-ena, combines with milk, cream or water, will be found a complete and unsurpassed food, pure, sweet, wholesome and nutritious, and one that will be easy to digest and assimilate. It makes blood, bone tissue and flesh in one harmonious growth. When it is remembered that the native Hawaiian child is thus fed from the day of his birth, that he remains free from the usual ills of childhood, and is remarkable for his perfect physical development, the value of Taro-ena as a nourishing infant food must at once be admitted.

Taro-ena is recommended as a grand diet for invalids and dyspeptics. It is endorsed by physicians as the most nutritious and easily digested food which can be used in cases of convalescence from fevers and all forms of wasting diseases, or whenever the ordinary foods cannot be retained. It has been used beneficially in a variety of conditions. In the vomiting of pregnancy, or any form of reflex vomiting, it is almost a specific. In all forms of gastric and intestinal operations; as a diet of adult or infant, where an easily digested, nourishing food is indicated, Taro-ena has proven its clinical worth.

Taro-ena is absolutely unlike any other invalid food in the important essential that it contains, placed there by nature, *a digestive ferment* peculiar to itself. In no other way, than by the presence of a natural ferment, can the wonderful digestibility of this food be explained. A brief examination of the various testimonials which have been received reveals that fact that Taro-ena may be taken into the most delicate stomach, even though all other foods have been immediately rejected. In other words, it has been found that Taro-ena will *stay down* when other foods are quickly repelled.

Again, Taro-ena is unlike other health foods in the important particular that it is a true nature made food and not an artificial food. Its nutritive properties are no more and no less than those possessed by cooked taro—which Taro-ena is. Hence, Taro-ena is not like the various foods in the market which have been artificially compounded in some chemical laboratory. In short, this remarkable food-plant contains in nature's pure proper proportion all the elements that go to build up a healthy human body, and it contains them in a form that the weakest stomach can digest and assimilate. It is a strong, and at the same time, a light food, containing nothing of an irritable nature, but possessing marked soothing properties that allay irritation of the stomach and intestines.

1906

THE NUTRITIVE VALUE OF UNPOLISHED RICE
OTTO CARQUÉ

ADULTERATION OF FOOD
SAMUEL A. BLOCH

FRUIT AND NUT DIET
O. HASHNU HARA

THIS NATION SUICIDING
CORA G. IVES, D.O.

GREEN SALADS AND VEGETABLES AS MEDICINE
ADAM CLARK

The Wonderful Benefits

... OF ...

DISTILLED WATER

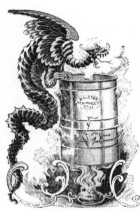

You don't know about them? Let us send you a copy of our booklet which treats the water question scientifically, gives you the best medical opinions upon the subject, and the testimonials of grateful people cured of disease by this simple but wonderful remedy.

DISTILLED WATER is now within easy reach of all, at little trouble and no expense, through the agency of that marvelously simple and efficient device.

——THE——

RALSTON NEW-PROCESS WATER STILL,

Price, - - - $10.00.

(Immediate delivery can be made where cash accompanies order.)

We are the oldest and largest domestic water still manufacturers in the United States. The Ralston was the first family still placed upon the market, and by frequently improving it we have easily kept it well in the lead. Buy only the Ralston. Cheap and spurious imitations will surely disappoint.

The A. R. Bailey M'f'g Co.,

4 CEDAR STREET, NEW YORK, U. S. A.

Ask for Booklet K.

When writing, please mention this paper.

Distilled water was highly recommended by the early Naturopaths.

THE NUTRITIVE VALUE OF UNPOLISHED RICE

by Otto Carqué

The Naturopath and Herald of Health, VII(I), 35-37. (1906)

Much has been said and written against the use of white flour as a cause of many diseases which man is heir to. The same argument can be used against the rice of commerce which has undergone a process which is called "polishing." Fashion demands rice having a fine gloss, just for appearance's sake. To supply this the rice is put through the polishing process which removes some of the most nutritious parts of the rice kernel, especially fat and some very important organic salts, *silicon,* generally contained in the outer coats of grains.

Rice is a word that preserves its etymology through all human languages. From the Sanskrit through the Persian, Greek, Latin, Spanish, French, to contemporary English, it has kept its root unchanged. It is a cereal of the grass family, with the name *Oryza Sativa.* It is indigenous in certain parts of India and in tropical Australia.

There is no record of its nativity in Egypt, Persia, Greece or Rome. So as far as it is known it is the first cereal used by man. Probably the Aryans carried it with them in their migratory marches from the cradle of the human race, in the earliest dawn of history. We know that it was introduced into China 3,000 years B.C. We know that it was grown in the valley of the Euphrates over 2,000 years ago, that the Arabs took it to Spain, and sustained by its marvelous nourishment, planted their victorious banners everywhere.

It was introduced into Italy in 1468. Sir William Berkeley first cultivated it in Virginia in 1647. To-day it is grown as a staple article of food by the millions of India, Siam, China, Japan and Africa. In the Mediterranean countries, and in the tropical and sub-tropical regions of Northland South America, it is cultivated as a principal means of subsistence.

Rice is not only the most important if all cereals, but by far the most important of all food products. It is almost the exclusive diet of 57 per cent, and the principal support of nearly 75 per cent of all the human race. Not only is it the most extensively used and the most widely distributed of the world's foods, but it is *the food that produces the greatest amount of molecular energy and physical endurance.* Rice is the chief diet (about 1 ¼ lbs. per day) of the wonderful Japanese soldiery whose strength and prowess compel the admiration and wonder of mankind to-day. It is eaten almost exclusively by the Indian and Chinese coolies, those marvelous men who can carry a load all day under a burning sun, that would stagger an American or European; who can carry that load at a speed sufficient to tire a horse; and who accomplish labors that no meat-eating Caucasian could begin to perform.

UNPOLISHED   RICE

With all the heart left on in milling, put up in double sacks, and delivered any place east of the Rockeys per 100 pounds $6.50. Parcels post shipments, 6 cents per pound with postage added, to your place. J. ED. CABANISS, Producer to Consumers.

BOX 12, KATY, HARRIS CO., Texas

The main reason for the superiority of rice over all other forms of foods is its ready digestibility, plain boiled rice being assimilated in one hour, while the other cereals, legumes and most vegetables require from three and one-half to five hours. Rice thus enables a man to economize fully 75 per cent of the time and energy expected in the digestion of ordinary food, setting it free to be used in his daily vocation, in the pursuit of study, or social duties and in the case of invalids and people of enfeebled vitality, adding it to the reserve force of the system. The perfect digestibility of rice makes it exceedingly valuable for a weak digestion. A rice diet is generally prescribed for any inflammation of the mucous membrane—whether of the lungs, stomach or bowels. It is self-evident that these statements particularly refer to unpolished rice just as it comes out of the hulls without the bran taken off. Unfortunately, the majority of people are still ignorant of the great difference between polished and unpolished rice.

Estimated according to the food value "rice polish," the parts removed by the polishing processes, is nearly twice as valuable for food as polished rice. This polish contains the germ and the cuticle and, like in all other grains and fruit, as it comes next to the skin, is the sweetest part of the grain or fruit. In a hundred pounds of polish there are besides starch—*11 lbs. of protein, 7.2 lbs. of fat, and 5.2 lbs. of mineral elements;* while in a hundred pounds of polished rice there are only—*7.5 lbs. of protein, 0.3 lb. of fat, and 0.4 lb. of mineral elements.*

The unpolished rice is on an average ten times as rich in organic salts as the polished rice of commerce. As the flavor is in the fats and organic salts, it is easy to understand the lack of commercial rice and why travelers universally speak of the excellent quality of the rice they eat in oriental countries. It is not so much the higher percentage of protein, as the greater richness in fat and mineral elements which makes rice such a nutritious food.

IMPORTANCE OF THE MINERAL ELEMENTS IN RICE

Of the mineral elements lost in the polishing process SILICON is especially valuable. Silicon in the form of silicic acid (silica) makes up a large part of the solid surface of our planet. It is indispensable for the growth of plants and is likewise important in the animal body. It makes muscles firm, for it protects them against chemical decomposition and has, consequently, an antiseptic action; it warms the blood by isolating and keeping together the electricity by its salty constituents. Sulfur and silica are found in the hair, making the latter a non-conductor of heat and electricity. IRON is contained in the haemoglobin of the blood; on account of its great affinity to oxygen it readily takes up the latter in the lungs and forwards it in the arteries and capillaries to all parts of the body; it is therefore of great value in keeping up the oxidizing process in the tissues, and consequently in the creation of animal heat and magnetism. SODIUM is found in rice in a higher percentage than in any other cereal; this element combines with carbonic acid which is constantly formed by the oxidizing processes of the body and discharges the same through the lungs. CALCIUM and MAGNESIUM and PHOSPHOROUS are also important and these elements are indispensable for building up our bones and teeth.

Fashion demands rice having a fine gloss, just for appearance's sake. To supply this the rice is put through the polishing process which removes some of the most nutritious parts of the rice kernel, especially fat and some very important organic salts, silicon, generally contained in the outer coats of grains.

The main reason for the superiority of rice over all other forms of foods is its ready digestibility, plain boiled rice being assimilated in one hour, while the other cereals, legumes and most vegetables require from three and one-half to five hours.

The unpolished rice is on an average ten times as rich in organic salts as the polished rice of commerce.

ADULTERATION OF FOOD

by Samuel A. Bloch
The Naturopath and Herald of Health, VII(4), 167. (1906)

There have been numerous newspaper items and magazine contributions on the adulteration of food, which have created much discussion, pro and con, of the baneful effects of the use of various chemical agents for the preservation of articles of food. We also know that the primary motive for the addition of adulterants to foods is for the purpose of giving a far greater profit to the manufacturers and canners for their goods than can actually be made by honest manufacture.

This swindling of the people has become so wide-spread that we can conscientiously state that THERE IS NOT ONE ARTICLE OF DIET THAT IS NOT ADULTERATED more or less. We do not mean to state that EVERY ARTICLE of food of all manufacturers is adulterated, but simply that there is no article of food that is not adulterated. There may be some very conscientious manufacturers, who place good, honest food on the market, but it is a difficult matter to find one that can exist. The honest food manufacturer and canner cannot sell his goods cheaply, and of course the dishonest manufacturer can undersell him, and he is compelled to either sell out his business or go into bankruptcy.

It is quite difficult to differentiate between a good staple article and one that is adulterated; and of course the working class is the greater sufferer, because of the perverse economic system; but at the same time the rich people are no more positive of buying a good article of food than the poorer class.

In some future issues of this magazine we will endeavor to treat each article of food individually, giving its proceeds of manufacture and methods and chemical agents used for its preservation and adulteration. At present we will only give you a list of dietary articles that are chiefly used in every home and in considerable quantities:

FOOD ARTICLES	WHAT IT IS ADULTERATED WITH
BREAD	Alum, sulphate of copper, potatoes.
BUTTER	Copper, other fats, starch.
CANNED VEGETABLES	Salts of copper, lead.
CANDY	Poisonous colors, coal-tar essences, glucose.
CHOCOLATE COCOA	Oxide of iron, foreign coloring matters, animal fats, flour, starch, earth.
CAYENNE PEPPER	Red lead, flour, cornmeal.

FLOUR	Alum, ground rice, corn flour.
HONEY	Glucose, cane sugar, paraffin.
LARD	Alum, caustic lime, starch, cottonseed oil, stearine.
PEPPER	Sandalwood, red sawdust, sand, rice, bean shells, cocoanut shells, ground olive stones.
MILK	Water, chalk, coloring matter, formaldehyde preservative, borax.
RED RASPBERRY JAM	Gelatine, timothy seed, aniline dye.
CANNED PEAS	Salts of copper to color green.
MUSTARD	Chromate and sulphate of lead, flour, turmeric.
FRUIT JELLIES	Artificial coal-tar essences, gelatin, apple jelly, aniline dyes.
PICKLES	Salts of copper, alum, acetic acid.
PRESERVES	Aniline colors, artificial coal-tar essences, pumpkins, apples.
SUGAR	Salts of lead and of tin, gypsum, marble dust, rice, flour.
TEA	Gypsum, china clay, soapstone, other leaves, gum.
VINEGAR	Sulphuric acid, acetic acid, hydrochloric acid, burnt sugar, water.
SPICES	Mustard hulls, gypsum, potato flour, bark, turmeric, charcoal, sand.
MAPLE SUGAR	Glucose, brown cane sugar, extract of hickory bark.
LEMON EXTRACT	Coal-tar dyes.
COFFEE	Dried hogs' liver, chicory, beans.
NUTMEGS	Sawdust, sand, clay.

It is quite difficult to differentiate between a good staple article and one that is adulterated; and of course the working class is the greater sufferer, because of the perverse economic system; but at the same time the rich people are no more positive of buying a good article of food than the poorer class.

FRUIT AND NUT DIET

by O. Hashnu Hara

The Naturopath and Herald of Health, VII(VI), 223-5. (1906)

PRACTICAL HINTS UPON NATURAL DIET, GIVING QUANTITIES AND FULL DIRECTIONS FOR THE DAILY MEAL

That men and women are ready and anxious to adopt a meatless and natural form of diet is very evident by the numerous inquiries one continually meets with as to the best way to *begin*.

Some are accentuated by ideas of pure blood, better health; some by the desire for greater spirituality; others, and these the truly humane, whose very soul loathe and revolt against the brutalities of the slaughter-house. But, no matter what the motive, we welcome them all.

But the trouble is, *what* quantities do we require? What foods, in plain English, must we take and replace meat, and how much of each kind? These queries remain unanswered, except by elaborate statistics, and the dietary of uncooked fruit and nuts, the best, purest and most natural of all has remained unexploited, or else overloaded stomachs have blasted its reputation wrongfully. Better far eat too little than too much is an axiom all should bear in mind.

For perfect health and strength and the "staying" power boasted of by meat eaters, nothing can beat a fruitarian diet.

To prove this we need only consider the results of this years' great international walking race, held last Whitsundtide, in Germany, when the competitors walked from Dresden to Berlin, a distance of 124 ½ miles.

Thirty-two competitors started from Dresden at 7:30 a.m. on May 18th, (1906), in bad weather. Of these men part were fruitarians and vegetarians (including the great Karl Mann, the world's champion walker, of Berlin), part meat eaters.

THE FIRST SIX TO ARRIVE IN BERLIN WERE FRUITARIANS AND VEGETARIANS, the third man, Martin Rehann, being only twenty years old.

Of course Karl Mann was first, having done the distance in twenty-six hours fifty-eight minutes, and fresh as a daisy at the finish, whilst the meat eaters, well-known and tried athletes, arrived utterly exhausted.

George Allen, the English (Leicester) hundred miles walker, is also a vegetarian, and we all know Eustace Miles.

These cases are officially attested, and anybody who likes can verify the statements for themselves.

Karl Mann only takes two meals a day, and he partakes of neither flesh, fowl, alcohol, coffee, tea, chocolate, etc., and when training, neither eggs, milk, cheese, butter, nor pulse.

NUTS AND FRUITS, THE TWENTIETH CENTURY DIET
ADVOCATED BY THIS MAGAZINE.

Specimen samples of our delicious preparations, Nut Meats, Dates, Prunes, Figs, Nut Butters, Nut Marmelades, Nut Food Combinations. Price Lists and Pamphlets, description and information, mailed postpaid upon receipt of 25c. in stamps, cash or P. O. Money Order. CORONA. The new and delicious Uncooked Health Food. Sample of "Corona" with circular and price list sent for 10c, in coin or postage. Address:

KOERBER NUT MEAT CO., 156 a Read St., New York City.

Vegetarian diets such as the fruit and nut diet were made popular by O. Hashnu Hara and health food companies were created to supply these demands.

We, personally, have two meals daily, the first at 12:30 p.m., the second at 6:30, working on the no breakfast plan, which I find splendid for health and a clear brain.

The fruitarian diet is fine, and, to my mind, more satisfying than vegetarianism, to say nothing of what it saves in household work.

However, to the point—it's no use preaching a fruitarian diet if I don't give you practical teaching as to rules, quantities, etc.

I read so much about the beauties of the diet, etc., in some fifteen or twenty American magazines, and not one practical hint, that I used to get quite mad, and I firmly believe any number of people would turn from a flesh diet if they only knew how to begin.

The ordinary individual has a tendency to over-eat himself six days out of seven, and to prevent this tendency I advise that a pair of kitchen scales be requisitioned and the proper quantities duly weighed out—indeed this is imperative.

I am allowing the same amount of nutriment for a woman as for a man, but at the same time the fair sex can from the day's allowance knock off a quarter of a pound of dried fruit and half a pound of fresh if necessary.

Personally I think the idea that women eat less than men has arisen because they too often eat *between* meals and men haven't the *chance* as a rule.

Every adult requires from twelve to sixteen ounces of dry food, *free from water*, daily. To supply this a quarter of a pound of *shelled* nuts and three quarters of a pound of any dried fruit must be used.

In addition to this from two to three pounds of any *fresh fruit* in season goes to complete the day's allowance.

These quantities should be weighed out and divided in half for the two meals, and will sustain a full grown man in perfect health and vitality. The quantity of ripe fresh fruit may be slightly increased in summer, with a corresponding decrease in the dried fruit.

When beginning the diet it is as well to use a little bread (wholemeal) and plenty of eggs, milk, cream cheese, and cream, until gradually weaned from cereals.

Strawberries, raspberries, cherries, plums, apples, pineapples, grapes, melons, currants, etc., can all be used in summer, and grapes, pears, apples, oranges, bananas, etc., in winter.

For the dried fruit, raisins, sultanas, prunes, dates, figs and plums, and for a change and stewing purposes we have splendid variety in Californian prunes, apricots, peaches, Bartlett pears, dried apples, bananas and plums.

The nut foods are almonds, walnuts, hazels, cashews, pine kernels, peanuts (these can be bought *ready shelled*), sapricia, pecan, butter nuts, hickory, brazils (excellent for constipation), Japan peanuts, chestnuts, and cocoanuts.*

All these should be got in by large quantities—by far the cheapest way—and the diet will be found to pan out a healthier, purer method of living, and infinitely more economical to those who consider such matters.

To cook *dried fruit,* wash it thoroughly in clean water, then place it in a dish with enough water to cover it, and soak ten or fifteen hours, then, leaving it in the water it has been soaked in, put it on the stove and let it simmer gently until cooked. When nearly done add sufficient sugar for the individual taste. The fruit cooked in this manner very nearly resembles fresh fruit, with the full flavor and taste.

Housekeepers generally don't know how to cook dried fruit, and it enters comparatively little into their menus. The above is an American recipe and may be adopted for all the dried fruits, though the dried bananas may be eaten raw or *steamed* in an ordinary potato steamer and eaten with fresh or whipped cream. At the same time the genuine fruitarian who has become used to the diet will not cook dried fruit, and it is certainly better in the natural state. It should be well washed in a colander and then dried lightly in a scrupulously clean cloth.

Some people advise *regularity* of meals. I advise only two daily, but it is *best* to eat when you are hungry. All the same you will be hungry if you follow the "no breakfast" plan, and able to relish your natural food with a natural appetite.

You will find your magnetic and vital power doubled—nay trebled—by the simple pure food. You will enjoy health such as you never had before, double working capacity, and be able to look God's creatures in the face without a blush.

Women who value their looks will adopt this diet rigorously, for even

*Cocoanut refers to coconut. *Ed.*

men, and old men at that, who have lived on it, and the two meal, non-breakfast plan, can boast a complexion like a wild rose.

Finally, if in addition to the fruit and nut, further nutriment is required, the best thing I know of is "Yungborn Wheat," a specialty which has been known in its crude state for centuries by all the fighting and most stalwart classes of the natives of India. It has wonderful properties for building up muscle and power for reducing fatigue. Moreover, like the rest of this diet, it *requires no cooking*, and is very nice to eat.

Better far eat too little than too much is an axiom all should bear in mind.

For perfect health and strength and the "staying" power boasted of by meat eaters, nothing can beat a fruitarian diet.

THIS NATION SUICIDING

by Cora G. Ives, D.O.
266 W. Newton St., Boston, March 5, 1906
The Naturopath and Herald of Health, VII(6), 230-231. (1906)

With a very few exceptions this is true of every one of you. You eat meat and milk daily that are loaded with formaldehyde and other poisons such as sulfuric acid, hydrochloric, boracic, etc. I know some tell us we have the new disease "adulteritis," but is not the time opportune that somebody or some organization set each individual thinking concerning what enters his stomach? The butcher tells us that he can't sell his meat unless it is bright red and fresh-looking, and as he must satisfy the demands of his customers he puts on a preservative, made of the most powerful acids. The good housewife desires bright jellies and preserves, so the canning companies resort to coal tar products as coloring matters; and, in order to keep corn, beans and tomatoes, other poisons are used in the form of a preservative.

Mr. Ballinger, of Keokuk, Iowa, representing one big canning company, says if the use of preservatives is prohibited it will mean a loss of $25,000,000 to $50,000,000 annually. As this is probably a conservative estimate, what must we be paying yearly for poison under the supposition that it is good food? Is it not time we stopped to consider our daily food and what enters our stomach? As the blame must partially rest on the individual consumer, and reform must begin in each home by the housewife using only pure foods, let us have them even if we must employ the present Chinese method of boycotting.

This is only one of the ways in which we daily shorten our lease of health and vitality. We insist on using tea, coffee and cocoa, which are unnatural stimulants, and absolute poison to many people. They bring on dyspepsia and heart troubles. Why will man persist in whipping up his overworked nerves by such stimulants?

Tobacco and alcohol in their many forms are others of this list of poisons which are causing degeneration and suicides in many families, not only of this generation but the succeeding ones.

Many who are not guilty of this evil become victims of the patent-medicine vender. Thousands of good people who use their voice and combined nervous energy in the cause of temperance would not drink a drop of beer or light wine but at the same time are using three times daily a patent medicine. I know an evangelist who gave a strong and eloquent sermon on the temperance cause, and later in the same evening, in a fireside talk, told how Peruna was helping his catarrh. Now Peruna has 28 per cent. alcohol—a much larger per cent. than beer. This patent medicine evil is in many forms, such as tonics for the old and young, headache powders, sleeping potions, soothing syrups for the helpless babe, and so on without number. The exposing of this evil by magazines and newspapers and legislation, is a grand good work. It will cause the individual to do some thinking about what enters his body.

Lastly, many people are undermining their good health and suiciding at the hands of their "regular" physician. They take a poison of some kind prescribed by the physician to counteract the acid in their blood which he tells them is causing rheumatism. Another one is taking something to deaden pain in some portion of the body, thinking he has cured the disease because there is no more pain. He fails to realize that the drug has desensitized his nerves for the time and has not removed the cause of his suffering. He very frequently becomes addicted to a drug habit as a result, then wonders why he feels so melancholy and has no interest in life, or in other words, is a nervous wreck. He fails to trace his early heart trouble to the drug which he used to temporarily allay his pain.

Now all the blame is not laid to the physician in these cases for it is the duty of the individual to think for himself, to know that nothing enters his stomach but wholesome food, and not too much of that. He should demand cures along drugless lines of healing. Many a physician would not give drugs if the patient did not demand them.

All these fights in the cause of pure food legislation—brought about largely through the influence of women's clubs—in the cause of temperance, against patent medicine and drug medication, are good, but the better way to get rid of an evil is to kill it by starvation. There are plenty of good, pure foods that are not adulterated, such as cereals, grains in the berry, nuts, fruit, and fresh vegetables. And as for meat we have ample proof that it is not necessary to maintain strength. Nut, beans, and peas are richer in the proteid element than meat, and are absolutely pure, in the fresh or dried state; so why not eat them? As the body is more supple and vigorous and has a much greater sense of freedom on these simple pure foods, let us eat them.

In order to live up to this standard of simplicity the individual must use his will power. He must have courage to follow the leadings of his own conscience instead of walking in the great procession.

The good housewife desires bright jellies and preserves, so the canning companies resort to coal tar products as coloring matters; and, in order to keep corn, beans and tomatoes, other poisons are used in the form of a preservative.

GREEN SALADS AND VEGETABLES AS MEDICINE

by Adam Clark

The Naturopath and Herald of Health, VII(6), 254. (1906)

We consider green vegetables to be far more valuable than a dose of medicine. They contain true medicinal properties in the form of salts for the body. Asparagus will purge the blood. It acts beneficially upon the kidneys. Spinach and dandelions also act beneficially upon the kidneys. Lettuce and cucumbers cool the blood. Celery tones the nerves and produces healthy sleep. Onions, leeks, and garlic increase blood circulation, promote digestion, and increase the flow of saliva and the gastric juices. Peas and beans are muscle-forming. Tomatoes act beneficially upon the liver. In fact, every product of vegetable, choose whatever one you will, possesses elements suitable for the body. Eat plenty of vegetables and less meat!

The secret of happiness is never to allow your energies to stagnate.

Every product of vegetable, choose whatever one you will, possesses elements suitable for the body. Eat plenty of vegetables and less meat!

AN APPEAL TO COMMON SENSE.

The Folly of Meat=Eating

A POWERFUL REPLY

to an Editorial of the New York and Chicago
Evening American & San Francisco Examiner

By Otto Carque,

Author of "The Foundation of all Reform".

The information contained in this 16 page pamphlet
whic h includes two valuable tables giving complete
analyses of the 12 mineral constituents of various
foods is worth at least a hundred times the price
charged for it.   The arguments of the author are
unanswerable and based on new and original scientific investigations.   Published the first time in this
country.   Indispensable to every student of nature.
Price Postpaid United States and Canada 10 Cents.
Great Britain 6 d.

Send orders to the

"Naturopath," 124 E. 59th St., N. Y.

Response to an Editorial of the New York and Chicago Evening American and
San Francisco Examiner by Otto Carqué.

Cause And Cure Of Ailments According To Natur-Therapeutics

Benedict Lust

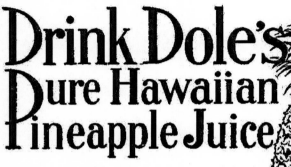

Drink Dole's
Pure Hawaiian
Pineapple Juice

A wonderful, Healthful, all-the-year-round Drink. Prescribed by physicians in throat, stomach and intestinal difficulties. A refreshing drink in fever convalescence. Druggists, Grocers and Soda Fountains supplied through regular channels.

Write for Booklet.

HAWAIIAN PINEAPPLE PRODUCTS CO., Ltd.
112 MARKET STREET, SAN FRANCISCO, CALIFORNIA

Ad for Dole's Pure Hawaiian Pineapple Juice.

Cause And Cure Of Ailments According To Natur-Therapeutics

by Benedict Lust

The Naturopath and Herald of Health, VIII(4), 97-98. (1907)

Spring Treatments

At this time of year the housekeeper delights in marketing. While in winter she had to be satisfied with poor substitutes for food she now finds a rich variety of eatables from which to select. Lettuce and spinach ought to be found on every table at this season of the year. These salads while containing considerable water and waste matter at the same time contain valuable nutritive salts and carbohydrates. The salts especially are essential for a health formation of blood.

People who do not favor vegetables always speak of their inferior value in albumen. This is more or less a fact, but one thing is not sufficiently considered, that is, that vegetables contribute a great deal to normal metabolic assimilation. The supposedly waste vegetable matter stimulates the activity of the bowels and this is a point of great value.

We are wrong in not fully appreciating lettuce. This salad contains about 1.41% albumen and 1.03% nutritive salts; consequently, it is a foodstuff to be appreciated.

Spring is the time for taking one of the best cures known to Naturopathy that is the salad-cure. Fields and gardens yield a variety of leaf-vegetables, such as garden and water-cress lettuce, common corn valerian, the tender leaves of the dandelion and so forth. Those affected with stomach troubles as well as all those who have transgressed the natural laws in any manner, ought at this season to take up a cure of this kind. Of course, the manner of taking the treatment depends on the individual.

Some people, if overfed, are able to live for weeks on salads and stale bread, at the same time strengthening their digestive powers and improving metabolic assimilation. The fresh, green salads contain a vital force which is lacking in dried, cooked or preserved vegetables. Besides, these salads are rich in nutritive salts which many foods do not contain. In order not to neutralize the beneficial effects of a treatment of this kind, the other foods consumed with these salads, should be well selected.

Potato-salad, made of old potatoes has practically no nutritive value. Instead of this kind of food I would advise rice, lentils, or white beans. All of these are rich in albumen. Oil should be used plentifully. The same is very nutritious and eases the evacuation of the bowels. Instead of lemon one may also take sour milk or cream. Avoid vinegar by all means.

As a matter of course all salads should be scrupulously cleansed in fresh water before reaching the table. Plants of this kind sometimes possess parasitical insects which develop into tape-worms where the stomach and bowels are not in good condition.

Another vegetable that is not sufficiently appreciated is the rhubarb. About 300 years ago this plant was introduced into Europe. The Arabs long since understood its curative value. Its original home was on the shores of the Caspian and the Black Sea, as well on the banks of the Volga. The roots of this plant are an effective purgative, while its stalks and leaves form a delicious dish. The stalks are peeled, cut into small pieces and cooked in sugar; the flowers are prepared like cauliflower.

It may interest our readers to know that many of the famous men of ancient times highly valued green vegetables. For instance, Erasistratus, Chrysippus, Diencles, Pythagoras and Cato maintained that nothing was of greater benefit to the stomach and the nerves than green vegetables; as well as in the cases of gout, rheumatism, etc. Salads produce healthy humors, and also milk in nursing women. It is reputed that the Emperor Augustus was cured of an incurable disease by eating lettuce. This plant increases the appetite and creates new blood.

Onions are good for the complexion. An onion eaten on an empty stomach, cleanses the bowels and promotes digestion.

Spring is the time or taking one of the best cures known to Naturopathy that is the salad-cure. Fields and gardens yield a variety of leaf-vegetables, such as garden and water-cress lettuce, common corn valerian, the tender leaves of the dandelion and so forth. Those affected with stomach troubles as well as all those who have transgressed the natural laws in any manner, ought at this season to take up a cure of this kind. Of course, the manner of taking the treatment depends on the individual.

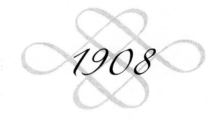

1908

Become a Vegetarian

And become stronger, healthier, happier, clearer-headed—and save money. Learn about Vegetarianism through THE VEGETARIAN MAGAZINE, (reduced fac-simile of cover shown here).

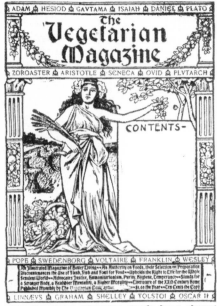

The Vegetarian Magazine stands for a cleaner body, a healthier mentality and a higher morality. Advocates disuse of flesh, fish and fowl as food; hygienic living and natural methods of obtaining health. Preaches humanitarianism, purity and temperance in all things. Upholds all that's sensible, right and decent. Able contributors. Has a Household Department which tells how to prepare Healthful and Nutritious Dishes without the use of meats or animal fats. Gives valuable Tested Recipes and useful hints on HYGIENE, SELECTION OF FOODS, TABLE DECORATION, KITCHEN ECONOMY, CARE OF COOKING UTENSILS, etc. Full of timely hints on PREVENTION AND CURE OF DISEASE. Gives portraits of prominent vegetarians, and personal testimonials from those who have been cured of long-standing diseases by the adoption of a natural method of living. TELLS HOW TO CUT DOWN LIVING EXPENSES WITHOUT GOING WITHOUT ANY OF LIFE'S NECESSITIES. EXPLAINS THE ONLY WAY OF PERMANENTLY CURING THE LIQUOR HABIT. WAYS TO INCREASE MUSCLE AND BRAIN POWER. Valuable hints on Child-Culture—how to inculcate unselfishness, benevolence and sympathy in children. A magazine for the whole family. Uniquely printed, well illustrated. Pages 7 by 10 inches in size. Published monthly. Sent postpaid to your address, 1 year, for $1; 6 mos., 50c; 3 mos., 25c; 1 mo., 10c.

A free sample of a back number on request. Address:

The Vegetarian Company, Inc.
No. 243 Michigan Boulevard, Chicago.

Ad for *The Vegetarian Magazine.*

DIET FOR CORPULENT PEOPLE

by Benedict Lust, N.D.

The Naturopath and Herald of Health, IX(2), 38. (1908)

Cause.—People of a quiet phlegmatic temper, of a one-sided business-diet, especially of beer and meat—of a sedentary occupation and doing too little physical work, are naturally, disposed to obesity.

Some time ago a farmer called at my office and told me that he had retired from work, in order to spend the rest of his life in leisure and well-being, but that he now felt sick and uncomfortable. I recommended him to resume his work in the open air and his former plain way of living and he would soon be all right again.

The man followed my advice and later on thanked me, for he was again healthy, contented and happy.

Then a gentleman, sitting beside me in a restaurant, busy with a large quantity of meat, a small piece of white bread and a bumper full of beer, asked me what he had to do to get rid of his big belly; he had already undergone many a treatment, advised by doctors and professors, without any result whatever. I told him to eat only black bread, drink no beer, but eat fruit and his "mortgage," as he called his belly, would soon vanish. "But I don't like that," he replied. Well, he was incurable.

Taste differs. I for my part, prefer a plain meal and a healthy body to a plate full of meat with a sick body. I know people, disposed to obesity, but living a harmonious life and on a vegetarian diet, are healthy, normal beings.

The view of various authorities that stout people should abstain from farinaceous dishes, is not correct; vegetarians eat many such dishes and I have never yet met any corpulent individuals among them, not even a disposition to obesity.

Symptoms.—Exorbitant laying on of fat, fatty degeneration of the heart, apoplectic attacks, dropsy, rheumatism and gout.

Treatment.—Avoid everything that contributes to the formation of fat, as fat meat, best none at all, sugar, butter, the yolk of eggs, no strong beers, no wine and brandy, at most, cider; drink as little as possible, if thirsty, lemon water; light black malt coffee, dry bilberry, currant or moselle wines (one glass a day).

The safest cure is: Live on twenty-five cents a day; do physical work for your living; for I have not yet seen a corpulent wood-cutter or a fat letter-carrier. These people have to work hard for their living.

Any one not willing to do so has to observe the following diet: In the morning light coffee or tea without milk and sugar, with black bread and a little butter. At noon, vegetables, especially green cabbage, lettuce, and so forth; in winter, dried vegetables; no legumes, peas and so forth, but rice hulled grains, and much fruit, especially the sour kinds. Never drink between the meals.

In the afternoon health-coffee. In the evening sour or skimmed milk, stewed fruit with black bread and little fat.

If the food is neither too salty nor too spicy, no thirst will come up. Smoking, too, provokes drinking. During the day nothing more than one glass water with lemon juice or light beer should be taken. Sleep not more than six or seven hours, never after a meal. Wash the body every morning with cold water; take much outdoor exercise; climb mountains from three to four hours at a quick, but not at a slow, pace; cut wood, ride the wheel; work in the garden from five to eight hours in such a way that your body becomes really tired. Breathe deep and sleep with open windows; take sun and airbaths.

Any one who follows conscientiously this prescription, will certainly not become fat, and he who is so will lose his surplus. But who will not do so, must for the lack of will-power go to destruction by his old way of living.

The safest cure is: Live on twenty-five cents a day; do physical work for your living; for I have not yet seen a corpulent wood-cutter or a fat letter-carrier. These people have to work hard for their living.

Vegetarian Method Of Life

by Benedict Lust

The Naturopath and Herald of Health, IX(5), 148-149. (1908)

Practical Suggestions To Beginners

The following advices are given in *Gesundes Leben* to those who have resolved to give up the meat diet for a more natural and healthful method of living.

1. Give up the eating of all meats, gradually but as quickly as possible, and substitute eggs, cheese, pastry, peas, lentils, nut dishes and good whole wheat bread. It is well to start slowly, but sure. All the above-named foods contain superfluously all that is required for the human body.

2. Eat rather less than you were formerly used to. Don't believe that you require greater quantities of food. Only what is thoroughly digested is feeding, and vegetarian food contains all the nourishments. Should you at first be inconvenienced through the lack of feeling satisfied, which is easily explainable through the absence of the usual irritation, it will soon disappear.

3. Avoid all spicy additions and try to obtain the required taste on simple dishes. Don't crave for great quantities and all such dishes that require long preparation. Shy all the artificial frying pan dishes.

4. Prefer rather dry and firm foods to pappy ones. The former are more easily digested, as they have to be properly chewed. With fluid foods always eat a little bread or a biscuit, so as to obtain the right proportion of saliva with your food. Chew everything very carefully.

5. Don't eat too much green vegetables and only when accompanied by appropriate dishes (pottages).

6. Persons whose daily occupation enforces sitting should have every day at least one meal consisting entirely of fruit with whole-wheat bread, and nuts form a fine substantial meal.

7. Cured or dried fruits, such as figs, dates, bananas, raisins, prunes, apricots, etc., are very nutritious and if dissolved in cold water and eaten with nuts form a fine substantial meal.

8. Should you have bad teeth, it is advisable to grind the nuts in a grinding machine to facilitate the digestion.

9. Don't fall into the common error of too great one-sidedness which impels to live only from potatoes, white bread and cabbage, or to drop all meats feeding on insufficient food which formed by dishes to the former meat diet.

10. Leave out all sorts of white breads and pastries and try to eat only such bread made from whole wheat flour, such as graham bread.

11. Don't let your fruit dishes be washed out; that means don't let the cooking water be wasted, and see that they are not prepared with spices, vinegar or salt. Instead of vinegar always use fresh lemon juice.

12. Shun absolutely all alcoholic beverages and tobacco, possibly also all coffee and tea.

13. Have great care to get plenty of physical exercise, such as swimming, gymnastics and other appropriate sports, by which you will fortify and strengthen the whole body.

14. Occupy yourself with dictating questions and read the phenomenal books of Dr. Haig, Dr. Bircher-Benner and other good books.

15. Should you suffer from indigestion, fast awhile and take physical exercise. Eat only when hungry.

16. If by the observance of such rules you are not making headway, you should consult a physician who is a vegetarian or an experienced naturopath.

Remarkable Discovery

by John Harvey Kellogg

The Naturopath and Herald of Health, IX(9), 269-270. (1908)

H. Kellogg, M.D., writes in the last issue of *Good Health*:

A few years ago Masson, of Geneva, in studying certain Bulgarian milk preparations discovered a new lactic-acid-forming ferment which excelled all other lactic-acid-forming ferments. In testing its properties he discovered that it possessed far greater quantities than any other known ferment. The eminent Professor Metchnikoff, of the Pasteur Institute, at once recognized the value of this new discovery, and after a careful study of the ferment, did not hesitate to recommend it as a most important means of combating many of the gravest forms of chronic disease, and especially that most inveterate of all human maladies, old age.

Professor Metchnikoff has long held the theory that old age, as well as many common chronic disorders, is due to poisons absorbed from the intestines. These poisons are formed by certain germs known as anaerobes. These germs are found in such great quantities in butcher's meat that Herter has given to them the name "meat bacteria." By the use of meat these germs are introduced into the intestine in great numbers. The poisons formed by these germs are extremely virulent, and when absorbed into the body gradually break down the liver, kidneys and other defensive organs, and so give rise to a large number of very common and very serious diseases. This chronic poisoning first makes its appearance in acute attacks, such as sick headache, nervous headache, loss of appetite, coated tongue, biliousness, bilious attacks, irregular action of the bowels, diarrhea, appendicitis, febrile attacks resembling malaria, and insomnia.

As the system becomes more and more saturated with these poisons through the gradual failure of the liver and kidneys and the constant multiplication of the bacteria, other more chronic symptoms appear, such as constant headache, mental confusion, neurasthenia, nervous exhaustion, gall stones, hemorrhoids, emaciation, browning of the skin, particularly about the eyes, neuralgia, pain and stiffness of the joints. After a time still worse conditions make their appearance, such as Bright's disease, sclerosis, or hardening of the liver, dropsy, chronic rheumatism and rheumatic gout.

Chronic autointoxication is unquestionably a factor in nearly all chronic disorders, and lays the foundation for tuberculosis, cancer of the stomach, ulcer of the stomach and other gastric disorders. Many women supposed to be suffering from disorders peculiar to their sex, are really suffering only from autointoxication, which is the natural result of the prolapsed of the colon and inattention to the hygiene of the bowels.

It has long been known that the conditions above mentioned may be greatly relieved by the use of buttermilk and kumyss, but these remedies have never gained very great confidence for the reason that, while they have seemed to succeed remarkably in certain cases, in the majority of cases the relief obtained has been very temporary, and often their use has been attended by complete failure. The reason for this was the fact that the lactic ferment of the kumyss and buttermilk is not able to live in the large intestine. This is the particular part of the alimentary canal in which the poison-forming anaerobes are found in largest numbers, especially in the cecum.

Metchnikoff's experiments show that the new lactic ferment has such great vitality that it is not only able to live but to flourish in the colon. Its great activity in the formation of acids enables it to kill off the anaerobes which can live only in an alkaline medium. Fortunately the new ferment is harmless, so that a person who is suffering from autointoxication may, by introducing into his alimentary canal a sufficient amount of the lactic ferment, drive out the poison-forming germs, or at least reduce their numbers to a very great extent. The importance of doing this will be realized when it is known that the poisons which they form are among the most highly toxic known. This is the reason why constipation produces headache, why diarrhea is accompanied by such terrible exhaustion. The headache and the prostration are simply results of the poisons which are absorbed from the infected intestines.

This ferment has been known for ages in Bulgaria and the Orient generally. In Egypt it is known as a leben. In these countries a milk preparation containing the ferment is prepared by sterilizing the milk and adding the ferment to it. It possesses the particular advantage that it does not produce alcohol as does the kumyss ferment, and when properly cultivated, it does not produce disagreeable flavors by decomposing the caseins and fats of the milk.

The use of the ferment has extended rapidly in France and Switzerland, and has lately been introduced into this country. For those who like milk and are able to digest it readily, the milk preparation requires considerable care and pains to prevent contamination. There are many, however—perhaps one-third or one-half of all chronic invalids—with whom milk does not agree. Such persons have been termed by Combe "casein dyspeptics." For the benefit of such cases a concentrated preparation of the new ferment has been devised. Pure cultures of the ferment are made in the bacteriological laboratory and in concentrated form are introduced into small capsules. Each capsule contains ten million or more units. One or two of these capsules taken after each meal in connection with a proper dietary—especially with the free use of such carbohydrates as farinaceous foods, especially rice, and, best of all, malted cereals and maltose in the form of malt extracts or maltose—develop rapidly, and by driving out the invading anaerobes stop the formation of poisons and give the body an opportunity to clear itself from the accumulated toxins, and thus establish conditions which render recovery possible. Those who like milk but do not like it sour may take it in its ordinary form with the meal. The capsules administered after the meal are fed by the lactose of the milk and other carbohydrates, and thus rapidly developing, are enabled to do the beneficent work.

This new method is based upon the discovery made some years ago by Metchnikoff that these lactic-acid forming ferments are a natural means by which the body is protected from the overdevelopment in the body of the meat bacteria. The intestine becomes infected through the free use of meat and eggs. The introduction of this ferment is, then, simply aiding the natural method of defense and hence is not a method capable of doing any harm. It is, of course, evident that a person adopting this method should discontinue the use of meat entirely, and should not use eggs freely. This new ferment in concentrated form is furnished in this country under the name of "Yogurt."

Professor Metchnikoff has long held the theory that old age, as well as many common chronic disorders, is due to poisons absorbed from the intestines.

Chronic autointoxication is unquestionably a factor in nearly all chronic disorders, and lays the foundation for tuberculosis, cancer of the stomach, ulcer of the stomach and other gastric disorders.

Metchnikoff's experiments show that the new lactic ferment has such great vitality that it is not only able to live but to flourish in the colon.

One or two of these capsules taken after each meal in connection with a proper dietary—especially with the free use of such carbohydrates as farinaceous foods, especially rice, and, best of all, malted cereals and maltose in the form of malt extracts or maltose—develop rapidly, and by driving out the invading anaerobes stop the formation of poisons and give the body an opportunity to clear itself from the accumulated toxins, and thus establish conditions which render recovery possible.

WHY WE FAVOR A VEGETARIAN DIET

by Dr. Henry Lindlahr

The Naturopath and Herald of Health, IX(10), 302-306. (1908)

We should exclude from our dietary the flesh of dead animals, because it doubles the work of our organs of *elimination* and overloads the system with animal *waste matter* and poisons. The following may serve to explain this more fully:

Two processes are constantly going on in every animal organism, a *building up* and a *tearing down* process. The red blood carries into the body the various elements of nutrition and comes back laden with poisonous gases, broken down cell material and devitalized food products. This debris is carried in the venous blood to the various organs of depuration and excreted as feces, urine, mucous, perspiration, etc. Every drop of venous blood and every part of animal flesh are contaminated with these excrements of the animal body. The meat eater, therefore, has to eliminate in addition to his *own* morbid matter that of the *animal* carcass.

Chemical analysis proves conclusively that uric acid and other uremic poisons contained in the animal carcass are almost identical with caffein and thein, the poisonous stimulating principles of coffee and tea. This puts flesh foods, meat soups and meat extracts in the same class with coffee, tea, alcohol and other poisonous stimulants. It explains why meat stimulates the *animal passions* and why it creates a craving for *liquor*, tobacco and other still stronger stimulants.

Not long ago we saw a father in high glee at the sight of his little two-year-old baby boy who was chewing busily at a piece of rare beefsteak, the blood running from the corners of his mouth. Daddy related to me proudly that baby liked his coffee already as well as anybody else in the family. Just imagine the tender, sensitive, *nervous* system of the little child, from the cradle up, over-irritated and over-stimulated with these powerful stimulants! Well-informed physicians tell us that over fifty percent of children are *sexual perverts* before they leave the public schools. Is it any wonder?

Did you ever notice on a saloonkeeper's free-lunch counter luscious fruits and vegetables? Not much! He knows very well that it takes strongly *spiced* and *salted* meats and fish to arouse the appetite for liquor and tobacco.

It must also be taken into consideration that the morbid matter of the dead animal body is foreign and uncongenial to the excretory organs of man; in other words, it is much harder for them to eliminate the waste matter of an animal carcass than that of their own bodies. Furthermore, formation of ptomains or corpse poisons begins immediately after the death of the animal. This is a serious matter since slaughtered "stock" is

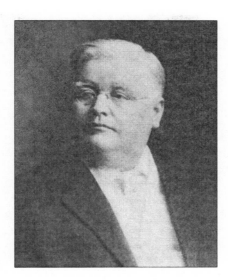

Dr. Henry Lindlahr.

kept under ice in refrigerators for many months and sometimes for a year before it reaches the kitchen, green and livid looking and sending forth suspicious odors which have to be doctored with chemicals and spices.

The nobler ones among carnivorous animals devour only freshly slaughtered prey, it remains for scavengers of the hog and hyena type and for man to feast on flesh long, cold and stark and tainted by the odors of incipient decay.

The foregoing statements will explain why even the best of meats are detrimental to health, but the danger becomes much greater when soup, roast, ham or sausage trace their pedigree to tuberculous or "lumpy-jaw" cattle or to scrofulous or cholera infected hogs. Raw meat is especially dangerous because it is often the cause of trichinae, tapeworms and of other parasitic infections.

The word scrofula is derived from the Latin word "scrofa" (sow), indicating that the ancients recognized the relationship between pork eating and scrofulous diseases.

Still other powerful influences tend to poison the flesh of slaughtered animals. It is now well understood that emotions of worry, fear and anger actually poison blood and tissues. Fear and anger of the mother poison her milk and through the milk her nursing babe. The bite of an infuriated man has often proved as poisonous as that of a mad dog. All of us have experienced the poisonous and paralyzing effects of worry and fear. Animals are instinctively very sensitive to approaching danger and death. Fear is one of their predominating characteristics.

Imagine, now, how excited they must be by emotions of worry, anger and fear after many days of travel, closely packed in shaking cars, hungry, thirsty, tired, scared and angered to the point of madness. Many die before the journey is ended; others are driven half dead with fear and exhaustion to the slaughter pens, their instinctive fear of death augmented by the sight and odor of the bloody shambles.

Think of the wounded deer and rabbit chased by hounds for many miles before death ends their agonies. Emotions of fear and anger thus aroused to the greatest intensity in the dying animal produce *chemical* changes which *poison* blood and tissues.

The otherwise sensible and hygienic Jewish ritual commands the faithful to slowly bleed to death the slaughtered animal in order to purify it of the "unclean blood." Such bleeding, however, removes only the comparatively harmless red *arterial blood*, while the disease laden *venous* blood is still retained in the carcass. The dubious purifying effect of the "bleeding" is more than offset by the poisonous effect of the prolonged death agony of the animal.

OVEREATING

But even the most wholesome foods will become injurious when taken in excessive quantities. Whatever we cannot properly *digest* and *assimilate* will ferment and decay and fill the system with waste matter and poisons. Many persons waste the best part of their vitality in order to eliminate noxious food ballast and then wonder why they are so weak in spite of a good *appetite* and rich *foods*. In such cases, when the organs of digestion are constantly overworked, they weaken and cannot transform the continuous oversupply of foods into the proper constituents for healthy blood and lymph; waste matter accumulates, ferments and decays, creating noxious gases and systemic poisons. Poisonous miasms thus created contaminate the vital fluids, cause corruption and obstruction in organs and tissues, and furnish a luxurious soil for all kinds of parasites, germs, and bacteria.

This is so simple and self-evident that we cannot comprehend how the "regular" profession can persist in "stuffing" continually the weak bodies of consumptives and other invalids with enormous quantities of food, under the impression that the patients are thus strengthened and built up. The profession does not seem to realize that the *stomach* and bowels of these poor sufferers are no less feeble and incapable of exertion than are their *arms* and *legs*.

Suppose one of these patients, hardly able to walk, complains of extreme weakness and is told by his physician to go home and chop a cord of wood daily. The patient would doubtless imagine there was a "loose screw" somewhere in the thinking apparatus of the good doctor. But when the latter tells him to go home and stuff his weak stomach every hour or two with eggs, meats, soups, beer, tonics, brandy and everything else imaginable, he goes home, does as advised, praises the wisdom of his doctor—and peacefully gives up the ghost. The good minister attributes his death to the inscrutable will of *Providence*. We rather suspect that he succumbed to an overdose of professional *ignorance*. It is not self-evident that the health and strength of the body do not depend upon the quantity *eaten*, but upon the quantity properly *digested* and assimilated? When will doctors learn that digestion and excretion are in themselves a great strain on vitality? Have they never experienced that "lazy feeling" after a heavy meal?

In severe disease and states of nervous and physical prostration, the ordinary functions are at a standstill—as is apparent from the extreme weakness and helplessness of the patient. Much less food, therefore, is needed than in times of healthy activity. Is it not evident that nature herself, in acute disease, protests against eating by loss of appetite, nausea and vomiting? But the patient may object ever so strenuously to the forced feeding; his whole organism may revolt against it, the wise doctor will insist that he must eat to keep up strength, so-called "sedatives" are given to paralyze the stomach into insensibility and down will go chicken soup, eggs and beef tea, in spite of nature's protest.

In acute *febrile* diseases, feeding is not only useless but actually harmful, because in such conditions, which we recognize as nature's healing and cleansing efforts, the normal activities of the organism, including the processes of digestion and assimilation, are at a standstill. All efforts are concentrated on elimination and the stomach and bowels also are called upon to assist in the general house cleaning. Instead of assimilating, they also are eliminating noxious poisons, which produce nausea, vomiting, diarrhea and catarrhal excretions. The digestive organs normally act like a sponge, but now the process is reversed, the sponge being squeezed. It is giving off old, filthy accumulations, thus aiding the "cleansing crisis." As soon as food is given, this beneficial elimination through stomach and bowels is hindered and interrupted; as a consequence, the temperature immediately rises and is followed by an aggravation of all symptoms.

The danger lies not so much in *underfeeding*, as in *overfeeding*. To *one* who dies from lack of food, *thousands* die from overeating. If the truth were known, we would be surprised at the small amount of food required to keep the body in perfect condition.

Cornaro, an Italian nobleman, when forty years of age, was given up by his doctors as dying from the effects of dissipation. He, at this time, instead of resigning himself to his fate, determined to enter upon a little experiment of his own: cut his food supply down to a few ounces a day, and before long regained health and strength. At one hundred years of age he wrote a book recounting his experiments and the wonderful effects of temperate living.

The only safe guide in eating is hunger, "not appetite"; this is nature's sign that more food is needed, and that the organism is in condition to take care of it.

If the doctors and friends of the patients better understood and applied this simple principle, a great many of those who are now carried to the grave would remain with us and enjoy life a little longer.

Arguments in favor of vegetarian diet are usually met with some such brilliant objection or criticism, as, "Why did God create cows and hogs, if they were not intended for us to eat?" To which thoughtful query we sometimes reply by asking the still deeper question, "Why did God create *you*, if you are not to be *eaten*?" Others tells us about the man who eats meats, smokes tobacco, drinks coffee and brandy and who is now over a hundred years old and in perfect health. All are certain that our arguments are mere theorizing and that nobody can actually prove the truth of our statement.

The fact that some people are accidentally so constituted that they can withstand the injurious effects of bad habits for many years does not imply that others can indulge with impunity in a similar manner nor that these hale and hearty ones would not be healthier and stronger without these poisons. It will be found that most of these rugged persons owe their iron constitutions to simple, natural surroundings and frugal fare in *early* life. Most of them were raised "on the farm," or came from the European peasantry, who are practically vegetarians. Even though these robust specimens of humanity did endure for a lifetime, the weakening influences of "high living," who can tell in how far they planted in their *descendants*, by their abnormal habits of life, the seeds of scrofula, psora and other hereditary taints with which, as the diagnosis from the eye reveals, all human beings are now more or less affected.

Careful observations disclose the interesting fact that the descendants of these hardy pioneers, when exposed to the degenerating influences of our city life, become extinct in the third, fourth or fifth generation.

If it were not for the steady influx of vegetarian stock from the villages of Germany, Ireland, Scotland and other European countries, the birth statistics of meat-eating America would make a poorer showing than those of France. Somebody will say, "This is due to race suicide, not to dietetics." Not altogether, for the same law holds true in the deeply religious country districts of Europe, where race suicide is unknown. There, also, the laborer or the schoolmaster living on black bread, vegetables and pure water have twice or three times as many children as the well-to-do citizen who lives in ease and luxury.

Orthodox science admits that the average length of life should be over one hundred years, while in fact it is now about thirty-seven. Man is the only animal falls far short of his allotted span of life, and what are even these few years for the great majority but from the cradle to the grave a *slow dying*? Very few ever know, for a single day, what it means to enjoy the full measure of abounding health, virile strength and elasticity of body and mind which nature intended for them.

There must be something wrong somewhere in man's habits of life to account for this discrepancy between the possible and the actual state of physical, mental and moral health.

"THE PROOF OF THE PUDDING IS THE EATING OF IT."

But we can offer still more direct and positive proof that meat-eating is injurious to health, and that it prevents the cure of serious chronic ailments. In evidence of this, we will present some typical incidents from our daily practice.

About a year ago there came under our treatment a woman whose head on one side was covered by a cancerous mass of large proportions. Her troubles started two years earlier, with an operation for the removal of a wen, "because it didn't look well." Neither she nor the learned surgeon, however, took into consideration that behind the wen lurked a constitutional sycotic taint, in consequence of which the scar left by the operation soon became inflamed, opened and began to discharge pus. Four different times the wound was operated on, but in spite of antiseptics, cauterization, skin grafting and everything else the surgeon's skill could do it would not stay healed. After the fourth operation, the growth became so large and so malignant that the surgeons were at the end of their wits. They said the growth had developed into a true cancer and dismissed her as incurable.

In this state she came under our treatment, improved rapidly, and after five months of natural living and treatment, when scrofula and drug poisons were thoroughly eliminated from her system, the growth had disappeared and the wound was covered with a healthy new skin.

Some time after this, however, she returned and reported that the wound had opened once more. On catechizing her, we found that—tempted by other members of the family—she had commenced to eat *meat*. Following our strict advice, she adhered more closely to her vegetarian regime, the wound immediately ceased to discharge and healed up once more. Several times after she had the same experience. Whenever she partook of meat and coffee for a few days, the wound would open and discharge.

Another case now under our treatment is that of a gentleman about thirty years of age. When we first attended him in his home, he had been in bed with inflammatory *rheumatism* for five months. He was unable to move a limb and his friends had given up all hope of his recovery. After four weeks of Nature Cure at home, he was able to come for treatment to our sanitarium; two months later he was apparently a well man. There was only an inflammatory condition in his right foot which made walking very painful. For three months, in spite of vigorous Nature Cure treatment, this painful lesion would not yield. Then we became convinced that something was wrong. We told him that somehow he must be violating the law. If our treatment was good enough to cure the worst of his condition, this comparatively insignificant symptom should also yield.

"Well, doctor," he answered, "I am living up strictly to directions, but I have been taking a little meat now and then, and I smoke one or two pipes of tobacco a day. I thought this could not harm me."

We explained to him that his system under the influence of Nature Cure treatments had become purified to such an extent that it was sensitive now, even to small quantities of poisons; that there was just enough uric acid and nicotine in the occasional piece of meat and pipe of tobacco to keep the weak part irritated and inflamed. He followed our directions more conscientiously and from that day on the inflammation subsided, and within a few weeks disappeared entirely.

Still another common occurrence in our practice confirms us in the opinion that meat-eating is neither natural nor necessary to man. People who have eaten meat regularly from childhood up adopt and follow under our advice a strictly vegetarian diet. After several months of meatless regime, they partake of some tempting roast or fowl, and they are very much surprised at the result of their experiment. They find that the tempting morsel does not *taste* as they had expected. Somehow it tastes "funny" (they are tasting the corpse!) and in many instances they experience unpleasant disturbances in the digestible organs, bad taste in the mouth, nausea, diarrhea and similar protests against unnatural food.

One may cease eating bread, *fruits* or vegetables for many years, but when these foods are again taken, there is never a sign of *protest* on nature's part; on the contrary, they are relished more than ever.

Persons who have broken and conquered the whisky or tobacco habit have similar experiences. A glass of whiskey or a cigar taken after long intervals of total abstinence nauseate them as much as when they first began to drink and smoke. They have to learn it all over again. Complaints like the following are quite familiar to us: "Why, doctor, this simple life is making me so *weak* that I cannot smoke a cigar without it turning my stomach inside out; it makes me as sick as a green school boy." These acute revulsions are not due to a weakening of the system, but to the fact that the nervous organism is once more *sensitive* and *strong* enough to *revolt* against noxious poisons and to forcibly eliminate them. But, after repeated indulgence, the sensory nerves become so weakened that they can no longer protest, and our backslider is then once more "strong enough" to enjoy his steak, smoke, coffee and liquor.

And what a glorious experience (for a while) this return to stimulants then becomes. His system under the purifying and relaxing influences of natural living has become so pure and sensitive that it fully responds to the powerful stimulants. Our recreant friend feels so strong and buoyant that he "floats on air." He wonders how he could live so long without these "wonderful tonics." But, by and by the scene *changes*. Brain and nerves become more and more paralyzed under the continual action of nicotine, alcohol and uric acid. Morbid matter accumulates and clots the wheels of life. Bleary eyes, trembling hands, weak heart, rheumatic joints, fagged brain and irritable temper soon tell the tale of, "Eat and drink what '*agrees*' with you." The last things of these backsliders are worse than the first, for only too often, weakened and discouraged by defeat, they lack energy and moral courage to make another stand, and physical, mental and moral *degeneration* are the inevitable results.

We have in our practice so many confirmatory experiences of this nature that we never undertake to cure a patient of serious chronic ailments unless he is willing to forego the use of meat and other poisonous stimulants, at least until his recovery has taken place.

In acute **febrile** *diseases, feeding is not only useless but actually harmful, because in such conditions, which we recognize as nature's healing and cleansing efforts, the normal activities of the organism, including the processes of digestion and assimilation, are at a standstill.*

To one who dies from lack of food, thousands die from overeating.

People who have eaten meat regularly from childhood up adopt and follow under our advice a strictly vegetarian diet. After several months of meatless regime, they partake of some tempting roast or fowl, and they are very much surprised at the result of their experiment. They find that the tempting morsel does not taste as they had expected. Somehow it tastes "funny" (they are tasting the corpse!) and in many instances they experience unpleasant disturbances in the digestible organs, bad taste in the mouth, nausea, diarrhea and similar protests against unnatural food.

THE SIMPLE LIFE IN A NUTSHELL

by John Harvey Kellogg

The Naturopath and Herald of Health, IX(10), 319-323. (1908)

The purpose of this article is to present a few simple rules, the careful following of which will promote to the highest degree physical and mental efficiency, mental and moral equipoise and equanimity, and will prolong to the greatest limit possible life and useful activity.

As space is too limited to permit of the presentation of arguments or reasons these rules are expected to be of chief service to those who are already persuaded of the correctness of general propositions of the simple life, or return-to-nature movement.

It is proper, however, to say for the encouragement of those to whom the ideas presented are altogether new, that of the various suggestions made, not one is presented which has not been thoroughly tried and tested in the experience of hundreds, even thousands, of persons neither is a single suggestion offered which does not rest upon a sound basis of scientific fact.

The simple life, or so-called return to nature, is not an innovation. It is a return to the 'old paths" from which the perversions of our modern civilization have gradually diverted millions of men and women, perversions that are responsible for the multitudinous maladies and degeneracies which yearly multiply in number and gravity.

GENERAL RULES

1. *Give attention daily to cultivating health.* It will pay. Study the conditions and the surroundings of the home and the business, and give careful thought to personal habits and practices with special reference to their bearing on health.

2. Recognize that health of mind and body is one of the most valuable of all personal assets, determine to make every reasonable effort to *maintain intact, and if possible to increase the capital of physical and mental health.*

3. *Give to the body* and its functions that *care and study* which you would accord to any other valuable and costly mechanism, so as to become familiar with its needs and the best means of supplying them.

EATING FOR HEALTH AND EFFICIENCY

4. *Eat only natural foods;* that is, those which are naturally adapted to the human constitution. The natural *dietary* includes fruits, nuts,

cooked grains, legumes, and vegetables. Natural food imparts to the body the greatest amount of energy and maintains normal conditions of life.

5. *Avoid meats of all sorts* (flesh, fowl, fish, including "sea food"). These are unnatural foods. They are all likely to contain deadly parasites of various kinds and always contain noxious germs, meat bacteria or "anaerobes," which infect the intestines, inoculate the body with disease, and cause putrefaction and other poison-forming and various morbid processes. These germs are not destroyed by ordinary cooking such as stewing, broiling, frying, roasting, etc.

6. Take care to *avoid an excess of protein,* that is, the albuminous element represented in lean meat, the white of an egg, and the curd of milk. An excess of protein promotes putrefaction, and thus intestinal autointoxication, the chief cause of "biliousness," colitis, appendicitis, gall-stones, arteriosclerosis, possibly cancer, Bright's disease, and premature old age. Ordinary bread contains a sufficient amount of protein, as do also rice and other cereals and the potato. Most nuts, also dried peas and beans, contain an excess of protein, and should be eaten sparingly. Most cases of acute illness, excepting contagious disorders are due to some form of autointoxication. The best remedy is fasting or a meager diet of fruits and cereals for a day or two.

7. *Eggs should be eaten in great moderation if at all.* They encourage autointoxication, and thus often cause 'biliousness." The yolk of the egg is more wholesome than the white.

8. *Cow's milk is not altogether suited for human food.* A large proportion of invalids—nearly half, perhaps—suffer from "casein dyspepsia," and cannot take milk without suffering from constipation, headache, "biliousness," coated tongue, of other unpleasant symptoms which indicate intestinal autointoxication. Ordinary butter is unfit for food. To be wholesome, butter must be made from sterilized, or boiled, cream.

9. Persons who are not subject to casein dyspepsia are often able to digest sterilized cream more easily than butter. Persons who suffer from hyperpepsia—"sour stomach"—may take sterilized butter and cream more freely than those who suffer from slow digestion. When butter or cream produces pimples on the face, a coated tongue, or a bad taste in the mouth, it must be diminished in quantity, or omitted altogether. *Nuts are an excellent substitute for butter and cream when a substitute is necessary.*

10. *Avoid poison foods.* Tea, coffee, chocolate, and cocoa are poisons.

The special poisons which they contain, impair digestion, damage the nerves and promote disease of the liver, kidneys, and blood vessels. *Cereal beverages and hot fruit juices are wholesome substitutes for tea and coffee.*

11. *Condiments*—mustard, pepper, pepper sauce, cayenne, capsicum, vinegar, hot irritating sauces and spices of all kinds—*must be wholly discarded.* They irritate the stomach, thus giving rise to gastric and intestinal catarrh, and damage the liver and kidneys.

12. *Common salt,* or chlorid[e] of sodium, *should be used sparingly,* if at all. According to Richet and others, the food naturally contains all the chlorid[e] of sodium actually required by the body, so that the addition of salt to the food is necessary only to please a cultivated taste. A safe rule is, the less the better.

13. *Food combinations should be such as to give the proper proportion of the several elements,—proteids, carbohydrates, and fats.* Fruits and vegetables as well as other combinations of natural foodstuffs, agree perfectly when mastication is sufficiently thorough to reduce the food to a liquid state in the mouth and when indigestible residues are rejected.

14. *The quantity of food should be adapted to the size of the person* and the amount of work which he does. Never eat to satiety. *Eat only when hungry,* never because it is meal-time, or because invited to eat. A person of *average* height and moderately active requires 200 calories of proteid, 450 calories of fat, and 1,350 calories of carbohydrates, or a total of 2,000 *calories,* or food units, daily. The total number of calories required is furnished respectively by about 28 ounces of bread, or 96 ounces of milk, or 62 ounces of potatoes, or 9 ounces of butter. One-fourth of each of these, or any other fractions which together equal unity, will aggregate 2,000 food units, or a day's ration. Be careful to eat enough.

15. *Food must be well relished to be well digested.* According to Pawlow "appetite juice" which is produced by stimulation of the nerves of taste by palatable food, is the most important factor in gastric digestion.

16. *Cane-sugar must be taken only in small quantity.* Large quantities give rise to gastric catarrh and indigestion. Sweet fruits, such as raisins and figs, honey, maltose or malt sugar, are natural and wholesome sweets.

17. A sedentary life tends to produce intestinal inactivity, that is, slow digestion and constipation; hence, *the ordinary daily bill of fare should supply an adequate amount of laxative foodstuff* such

as *sweets* (not cane-sugar syrups), *sweet fruits,* especially *figs* and *prunes, acid fruits* and *fruit juices, fats, fresh vegetables,* and *whole grain preparations.*

18. Some *fresh, raw food should be eaten daily* in the form of fresh fruit or fruit juices, nuts, or salads. Raw cereals are indigestible. The cellulose of fruits, and of young buds, leaves, and shoots is digestible in the intestine. Fresh vegetables and whole grain cereals are needed to supply alkaline and earthly salts. The blood and all living cells require these salts, as well as the teeth and the bones. The free use cane-sugar and meats leads to lime starvation, being greatly deficient in salts.

19. Avoid complicated dishes of great variety at one meal, but vary diet from day to day, as the appetite may indicate.

20. *Eat at regular hours,* so as to maintain the normal intestinal rhythm which secures the daily movement of the bowels. Rather than omit a meal entirely, eat some fruit, or drink a glass of fruit juice, buttermilk, or some other simple nutrient which will keep up the peristaltic procession and rhythm. Never take food into the stomach when remains of a precious meal are present.

21. The best meal plan is to *eat twice a day.* Eight to nine a. m., and three to four p. m. are the best hours; or eleven a. m. and six p. m., if the retiring hour is necessarily very late.

22. *If three meals are eaten, the heartiest meal should be taken at midday.* The breakfast should be substantial, *the evening meal very light,* especially avoiding pastry, fats, rich sauces, and hearty foods. The evening meal should consist chiefly of ripe or cooked fruits, liquid foods, and such cereals as boiled rice or cereal flakes.

23. *Avoid iced foods and drinks.* Very cold foods or drinks, if taken at all, should be swallowed slowly and in very small quantities.

24. *Chew every morsel until reduced to liquid in the mouth,* rejecting and returning to the plate skins, seeds, and other tasteless woody residues. Thorough chewing develops "appetite juice" in the stomach and combats intestinal autointoxication, the most prolific cause of disease. Give preference to dry foods. Sip liquids slowly, taking care to insalivate thoroughly.

25. *Take three pints of water a day,* including liquid food. Do not drink much at nor immediately after meals. Take a few sips whenever thirsty. *Drink a glassful of water on rising in the morning, on retiring at night, an hour before each meal, and two or three hours after eating.* If digestion and bowel action are sluggish, sip half a glassful of cold water half an hour before meals.

EXERCISE FOR HEALTH

26. *Live as much as possible in the open air.* If compelled to work indoors, be sure that the living and work rooms have an ample, continual supply of fresh air. The lower the temperature the better, so long as the body is kept comfortably warm. Temperatures above 70° are depressing. The breathing of cold air is a continuous tonic; every breath is a tonic bath, a vital lift. A thousand breaths an hour count greatly toward health or disease, according as the air breathed is pure and cool, or impure and hot.

27. *Working in the open air is one of the best forms of exercise,* especially working in the garden, digging, hoeing, pruning, etc. Do some good, hard muscular work every day, enough to produce slight muscular fatigue; but avoid exhaustion. Swimming in water at 76° to 80° is the best of all special health exercises. Rapid walking and hill-climbing are excellent.

28. One need not live a sedentary life because his occupation is sedentary. *Always sit erect, with the chest held high and small of back supported.* Sit little as possible. Standing and lying are more natural and healthful positions than sitting. One may exercise while sitting at work by stiffening the muscles of first one limb a few seconds, then the other. All the muscles in the body may be exercised in the same way.

29. *Deep breathing aids digestion, encourages liver and bowel action, develops the lungs, and purifies the blood.* The only directions needed are: *Hold the chest high and breathe as deep as you can* ten or twenty times every hour, or oftener. The best "breath" gymnastics are swimming, hill-climbing, and rapid walking or running. Always breathe through the nose.

30. In walking, *always hold the chest high* and carry it well to the front. Swing the arms moderately and *walk fast enough to hasten the breathing a little. Nine miles a day at three miles an hour is the proper distance* for the average adult. Most busy housekeepers and farmers do more than this.

31. If the abdominal muscles are weak, develop them by simple exercises, such as walking on tiptoe with chest held high, and running round the room on all fours; lie on the back, hold the legs straight and raise them to the perpendicular, repeating thirty or forty times three times a day. Lying on the back, raising the body from the lying to the sitting position with the hands placed upon the back of the neck. Repeat ten to twenty times three times a day, gradually increasing the number.

32. If the abdominal muscles are weakened, so that the lower abdomen bulges forward, a tight flannel bandage, or more substantial support, should be worn about the lower abdomen when on the feet, until the muscles have been strengthened by exercise.

THE TOILET

33. *Cleanse the mouth and teeth thoroughly before and after each meal and on rising and retiring.* A foul tongue and decaying teeth indicate mouth infection.

34. Take a warm cleansing bath before retiring twice a week in winter. Apply olive oil or fine Vaseline after the bath.

35. Take a short cold bath every morning on rising. This is an excellent tonic. Or take a cool air bath, rubbing the skin with a dry towel. A very short hot bath (half a minute at 110°) may, if necessary, be substituted for the cold bath.

36. The hands, nose, and the scalp also require sanitary attention. For the hands use a good strong soap and rinse well with soft water.

37. The bowels should move thoroughly at least once a day, most naturally soon after breakfast. Putrid, foul-smelling stools are an indication of intestinal autointoxication, and are due to an excess of proteid in the form of meat, eggs, or possibly milk. Such a condition always breeds disease.

SLEEP AND REST

37. *Sleep eight hours every night.* If not strong, or if neurasthenic, take a nap before dinner.

38. *Surroundings at night should be quiet.* Sleep amid noise is not refreshing. Lie on the right side, or slightly turned toward the face. The bed should be neither too hard or too soft. Avoid feathers. The covers should be dry, warm, and porous. *Avoid overheating by excess of clothing.* Use a small pillow or none at all.

39. Always breathe outdoor air when asleep by means of wide open windows, the window tent, the air tube, or a sleeping balcony. Do not sleep within two hours after eating.

40. Make the weekly Sabbath a day of complete rest from work. Take a halfday off in the middle of the week if possible. Recreate in the open air an hour or two daily.

CLOTHING

41. *The clothing should be loose, comfortable, light, and porous.*

Restrictive clothing is necessarily damaging, for the trunk of the body is continually changing in form and size. Wear porous, cotton or linen underclothing next the skin. *Avoid waterproofs except for temporary protection.* Clothe the extremities so as to keep them warm under all conditions.

MENTAL HYGIENE

42. *Do not worry.* Horace Fletcher has shown us the pernicious influence of "fear-thought." The Power that made us can and does take care of us. There is no need to worry. The intelligence that controls and energizes heart and lungs can rule our destinies and with our co-operation will lead our lives in ways where "all things work together for good" to us. Worry kills. Hope inspires, uplifts. Cheer up.

43. Do not become self-centered. Avoid thinking or talking about ailments or other unpleasant things. Let your ideals be altruistic.

44. Exercise self-control and restraint in all things. Work uses energy moderately, the passions and the emotions enormously.

45. Study the dreams and take a vacation when you dream about your work.

SUGGESTIONS

46. *For constipation, knead the bowels well* with the hands night and morning. Eat laxative foods, especially fruits and nuts, and whole-grain "cereals." Avoid oatmeal mush.

47. *For a cold,* take a hot bath on retiring; drink abundantly; eat little but fruit for a day or two; and stay out of doors. Live in the fresh air and avoid colds.

48. *If sleepless or nervous,* take a warm bath at 102° F. for one or two minutes then cool to 93° to 95°; continue after half an hour to two hours if necessary.

49. *For "biliousness,"* clear the stomach and bowels, fast or eat fruit exclusively for a day or two, and adopt a strict antitoxic diet, avoiding meat, eggs, animal fats, and perhaps milk.

50. *The* best foods in the order of excellence, *antitoxic foods in italic: Fresh, ripe fruits, cooked fresh fruits, cooked dried fruits,* nuts, cooked cereals—*rice, zwieback, toasted corn flakes,—potato, cauliflower and other fresh vegetables* (if fiber is rejected), *honey, maltose, malted nuts, yogurt, buttermilk,* sterilized *milk* and cream, peas, beans, lentils, *raised bread,* sterilized butter.

– J. H. KELLOGG, in *Good Health.*

WHY PEANUTS ARE HARD TO DIGEST

by Benedict Lust

The Naturopath and Herald of Health, IX(11), 355. (1908)

The peanut, though not a nut, is classed with nuts, and is in universal use. Unfortunately, as commonly sold and eaten it has been proved to be hard to digest and very difficult for many people to eat at all.

Nor does peanut butter, if made from roasted peanuts, agree with some people. The digestibility of the peanut butter depends upon how it is made. If it is made from roasted peanuts, it is not good because roasting sets free the fat of the peanut, which is burned upon the surface, and the peanut is really fried and becomes indigestible. But peanut butter prepared in the proper way is entirely wholesome. The proper way is heating it at a temperature of perhaps 240 degrees, not highly, so that it is thoroughly cooked, slightly browned, but not roasted in any sense.

NATURAL — — HEALTHFUL

L. Lust's unroasted

RAW PEANUT BUTTER

A boon for the Uncooked Food Dietist. Free from the dry parched taste so common in all roasted Peanut Butter. Highly Nutritious, rich in protein and nutritive salts. Will keep for months. (2 lb. tins only) 65 cents, postpaid 75 cents; 6-2 lbs. tins (12 lbs.) prepaid $4.25.

L. LUST'S HEALTH FOOD BAKERY, Inc.

CORNER 105th STREET AND PARK AVENUE
NEW YORK CITY

Agents solicited

Louis Lust, Benedict's brother, established a bakery in NYC that expanded into health food products such as raw peanut butter.

1909

Mother's Milk

is undoubtetly the best food for infants. When this, however, is not procurable the best substitute for it only should be used. The best substitute for mother's milk is one that contains all the ingredients of the same. Cow's milk would be excellent if it was not for the lack principally of fats. These are supplied in the proper proportion and of the proper character by

Dr. Lahmann's Vegetable Milk (Pflanzen=Milch)

Cow's milk mixed with „Vegetable Milk" is an exact reproduction of mother's milk. It is as palatable, as digestible, and as nutritive as mother's milk.

————Mrs. E. F. HENDERSON of Chestnut Hill, Mass., (now a customer of four years standing) writes: "My baby has been fed on it (Vegetable Milk and Cow's Milk) and has been **invariably well** and particularly **strong and muscular."** Thousands of others have since sent similar testimonials. **Price per can (sufficient for one week), 60 Cents, Postage 15 Cts., Price per doz. cans $6.50. Express prepaid $7.00.**

Dr. Lahmann's Nutritive Salt Health Cocoa
(Nährsalz=Cacao),

is perfectly digestible for the weakest invalid. Its exquisite aroma makes it a luxury for the richest table, while its purity and economy render it superior to tea and coffee for every home. **1 lb. (100 cups) $1.00, ½ lb. 50 cts.** Postage 18 cents per lb.

Dr. Lahmann's sweetened Chocolate,

for all uses the best and most exquisite.
Per lb.: No. 1 70c. No 2 60c.
Postage 18c. per lb.

Dr. Lahmann's Nutritive Extract,
(Nährsalz=Extract)

renders all foods more digestible by adding the parts lost in the preparation of the food. An excellent remedy for indigestion.
Price per Jar $1.00. Postage 10c.

Dr. Lahmann's Eating Chocolate,
25 Cents per Package.

Dr. Lahmann's Cocoa with Oatmeal Addition, ½ lb. 45 Cents.

Dr. Lahmann's Oatmeal and Nährsalz· Biscuits, 15 Cents.

Dr. Lahmann's Japan Soya Sause $1.00

Sole Importer and Agent for the U. S.: **Benedict Lust, 124 E. 59th St., New York.**
Descriptive pamphlet on receipt of 2 Cents stamp.

FOR SALE BY ALL NATUROPATHIC SANITARIA AND N. D'S.

Dr. Lahmann developed a vegetarian milk substitute made of ingredients that he never revealed.

Nutritive Value Of Oats

Author Unknown

The Naturopath and Herald of Health, XIV (2), 103-104. (1909)

Two experiments in cattle-raising taught me the nutritive value of oats. A friend of mine bought at an auction an old miserable jade for $25, too high a price for such a worn-out nag. If a horse-butcher had been around, he would have chopped up the bones and skin and converted them into steaks and sausages. Advised by a peasant, an expert in horse-raising, my friend treated his Rosinante to oats, beginning with small rations, increasing them day by day, and finally sending the horse to pasture. And O! Wonder! After a short time the horse improved and became such a fine specimen that anybody who had seen it first could not recognize it. This metamorphosis had been affected by oats.

The second experiment I made on my own farm, composed of one goat, sixteen hens and one rooster. One spring the hens were slow in lay-ing eggs, though they were well fed. Besides the **offals** from the kitchen, they had been treated to maize. Annoyed at the poor results in the egg-production, we in a rare family council decided to kill them. Two of them had not only died by the knife, but had also been boiled to soup. As their meat was fat and tender, we were well satisfied with this decision.

Then I began to ponder, if our way of feeding them was really the right one, if maize is egg producing. Then I decided to try oats, though this food is a little more expensive. After a fortnight we were satisfied with these results. Formerly sixteen hens had scarcely laid seven eggs a day, and now fourteen hens gave us nine eggs a day. Then, further execu-tions were naturally suspended.

Such illustrations from animals are not always transferable on human beings; but we are well entitled to recognize the nutritious value of oats.

According to Petersen albumin, most necessary for the formation of blood is found in the following proportion. In

1 kilogramme oats .... 140 grammes
1 kilogramme peas .... 220 grammes
1 kilogramme beef .... 200 grammes
1 kilogramme potatoes .... 20 grammes.

Seven times more albumin is contained in oats than in potatoes; it stands almost on a par with meat and legumes; therefore its high value for forming new blood and new tissues. That is the reason why physicians always prescribe gruel in all serious diseases.

The nutritive value of food does not depend on albumin alone, but also on its quantity of carbohydrates; these substances not only contribute to the formation of blood and tissues, but they also maintain the vitality and are, so to speak, the fuel which keeps the machine of the body going. According to Petersen carbohydrates are contained in

1 kilogramme oats .... 630 grammes
1 kilogramme peas .... 530 grammes
1 kilogramme beef .... 0 grammes
1 kilogramme potatoes ... 200 grammes

We see that meat contains no carbohydrates at all; it is therefore not sufficient for our sustenance. Dogs have been fed to death by lean meat; but nobody ever died of oat-meal or gruel; on the contrary, the human body can subsist on it and keep up strength and health.

Though the kind of food we take is of importance, the most essential point is the digestion. Legumes, though containing much albumin, are hard to digest, and therefore are not to be recommended to delicate people, but in oats we have both albumin and carbohydrates in so light a digestible form that it can easily be digested; and it is worthy of notice that the nutritive substance of the oats does not pass over into any detrimental combination; as, for instance, the albumin of the meat does, which passes over in creatin[e] and so forth. Besides the qualities just mentioned, the oats are rich in mineral substances.

These mineral substances give life to the dead matter of the contents of the tissues, therefore Biochemy calls them "function organs." The Naturopathists value this substance highly and maintain that without it a real nutrition were not possible; they are therefore called "nutritive salts."

Such mineral substances or nutritive salts are found in

1 kilogramme oats .... 30.2 grammes
1 kilogramme peas .... 25.8 grammes
1 kilogramme meat .... 11.0 grammes

Again we find oats on the first line of vitalizing influence, of which I have spoken in the beginning of this article. Our forefathers realized the value of oats in all forms and shapes, which were then standard dishes, but with the introduction of potatoes, coffee, maize, tea they have become neglected and despised to the detriment of the health of the people.

I trust that oats will again come to honor not only in artificial preparations as crackers and cacao, but as daily food in the plain old-fashioned style; besides all these merits it is also the most economical food.

THE NATUROPATH.

DEAR SIR:

Is the following diet sustaining as a body and brain builder?

Breakfast: Oatmeal, milk, some fruit.

Dinner: One pint milk, rye bread, new eggs, 2, beaten in sugar, bananas, figs, dates, grape-nuts with cream.

Supper: The same as dinner.

I also eat stewed prunes, baked apples and other fruit. Very seldom meat. Drink a cup of cocoa every night, also a tablespoonful of olive oil.

Plenty of water between meals. Cold bath (natural bath, just) and exercise every morning and night.

Yours truly,
W. F. J.

W.F.J. —Yes, the diet as you suggest here is complete all around. I do not see why a man could not live on this diet. Unless a man works in the open air and has lots of physical exercise it would be too rich. The diet is very good for a beginner in natural eating. Gradually he will wean himself off from quite a number of these foods, such as oatmeal, eggs, sugar, etc., and leave meat out entirely. The use of cocoa is not recommended unless Dr. Lahmann's or Bilz's Nutritive Salt Cocoa is substituted. Ordinarily cocoa is detrimental to health in the long run like coffee and tea. These two cocoas are the only ones which are pure and made soluble with vegetable and fruit extract. After living on this diet, cutting out all stimulants, salt, sugar, etc., the drinking of water will not be necessary any more. The exercises and the natural bath should be continued.

FRESH SHELLED NUTS
ALL KINDS
at *Wholesale Prices*

	Per Pound
English Walnuts	$0.38
Pecans (Halves)	.52
Almonds (Large)	.56
Brazil Nuts	.41
Cachew Nuts	.24
Butter Nuts	1.50
Cocoanuts (Grated, Sweet'd)	.15
Peanuts (Spanish, Raw) . .	.07½
Chestnuts (Dried)	.10
Black Walnuts	.45
Filberts (Whole)	.35
Almonds (Small)	.40
Hickory Nuts	.55
Pignolia Nuts	.35
Paradise Nuts	1.00
Pistaschio Nuts	.55
Peanuts (Virginia, Raw) . .	.07½
Chinese Leechie Nuts . . .	.35

Special prices on unbroken cases upon application. As the prices are low, please order at least a 5-pound assortment. They are fresh shelled and will keep. Prices quoted are F. O. B. Chicago. Money must accompany order.

V. F. SIMON, Foodologist
1505 E. 63rd ST., CHICAGO, ILL.

Nuts for a vegetarian were indispensable as a rich source of protein.

THE PRACTICAL NATUROPATHIC VEGETARIAN KITCHEN: COOKED AND UNCOOKED FOODS

by Mrs. Louise* Lust
The Naturopath and Herald of Health, XIV(2), 98-99. (1909)

The preparation of food is a science as well as an art. As a practising Naturopath and instructor of dietetics for about eighteen years, I have found the need of a simple instruction in wholesome vegetarian cooking with reference to dietetics in health and in disease. This need has been expressed by many of my patients and others who are interested in hygiene. Strange to say that there are upwards of seventeen hundred works extant on the subject of diet and cook books. And yet dyspepsia prevails. Good housekeeping is the science of combining perfect cleanliness with economy and comfort; of giving to the inmates of the house healthy bodies through the preparation of wholesome and palatable food, careful and intelligent attention to sanitation and the laws of hygiene. It also includes the fine art of homemaking in the highest and truest sense.

Not every woman may be a good cook. But the poorest may be improved, if she has a genuine love for her work. While the woman who has the aptitude as well as the fondness for cooking may make herself almost any kind of a success as a cook. Management, or in other words, domestic economy, is the real secret of inexpensive living. Food and nourishing food need not cost much if common sense is expended, as well as cash.

In the matter of diet, it is balance we want. We are learning slowly that the proper combination between acid and alkaline food shall answer this purpose; their reaction on each other, when realized and rightly understood, may give incalculable help in all our considerations with regard to food. Sufficient alkaline material is necessary to keep the acid in the blood in complete solution, and some acid is needed to neutralize any excess of alkalinity. To-day so many of us are poisoned with acid waste in the body or blood that we are apt to lose sight of the second proposition, and to conclude immediately that acid is altogether bad. But it is just as essential that the body shall not be poisoned with alkaline waste, as that it shall not be poisoned with acid waste. The uric acid is really present almost throughout the whole vegetable kingdom. And in choosing substances for our food, the only course that is open to us is to take those substances which contain least of it, and avoid those which contain most of it; or to

---

*Louisa Lust adopted different spellings to her name. Sometimes she used Louise Lust.

get the proper combination of food. Indeed, nature seems to produce no food quite free from acid. If this so-called poison then is of so much universal occurrence, "can it be altogether bad?" If we possessed the powers of out great-grandparents, before riches and luxury and overfeeding spread wide, their consequences which we are reaping to-day in weakened eliminative organs, this extra care on our part would largely cease to be needed. Let us, however, regain the balance of a well combined diet, leaving flesh foods out of the question; for it may be asserted that few who have thoroughly succeeded with a non-flesh diet will ever again resume the use of flesh as food; leaving these foods out of the question, no one can say to another: "You must do this and you must not eat that." General principles may be laid down, and some knowledge of cause and effect given, but it is better to leave details to the individual's own experience.

If the liver gets more work than it can do, it first gets clogged, then the blood gets over-balanced with waste, and the body is poisoned. There is a feeling of general heaviness, and the action of the heart, if the over-dose of alkaline material is large, may for a time be seriously depressed. Let us regain the balance by a little extra acid in the shape of fruit, and imitating nature, see that the acid is not too strong, and matters will soon right themselves again. One conclusion seems plain—that the grains, the pulses, peas, beans, lentils, fresh vegetables, salads and fruits, are the best foods for non-meat eaters. "Moderation in all things is the tempo which governs life in all the variations of that delightful theme, when rightly and intelligently played." A wise physician said: "We live on one-fourth of what we eat, and eat the other three-fourths at our peril." In all cases of sickness the lighter the diet is, the better chance will the patient generally have of recovery. The more inflammation and fever exists, the more fruit and cooling drinks should be given, and less nitrogenous and starch matter. Ample nourishment can be provided by nut products, dried and fresh fruits, and vegetable soups. One of the greatest evils to be avoided by those who are nursing the sick, is that of overfeeding. When nature is doing her best to meet a crisis, or to rid the body of poisonous germs, or impurities, it is a mistake to cause waste of vital energy by necessitating the expulsion of superfluous alimentary matter. Drugs and stimulants are not required. Beef essences are superfluous. The great healing agent is the life force within. The wise physician will see that this power has a fair chance. He will help the patient to overcome physical malady by encouraging the exercise of hygienic common sense, and hopeful mental influence. He will advocate pure air, pure food, and pure water, and the removal of the cause of the malady in question. Much of the suffering endured by sick persons is simply the result of erroneous diet. Care should be exercised lest the sick partake too freely of starchy foods, especially if such are badly or insufficiently cooked. Bread should be well baked, zwieback or bread toasted will be more easily assimilated. The entire wheatmeal in a cooked form, so that the starch is already transformed into "dextrine" will be found nutritious, easily digested, and slightly laxative. In my book will be found numerous well-combined, cooked dishes. Cooking, baking and stewing do not, if properly cooked, destroy the life principle of the vegetation, but they change its soil properties—the salts and the acids.

The ideal diet is the nut and fruit diet; but I know through experience the difficulty we meet with most people in adapting themselves suddenly to such a simple style of living, as nature would dictate. A step at a time, slowly but surely, is the wisest in the end. The first step must be abstinence from meat and the adoption of a vegetarian diet. In time the perverted taste will be restored to its natural condition, until it is fruitarian in its nature. Raw food or a fruitarian diet will also solve the servant question considerably. Another important reason for a raw diet is the ignorance of most people concerning food value, which knowledge is necessary to keep the human body in health. It seems difficult to make persons who are trying to live as vegetarians to choose a properly combined diet, they having made blunders come to the conclusion that vegetarianism does not suit everybody, and return to the flesh pots; and I must emphasize again: "This only happens to those who have not a properly balanced diet." And for this reason I will give you numerous recipes for vegetarian diet and a little practice on the individual's part will develop wonders.

—Mrs. Lust, in the *Naturopathic Cook Book*.

As a practising Naturopath and instructor of dietetics for about eighteen years, I have found the need of a simple instruction in wholesome vegetarian cooking with reference to dietetics in health and in disease.

Sufficient alkaline material is necessary to keep the acid in the blood in complete solution, and some acid is needed to neutralize any excess of alkalinity. To-day so many of us are poisoned with acid waste in the body or blood that we are apt to lose sight of the second proposition, and to conclude immediately that acid is altogether bad. But it is just as essential that the body shall not be poisoned with alkaline waste, as that it shall not be poisoned with acid waste.

UNBLEACHED FLOUR

by Charles Cristadodo

The Naturopath and the Herald of Health, XIV(5), 308. (1909)

Less than ten years ago the United States Department of Agriculture sent Prof. M. A. Carleton to Russia to investigate the durum wheats grown there. He returned with selected seed and the trip cost $10,000. The Dakotas and some other States began growing durum wheat. Last year the crop amounted to 60,000,000 bushels, worth $40,000,000 to $50,000,000. Much of the wheat is exported to France for French bread, so crusty and nutritious. Some goes to Italy for macaroni, and in this country some goes to the macaroni manufacturers, and the balance the millers use to blend with other flours.

Four years ago the United States Department of Agriculture clearly demonstrated in an exhaustive, careful test the superiority of durum flour as a bread flour over the heretofore acknowledged superlative flour from Minnesota spring wheat.

Four hundred loaves were baked, 200 from each kind of flour, by the most careful and skilled baker in Washington, D.C. Two loaves were sent out to parties to the number of 200, with requests to report upon each of the two loaves. Of the scientists, bakers, millers, housekeepers and to whom the loaves were sent 74 per cent. of those who answered gave the palm to the durum loaf.

The United States Department of Agriculture summed up the replies about as follows: The durum loaf was better colored; the durum loaf more moist, and the general opinion of the durum flour loaf as against the other was in favor of the durum flour loaf.

And but a few weeks ago the publisher of a New York baking paper arranged with Mr. Schinkel, one of the most experienced bakers in the United States, to make a similar test to that made by the United States Department of Agriculture.

Mr. Schinkel used equal quantities of durum and Minnesota spring wheat flour. Every condition of equality as to treatment and manipulation was looked after carefully.

Here is about what Mr. Schinkel reported in a preliminary report:

That durum flour yielded 16 pounds more dough to the barrel than did the Minnesota spring wheat flour; durum had a higher water absorption; the grain of durum was even, close and fine; the durum loaf had a rich, creamy color which was very pleasing and looked as if milk and malt extract were used, although neither were used. The durum loaf, on the whole, presented a much better appearance, the rich brown crust giving an impression of richness and solidity. Sugar need not be added to durum flour. It is particularly rich in sugar, which explains the brown and good

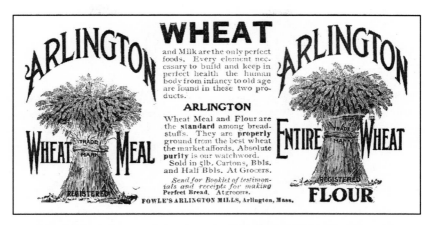

Many ads were placed in *The Naturopath and Herald of Health* advertising different wheat products.

appearance of the loaf. The durum loaf had a very agreeable taste and was fully as satisfactory.

Agreeable to eat and still moist, even after the fourth day. It yielded 333 pounds of dough to the barrel, 16 pounds more than Minnesota spring wheat flour.

As to the Minnesota spring wheat flour loaf, it provided a larger looking loaf; was white, as usual. It could no longer be eaten when the durum loaf was still moist and palatable. It had a better expansion in the oven than the durum loaf.

So he who runs may read. The report of Mr. Schinkel even goes further than the favoring reports made to the United States Department of Agriculture, extolling the durum loaf. Facts are stubborn things, meet them as we may, and the facts indicating clearly the superiority of durum flour for bread over the heretofore considered best flour for bread in the country cannot be gainsaid when emanating from the United States Department of Agriculture, and also from one of the best known and most experienced bakers, perhaps, in the United States, Mr. Adolph Schinkel, of New York.

> *Four years ago the United States Department of Agriculture clearly demonstrated in an exhaustive, careful test the superiority of durum flour as a bread flour over the heretofore acknowledged superlative flour from Minnesota spring wheat.*

SUBSTITUTES FOR MEAT AND THEIR VALUES

by Edwin C. Wilson

The Naturopath and Herald of Health, XIV(9), 569-572. (1909)

The recently converted Food-Reformer often asks the question, "What shall I eat in the place of meat?" and in answer thereto, he has almost invariable been told to "eat nuts, eggs, cheese, macaroni, legumes, etc." So far so good, but what quantity of each of these foods very often cannot be easily determined; and indeed it varies so with different people, that it is almost impossible to lay down any hard and fast rule. What I wish to do therefore, is to give the actual values of various meat-substitutes, so that each person, by comparing their nutritive qualities with those of beef and mutton can ascertain individually the correct quantities required.

Taking a standpoint from lean beef and moderately fat mutton, I will endeavor to give an idea how to find from the various tables used, the requisite amounts of the various articles of food named.

The composition of Meat is as follows:

	Protein	Fat	Starch
Lean Beef	19.3	3.6	0.0
Moderately Fat Mutton	14.5	19.5	0.0

Now supposing you are in the habit of eating 8 oz. of Meat daily and you wish to substitute cheese and macaroni for same.

	Protein	Fat	Starch
A Combination of Beef plus Mutton	16.9	11.5	0.0
Macaroni and Cheddar Cheese	19.2	16.5	37.5

It will then be seen at a glance that the latter being richer in all three elements, less will be required, say, 3 oz. of each; and moreover other starchy foods, such as white bread, etc., can be slightly diminished in quantity, as there is a good proportion of starch matter in macaroni and none in meat.

It is easy to understand that more errors are likely to be made by over-eating in connection with the Reformed Dietary, than otherwise, but such errors can easily be obviated if a little study and thought is given to the subject combined with a little common sense.

NUTS AND THEIR PRODUCTS

Here we have what is undoubtedly Man's natural Meat. Rich in Protein, Fat, Mineral Salt, and a small amount of Starch they are indeed an ideal type of food, and on that at the present time is not properly appreciated.

I give below the analyses of the three which are richest in the three necessary elements.

	Protein	Fat	Starch
Almonds	23.5	53.0	7.8
Pine Kernels	9.3	71.5	14.0
Chestnuts	6.2	5.4	42.1

Protein being found in greatest proportion in Almonds, Fat in Pine Kernels, and Starch in Chestnuts.

All nuts are fit to eat in their natural state except Chestnuts, which should be boiled, roasted or baked in order to cook the starch contained therein. Some people object to nuts on account of their being unable to masticate them properly through having defective teeth. This can, however, be over-come by flaking the nuts in a nut-mill, or they can be ground to a paste in a Nut-Butter-mill and eaten as butter.

Regarding Nut Products, we will first consider Nut Meats. These "meats," which have now been in the market a considerable number of years, are greatly appreciated by those that use them, and if properly cooked they closely resemble roast or boiled meat.

They have the appearance of meat, they smell like meat, and they taste somewhat like meat. They are put up in ½-lb., 1-lb. and 1½-lb. tins, are free from any danger of "ptomaine poisoning," and are guaranteed free from germs and uric acid.

The most well-known brands are Protose and Nuttose (International Health Association): Nutton, several varieties (Winter's Birmingham); Meatose, F.R. Nut Meat and Vegola (London Nut Food Co.); Brazose (Pitman's, Birmingham); Fibrose (Mapleton's, Wardle, Lancs).

All these preparations will be found digestible, pleasing to the palate, and, moreover, very economical.

I give the composition of the four most important varieties as follows:

	Protein	Fat	Starch
Protose	25.50	14.00	2.80
Nuttose	17.10	27.80	14.20
Nutton	20.00	11.00	12.20
Fibrose	14.55	5.40	71.40

For the invalid, the dyspeptic, and the thin, there are preparations that are unfortunately not yet widely known. Amongst other are Bromose, Prunus, Nutrogen and Malter Nuts. The two former are put up in handy caramel form and the latter in fine powder. They can be eaten dry or will readily dissolve in hot or cold water, milk, barley water etc., and as they are self-digesting and delicious in flavor they are indeed a boon to both strong and weak. They will, if necessary, entirely take the place of meat and cheese, and are guaranteed to make good blood, fat, and muscles, and are an excellent substitute for Cod Liver Oil.

I give below their compositions, and would mention the fact that the starch is predigested and the fat perfectly emulsified:

	Protein	Fat	Starch
Malted Nuts	23.7	27.6	43.9
Prunus	26.4	32.5	24.5
Bromose	19.6	24.0	39.4
Nutrogen	23.6	27.2	39.6

I must also add a word about Nut Cream. It is not usually known that Milk and Cream can be made from Nuts, yet so nice are these products that once tried they generally become appreciated. Messrs. Mapleton are now producing three varieties, viz. : Almond, Coconut and Hazel, also a Nut Milk. Two or three tablespoonfuls of cream beaten up in a pint of water and stirred over a slow fire until it thickens will make a custard for stewed fruit, plum pudding or trifle that is far richer than egg and milk and more tasty. The comparative value of Almond Cream as against Devonshire Cream will be seen from the following:

	Protein	Fat	Starch
Almond Cream	20.8	54.8	17.2
Devonshire Cream	4.0	65.0	0.0

LEGUMES

Under this heading we have Lentils, Peas, Haricot, and Butter Beans, and Pea Nuts. The last of these, sometimes called the monkey nut, is perhaps the most nutritious food produced by Nature. It is practically composed of Protein and fat, the amount of starch being under 2 percent. That it is in itself a perfect food has recently been demonstrated by an American doctor, who lived entirely on them for 60 days, and felt all the better for it. Moreover, at 4 [dollars] per lb., shelled, they may be called cheap. They require cooking, and the best method is to grind them to a paste, flavor with "Marmite," pepper and salt, etc., and bake in an oven at a low heat, for from two to three hours, and the result will be a very tasty dish.

Chemistry shows them to be made up as follows:

	Protein	Fat	Starch
[Pea Nut]	28.3	46.2	1.8

Lentils, as will be seen by their analysis are very nutritious and a great many people make the error of eating too great a quantity at one time, thus setting up fermentation and all its attendant troubles.

They are a fine food for brain workers, and, with the addition of fat, supply all the elements of nutrition.

	Protein	Fat	Starch
Lentils	25.9	1.9	53.0

Dried Peas and Beans are closely allied to Lentils, containing as they do the same proportion of Protein and starch and a little more fat. The great value of these foods, their cheapness and the numberless different ways of preparing them for table, commend them to everyone as articles of diet of the first order. (See recipes in *Comprehensive Guide Book*.)

When in season, Peas and Haricot Beans should always be eaten in the normal state, viz., freshly gathered. They are then soft, succulent and easily digested and most enjoyable.

Cheese

I am not going to say much regarding Cheese, as its value is so well known and it is such a popular favorite that to do so would be waste of time. That it is a perfect substitute of meat is ungainsayable [sic], bread and cheese being capable of sustaining both the laborer and brain worker alike.

I give below the analyses of two well-known brands, others being very similar in composition.

	Protein	Fat	Starch
Cheddar Cheese	28.4	31.1	0.0
Roquefort Cheese	26.52	30.1	0.0
Cottage-cheese	20.9	1.0	4.3

I should like to point out that many people in making cheese the staple article of diet, find it indigestible. If, however, instead of eating it raw, it is taken cooked with rice, tapioca, macaroni or barley, they will find that difficulty at once overcome—or it can be flaked in a nut mill.

Cottage-cheese, the analysis of which is given above, can be made at home by anyone who cares to take the trouble. To one gallon of boiled milk, add the juice of three lemons or three tablespoonfuls of French white wine vinegar. Strain it, when curdled, through a fine muslin cloth and let it stand aside for two days. It is then ready for use and has a very delicate flavor.

Eggs

Eggs, if perfectly fresh, are without doubt a most useful and valuable animal product, being—like cheese—almost entirely free from uric acid. In composition they greatly resemble nuts, but are free from starch. The white is composed of albumen (protein) and water, and the yolk, albumen, fat, and water. As a whole they are constituted as follows:

	Protein	Fat
Hen's Eggs	14.0	10.5

CEREALS

When placing cereal foods under the heading of meat substitutes it must not be supposed that white bread, tapioca, semolina, barley, sago, etc., are meant. These and similar foods are practically all starch and should only be used as mediums whereby quantities of fat and protein can be taken. Brown Bread, Wheatmeal Biscuits, Rice, Oatmeal, Macaroni and Granose Flakes and Biscuits are, however, substances of a very different character. They represent foods rich in bone and muscle forming elements, of great sustaining power and are well supplied with valuable organic salts.

I give them according to their respective values:

	Protein	Fat	Starch
Oatmeal	15.6	6.1	63.6
Granose Flakes and Biscuits	15.4	2.3	75.0
Macaroni	11.7	2.0	75.0
Brown Bread and Wheatmeal Biscuits	8.7	1.2	64.0
Rice	7.8	0.4	79.0

It should be noted that the Rice mentioned is the once milled and unglazed variety as used in China and Japan by the working classes. The protein found in Rice is nearly all contained in the cuticle or outer layer of the cereal, and this is eliminated by the second and third milling, which is done to make it look white, but which robs it of the best part of its good qualities. The difference between once-milled and thrice-milled Rice is much the same as that between Brown and White Bread.

BEEF TEA SUBSTITUTES

Regarding substitutes for Bovril, Beef Tea, etc., Malted Nuts, Bromose and Prunus, already referred to, when dissolved in water are perfect substitutes for beef tea for the sick room; Almond Cream is also a food that will be retained by the feeblest stomach.

A broth made by stewing Brown Haricot Beans in water for about three hours and serving with butter, pepper and salt, etc., is far more nutritious than Beef Tea, Mutton, or Chicken Broth, and will be found very strengthening on account of the iron it contains (see *Comprehensive Guide Book* for recipe).

In addition, I would mention Marmite, Odin, Carnox, Nuxo, Mapleton's Nut Extract and other similar preparations, which will be found quite as nice in flavor and far more economical than any of the so-called Meat Extracts, and more nourishing.

I should like to say one thing before closing. What information I have given here, properly used, should be helpful to those commencing to live on a non-flesh diet. But, I hope that none will adopt the custom of having every meal weighed and worked out, because such action would be likely to make one a nuisance to those around and a faddist into the bargain.

All nuts are fit to eat in their natural state except Chestnuts, which should be boiled, roasted or baked in order to cook the starch contained therein. Some people object to nuts on account of their being unable to masticate them properly through having defective teeth. This can, however, be overcome by flaking the nuts in a nut-mill, or they can be ground to a paste in a Nut-Butter-mill and eaten as butter.

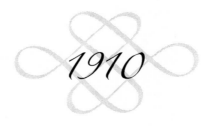

1910

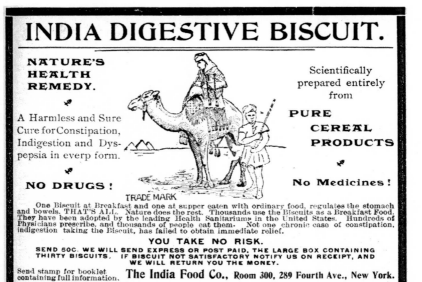

INDIA DIGESTIVE BISCUIT.

NATURE'S HEALTH REMEDY.

A Harmless and Sure Cure for Constipation, Indigestion and Dyspepsia in everp form.

NO DRUGS !

Scientifically prepared entirely from

PURE CEREAL PRODUCTS

No Medicines !

TRADE MARK

One Biscuit at Breakfast and one at supper eaten with ordinary food, regulates the stomach and bowels. THAT'S ALL. Nature does the rest. Thousands use the Biscuits as a Breakfast Food. They have been adopted by the leading Health Sanitariums in the United States. Hundreds of Physicians prescribe, and thousands of people eat them. Not one chronic case of constipation, indigestion taking the Biscuit, has failed to obtain immediate relief.

YOU TAKE NO RISK.

SEND 50C. WE WILL SEND EXPRESS OR POST PAID, THE LARGE BOX CONTAINING THIRTY BISCUITS. IF BISCUIT NOT SATISFACTORY NOTIFY US ON RECEIPT, AND WE WILL RETURN YOU THE MONEY.

Send stamp for booklet containing full information. **The India Food Co.,** Room 300, 289 Fourth Ave., New York.

Products made from cereals provided fiber to the diet.

THE MAGNETIC PROPERTIES OF FOOD

by Henry Lindlahr, M.D.

Copyright by The Nature Cure Publishing Co., Chicago.

The Naturopath and Herald of Health, XV(2), 103-105. (1910)

In compliance with our promise in the first number of this volume we will give a table of standard foods, together with the qualitative and quantitative analyses of all the elements which they contain in appreciable quantities. Each one of these analyses represents the average result of many separate experiments and has been tested and verified by different investigators.

These diagrams are compiled from the analytical tables on natural dietetics of the five greatest German authorities on food chemistry, viz., Doctors Lahmann, Koenig, Schuessler, Hensel and Bunge. These compilations will always form an indispensable basis for the rational and scientific study of food chemistry.

In fact, it is impossible to arrive at an intelligent understanding of truly scientific dietetics without a knowledge of the facts and principles disclosed in these tables.

Among other things a study of these tables will disclose the facts that foods classified in *The Great Psychological Crime*, on pages 280-1-3, as positive are rich in the four, most important positive mineral elements found in the human body, namely: Iron, Sodium, Calcium and Magnesium, while those groups of food classified by the author as negative are found to be sub-normal in their percentages of these positive mineral elements. The coincidence is a most remarkable one.

In order to fully understand the subject of food magnetism we must first consider what we mean by positive and negative magnetic qualities.

Positiveness is synonymous with vigorous health and strength; negativeness with a lack of these qualities. We define health in our Catechism of Nature Cure as follows: "WHAT IS HEALTH? Health is normal and harmonious vibration of all the elements and forces comprising the human entity on the physical, mental and moral planes of being, in conformity with the constructive principle of individual life."

"Free, harmonious and vigorous vibration of all the parts, particles and forces composing the human organism; depends, first on inherent vitality; second, on the rapid combustion of food and waste; third, on the prompt elimination of all effete matter and poisons from the system; fourth, on the textile strength and normal density of all tissues."

We will now consider in how far "positiveness" or "normal function" is dependent on the positive mineral salts in the food and drink of man.

IRON

Iron in the form of Haemoglobin is all important as a carrier of oxygen from the lungs into the various parts of the body. Combustion is impossible without oxygen, and digestion is simply a slow process of combustion. Without combustion there can be no heat production nor any cremation and elimination of waste matter. Furthermore, it has been discovered by German scientists that iron moving rapidly in a salty solution (sodium-chloride in the blood) produces electric and magnetic currents. Therefore iron is one of the most important positive "working" elements in the body.

SODIUM

Carbon, Oxygen, Hydrogen and Nitrogen are the four unstable negative gaseous elements in the human body. Three of these—carbon, oxygen and hydrogen—make up the various fuel materials, such as fats, oils, starches and sugars. They are to the body what coal is to the engine; they liberate heat and energy. Similar to coal, they give off, in the process of combustion, a great deal of coal gas or carbon-dioxide (CO_2), and if this poisonous gas is allowed to accumulate it will extinguish the fire in the furnace or the life in the body.

On sodium, a positive mineral element, depends the elimination from the body of the carbon-dioxide. It accomplishes this in the following manner: Sodium circulates in the body as di-sodium phosphate; that is, in molecules which contain one atom of phosphorus to two atoms of sodium. This combination, however, is a loose one. One forms a stable union, but the second atom of sodium is only a loose addition. As soon as this unstable sodium finds a more powerful attraction it leaves the phosphorus and joins the stronger affinity. Such an affinity for sodium is carbon-dioxide (CO_2).

These two, when they meet in the blood, form sodium-carbonate, but this union also is not a true and lasting one, for when the pair reach the lungs the airy CO_2 deserts its mate and passes through expiration, into the open air. The sodium now reunites with its old friend phosphorus, but on its travels back into the body, repeats the same trick when it meets again with CO_2.

If sodium is lacking in the blood, CO_2 accumulates and gradually asphyxiates the process of combustion on which depend digestion, reduction of waste and heat production. This becomes visible outwardly by loss of appetite, malnutrition, loss of weight, coldness of hands and feet, blue color of lips, nails and skin; in fact, by the prominent symptoms of consumption.

In other cases partial oxidation of food materials and tissue waste, under the influence of carbon-dioxide poisoning, causes fatty degeneration. The food materials, instead of being turned into heat and energy, are changed into fatty deposits.

Just as insufficient draft in the furnace turns coal into partially consumed clinkers, so in the body partial combustion turns the starchy foods into fat, instead of reducing them into heat and energy. Therefore it happens that the excessive consumption of starchy food, lack of exercise and fresh air causes fatty degeneration. People thus afflicted often complain: "I eat so little, yet everything seems to turn into fat." This is literally true for the reason just stated. The cure in such cases consists in prompt elimination of the carbon-dioxide and better oxidation, by increased muscular activity, by fresh air, deep breathing and by the increased use of sodium in the organic form, in fruits and vegetables.

Thus we are presented with the paradoxical fact that carbonic acid poisoning may cause, according to individual constitutional peculiarities, in one person, destruction of tissues by tuberculosis and in another person an excess of fatty deposits. In fact, many cases of tuberculosis are preceded by fatty degeneration. This connection between the two is now plain.

CALCIUM (LIME)

Lime in connection with silicon, phosphorus and magnesium makes up over 50 per cent. of the bony structures of the body; it imparts textile strength to all the tissues. If lime, silicon and magnesium are lacking in the daily dietary, rachitis and scorbutic diseases, scrofula, tendency to bleeding (Haemophelia), Osteomalecia and premature decay of teeth and diseases of the hair will be the inevitable results. Like other positive alkaline mineral elements, it also serves as a neutralizer and eliminator of poisonous acids.

MAGNESIUM

Magnesium, another of the alkaline elements, is similar to sodium and lime as an eliminator of destructive acids. It is also concerned in the production of electro-magnetic currents in the circulating blood.

THE RELATION OF POSITIVE ALKALINE SALTS TO NEGATIVE PROTEID FOOD MATERIALS

All proteid foods are composed of the unstable negative gaseous elements C. O. H. N., and of the negative earthy elements phosphorus and sulphur. Being very rich in acid producing nitrogen, phosphorus and sulphur, these foods form in the process of digestion a great deal of uric, phosphoric, sulphuric and hippuric acids. These acids, if not promptly neutralized by the positive alkaline mineral bases (especially sodium), accumulate in the system and actually destroy the living tissues. To make this clearer, if sodium, for instance, is lacking in the blood the destructive acids attract and combine with the alkaline mineral elements which form the solid basis of bone and muscles and thereby cause the weakening and breaking down of these tissues.

This fact is strikingly illustrated in the English *Banting Cure*, for the reduction of fat and flesh. This cure consists mainly in an excessive lean meat diet with the exclusion of fats, starchy foods and sugar. Such a purely proteid diet produces large amounts of uric and sulphuric acids and is utterly deficient in the acid binding alkaline bases (sodium and magnesium), the acids therefore break down and destroy not only the fat, but also the muscular tissues. Reduction of fat and flesh by such means, however, is a destructive disease process. This explains why people undergoing such cures become weak and nervous and develop various forms of uric acid diseases, such as rheumatism, heart disease, calculi (stones) in kidneys, bladder, etc.

We can now understand why people, living almost exclusively on "strengthening" meats and eggs grow livid and thin, while the German peasant girl, reared on coarse bread, roots and vegetables, is plump and strong, and why she loses her milk-and-blood complexion after a few years of American "high living."

The positive mineral elements are prominent not only in the blood, but also in the digestive juices of stomach and pancreas, in the bile and all other important "working" secretions in the body, concerned in the processes of digestion, assimilation and elimination.

POTASSIUM

So far we have not said anything about the positive mineral element potassium. It serves principally as a solid basis for the muscular parts of the body, as lime does for the bony structures. It belongs more to the passive or tissue building material than to the active working elements, and hence it does not contribute as much to the positiveness of foods and medicines as the other four positive mineral elements.

This brief survey of the positive mineral elements and their functions in the body now explain why foods rich in these "organic salts" exert a positive influence on the human organism and its functions.

It becomes evident now that an excess in the daily dietary of proteid and starchy foods and a simultaneous shortage of mineral salts will inevitably clog the system with waste matter and destructive poisonous acids and alkaloids.

A glance at our analytical tables will reveal the remarkable correspondence between these conclusions of German *Natural Dietetics* and the magnetic classification of foods as given in the *Great Psychological Crime*.

The Vegetarian Kitchen: Suggestions For Cooking Vegetables

by Mrs. Anna Lindlahr

The Naturopath and Herald of Health, XV(2), 107-108. (1910)

DO NOT OVERCOOK. Cook the vegetables no more than is necessary to comply with the recipes. Avoid frying or boiling foods violently. As a rule it is better to cook vegetables slowly and conserve the life force or life energy of the living plant, which is lost in proportion to the heat applied in cooking.

FRIED FOODS, the same as soups, are tolerated rather than advised, not only because of the waste of life-energy and plant magnetism due to the rapid cooking and intense heat to which the foods are applied, but also because of the grease which the heat causes to permeate the food, coating over every food particle with a film of fat, rendering it practically impermeable to the digestive juices of the mouth and stomach; for fats are not digested until they reach the intestines. Therefore the fried foods containing starches, proteids and sugars cannot be assimilated until the fats are digested by the fluids of the intestines, thereby partly doing away with salivary and gastric digestion and entailing upon the intestines the work that should take place in the mouth and stomach. In time this additional work thrust upon the intestines will cause defective digestion.

ALWAYS USE BUTTER OR SOME PURE VEGETABLE FATS, such as olive oil, cooking oil or ko-nut lard* in cooking. Never use lard, suet, bacon grease or other dead animal products.

BE AS MODERATE IN THE USE OF SPICES AND SALT as is consistent with the recipes and good cooking. PEPPER especially should be avoided. The pepper called for in these recipes is not at all essential, but is mentioned for the convenience of those who desire it. Butter and salt are, of course, more permissible, but even these, especially the salt, should be used moderately.

Proper food combination in accord with our food tables renders superfluous the coarse inorganic mineral salt, because the raw fruits and vegetables as shown by our analysis contain all mineral salts needed by the human organism in the greatest abundance—refined and made "organic" in the wonderfully complicated molecule of the living cells of plants and animals, for only in this refined organic form are minerals fit to be absorbed by animals and human bodies.

Learn to appreciate the natural flavors of the natural foods. Spicing and salting will then become largely or wholly superfluous. Under the influences of unnatural living and diet, our sense of taste has become so depraved and paralyzed that it is sensitive only to the stronger tasting

---

*Anna Lindlahr used coconut oil and called it ko-nut lard. *Ed.*

substances, such as salt, spices, sugar, butter, meat juices, liquors, etc., and it has become necessary to saturate our food with these substances before we can "taste" and enjoy it. Such tastes cannot appreciate the delicate flavors of the natural foods which are entirely lost in the presence of the seasoning.

But as we "Return to Nature" in eating and other habits of life our senses and tastes become more acute and normal and the delicious flavors of the fruit and vegetable become a reality and a pleasure beyond the dreams of the most exacting and fastidious epicure. Spicing, seasoning and artificial preparing then become not only a sacrifice of desirable flavors, but a substitution of objectionable ones. Until this condition obtains, no one can realize what it means to have natural senses and to really "enjoy eating."

AVOID ALL METHODS OF PREPARING VEGETABLES WHEREBY THE ORGANIC SALTS ARE LOST. Do not reject the water in which they are cooked. Cook vegetables in their own juices; that is, steam or cook them in just enough water to make a sauce to serve with the vegetable. Where it is impracticable to serve the cooking water with the vegetable, as in the case with potatoes, corn on the ear, etc., the water can be saved and be used in making soups and soup stocks, and thus the organic salts are conserved.

As vegetables and sometimes fruits are ordinarily prepared—cooked in a lot of water, drained and the water rejected—the most important parts of the vegetables, viz., the mineral elements (organic salts) are dissolved from the vegetable by the water and thrown into the sewer. The tasteless wood-fibre and straw (cellulose) which remains must need [to] be spiced, salted, seasoned and saturated with meat juices and butter to be made "palatable." The finest flavors are those of the vegetable itself when properly preserved by common sense cooking or preferably not cooked at all. When the ideal dietetic conditions obtain, man will eat only those foods that appeal to the senses of sight, smell and taste in their natural unaltered conditions.

As a rule it is better to cook vegetables slowly and conserve the life force or life energy of the living plant, which is lost in proportion to the heat applied in cooking.

Proper food combination in accord with our food tables renders superfluous the coarse inorganic mineral salt, because the raw fruits and vegetables as shown by our analysis contain all mineral salts needed by the human organism in the greatest abundance.

Raw Food Diet

by Mrs. Anna Lindlahr

The Naturopath and Herald of Health, XV(4), 239-240. (1910)

A man may eat in due proportion and in highly refined preparations all the fifteen elements found in his body; he may also take a sufficient amount of air and water, yet he will surely die. German experiments have demonstrated that even proximate food elements, when chemically pure, will not sustain animal or human life. Animals fed on chemically pure white starch, albumen, sugar, gluten, etc., will die sooner than if they receive no food at all. This clearly indicates that not the various elements in and by themselves sustain animal and human life, but that life and energy depend on something else which adheres to the complicated organic molecules which are formed in the living cells of plants and animals.

What is this mysterious something which builds up and sustains animal and human bodies? It is **sun energy**.

Cold makes ice. During the formation of the ice molecule, cold becomes fixed or latent in it. When the ice molecule disintegrates under the influence of heat, cold is liberated. The heat which gives warmth and comfort to our home this wintry night is sun warmth stored up in the plant and tree molecules of primeval forests. In similar manner have sun warmth and energy elaborated the organic vegetable molecule from the elements of earth, water and air, but at the same time these sun forces have become absorbed in that which they were building. Thus the molecules of plant and fruit have become charged with the warmth and the electromagnetic currents of the great life-giver. These forces are liberated again when the molecules disintegrate under the action of digestive ferments, thus furnishing heat and energy for the building up and sustenance of animal and human bodies.

When in the process of digestion and assimilation these electromagnetic forces have been liberated and absorbed by the body, nothing remains of the erstwhile foods but poisonous excrements, which, if not promptly eliminated, become destructive to the organism; the organic has become inorganic; when the life principle is taken away from food nothing remains but poison.

Vegetable and animal foods are, therefore, foods only by virtue of the solar energy locked up in their molecules. As soon as these vegetable molecules disintegrate by any process whatsoever, their vital energy is dissipated and lost. This explains why boiling, baking and frying wastes food energy; why fermentation changes wholesome foods into poisonous alcohol. The Great Wisdom which built this wonderful entity called "Man" knows also how to feed him. The meddling art of cook, chemist and distiller, therefore, seldom improves upon Nature's foods, and the chemist's dream that all foods will some day be made in his laboratory and handed out in a tablet form will always remain a dream.

DINNER MENU
Served to the Sanitarium Family, Sunday, January 9, 1910.

SOUP
Clear Vegetable Bouillon

RELISHES
Green Onions
Water Cress

SALAD
Fruit Salad

VEGETABLES
Barley Sausage, with Brown Gravy
Wax Beans
Mashed Turnips
Baked Potatoes

DESSERT
Sago Pudding, with Grape Sauce
Fruit
Japanese Oranges
Apples
Figs
Assorted Nuts

RECIPES [FOR ABOVE]

CLEAR VEGETABLE BOUILLON

Take turnips, carrots, celery, parsnips, onions, cabbage, parsley, leeks, tomatoes and any other vegetables you may have. Scrape, wash and cut in pieces; add cupful of lentils or beans. Add enough water and let boil from two to three hours. Strain, add butter and season.

From this can be made any of the clear soups, such as rice, noodle, tapioca, etc.

FRUIT SALAD

Peel two oranges, two bananas, one grape fruit, and cut in dice; half cup Malaga grapes stoned and cut in half, about one-half cup pecans. Mix well with Mayonnaise dressing. Serve in half orange shell on lettuce.

Mayonnaise Dressing

Prepare as follows: Take the yolk of one egg, one teaspoonful each of salt, sugar and mustard, and stir together (always in one direction), and the while adding a cupful of olive oil, drop by drop, and lastly in the same manner the juice of two lemons; keep in cool place.

Barley Sausage

Cook about two cups barley in slightly salted water. Let it be very stiff. When cool add two well beaten eggs, one grated Spanish onion, season with sage. Shape into small sausages and brown in butter.

Brown Gravy

Put a large piece of butter in a skillet and let brown with one sliced onion and tablespoon of sugar. Then add one-half cupful of flour; keep stirring about five minutes. Add sufficient soup stock to make of the right consistency, also one-half pint of sour cream: Season and strain.

Wax Beans

Cut wax beans into long strips, wash, put on to cook with enough cold water to cover. Season with chopped parsley, little salt and thicken with a little flour and melted butter stirred together.

Mashed Turnips

Peel, wash and slice yellow turnips. Let cook until tender, then mash through colander. Add butter and a little cream. Salt.

Sago Pudding

Put two quarts milk in double boiler. Stir in one-half cup of sago and piece of butter, two tablespoonfuls of sugar. Let boil until clear, then mix with the beaten whites of four eggs.

Grape Sauce

Pick and wash Delaware grapes, add a little water and let cook about one-half hour. Sweeten and let cool. Thicken with corn starch if desired.

Vegetable and animal foods are, therefore, foods only by virtue of the solar energy locked up in their molecules.

STANDARD FOODS

by H. Lindlahr, M.D.
Copyright by The Nature Cure Publishing Company, Chicago.

The Naturopath and Herald of Health, Vol. XV(5), 259 -263. (1910)

Potatoes are an exception to this rule. While they are very rich in starchy elements they are comparatively poor in the positive mineral salts. Therefore they are insipid to the taste without a large amount of table salt, but radishes, cucumbers, carrots and other positive roots are perfectly palatable without any addition of table salt.

We have already called attention to the interesting fact, demonstrated by our analyses of two different kinds of potatoes, that the richness of the soil in mineral elements determines the degree of positiveness of the foods grown in it. This law applies, of course, to all products of the soil.

GRAINS, NEGATIVE

All grains are exceedingly negative. While they contain large amounts of proteid and starchy materials they are very poor in the positive mineral salts, and what little they possess of these important elements is stored in the hulls and in the dark outer layers. In order to comply with the popular demand for white flour and rice these outer layers are removed in the milling processes. Bran and rice polish are therefore exceedingly rich in mineral salts and very valuable foods for our domestic animals. The latter wax strong and fat on the "refuse" of the mills, rich in organic salts, while the farmer grows thin and dyspeptic on his "fine white flour." Oriental nations use unpolished rice, which is much richer in flavor and better fitted to sustain life than our refined but impoverished mill products.

CONCLUSIONS

Let us see, now, whether, after this brief survey of our food tables, we can explain some of the mysteries and perplexities of dietetics. We can understand now why our American vegetarians, living largely upon devitalized leguminous and grain products, with a liberal allowance of peanuts and olive oil, often fare worse than people living on the mixed meat diet, and become "warning examples" to the latter. Still more harmful is, in many instances, the "fruit and nut" diet. It is only a naturally very positive "animal" constitution that can afford to live on such a negative diet. Many of these fruit and nut enthusiasts expressly exclude from their dietary all things growing in and under the ground, "because they are coarsening and tend to develop the animal nature." They forget, in their endeavor to make by the diet route, short cuts to masterhood and godhood, that in these physical material surroundings of ours most of us need in our daily business a considerable amount of the positive animal magnetic qualities.

Negative food combinations, excessive fasting, concentrating in the silence, yogic breathing exercises, subjective psychism and a lot of other occult hocus pocus lead many misguided enthusiasts into physical and mental breakdown and not a few into obsession and insanity.

It is a pity that so many fake occultists use the pure and simple teachings of common-sense German "Nature Cure" as a bait and a cloak for their ridiculous and sometimes pernicious mystical pretensions.

These charlatans know full well that people are so hungry for the simple truths of Nature Cure that they will swallow with them any amount of dangerous occult impositions.

A look at the mineral constituents of grain and rice also answers effectively the common argument of the anti-vegetarian, "Look at your vegetarian nations in the Orient, the Hindus and Chinese. Would you lower us to their physical and mental level by the adoption of a vegetarian diet?" The answer to this is now plain.

Grains and rice rank lowest in the scale of negative foods and it is therefore no wonder that people living almost exclusively on these staples should be sub-normal physically and mentally. No wonder they are no match for the bloody beefsteak-consuming Briton and German.

A rational vegetarian diet properly combined, consisting of dairy products, the positive vegetables, and the medium positive fruits with just enough of starchy and proteid foods to supply the needs of the body for tissue building and fuel material, will be found to be an ideal diet for human beings fully sufficient to keep them in health and strength under the most trying circumstances.

We admit that there are cases of physical and nervous breakdown in which magnetic conditions have become so negative that the raw meat diet is, at least temporarily, of great advantage to supply the lack of animal magnetism until the system of the patient is put in such condition that it can manufacture and supply once more its own magnetic forces. The animal magnetism attached to flesh foods, however, is only borrowed, and is contaminated by the poisonous waste matter of the dead animal carcass. Therefore we have seen people cured by the Salisbury raw meat diet out of nervous prostration, but at the same time cured into rheumatism, heart disease, calculi in kidneys and bladder, and into other uric acid diseases.

Nature Cure follows a wiser plan. By its stimulating methods of natural treatment and eliminating yet positive vegetarian diet, it puts the organism of the patient in such a condition that it can generate its own positive magnetic forces.

WHAT ABOUT THE MILK CURE?

The Milk Cure has become quite a fad among certain food reformers and diet specialists. Even our wise Ella Wheeler Wilcox claims that she can cure almost anything from gripe to incipient cancer by a strict milk diet.

If she had opportunity to try her cure on a mixed assortment of cases, and watched the results for some time after the experiment, she would soon find out her mistake.

Some will say, "Your own tables give milk as Nature's perfect normal food. Furthermore, it comes from the live animal magnetism. What, then, is wrong with the milk cure?"

Milk is Nature's most perfect food for the new born. The digestive organs of the young animal are specially adapted for the digestion of milk.

The liver, which is a filter for fluid food, is, in proportion, three times as large in the infant as in the adult; the stomach is almost a straight tube and the bowels and intestines are very active. All this facilitates the disposal of large quantities of fluids.

Everywhere in Nature, however, we notice the change from fluid to solid food simultaneously with the growth of the individual.

The reason for this is that for the adult organism milk contains too much fluid in proportion to solids. Too large a proportion of fluids in the food of adults overworks the liver and kidneys and there is not enough woody fibre, cellulose, etc., to furnish the intestines sufficient solid material to work upon and to properly stimulate the peristalsis of the bowels.

For these reasons a strict milk diet has a tendency to cause distension of the stomach, fermentation, biliousness and constipation, especially when the bowels are sluggish and the stomach weak and relaxed.

Too much fluid of any kind dilutes the blood, lymph, digestive juices and all other secretions of the body and weakens their action, because the proportion of water to organic salts is greatly increased. This brings us to a consideration of water drinking and flushing which have also become popular fads with the public and with doctors.

Many physicians actually seem to understand that Water Cure means the absorption of large quantities of warm and cold water by way of the mouth or rectum. The universal slogan has gone forth, "Flush out the system!"

TO DRINK OR NOT TO DRINK

Doctors, health magazines, books on Nature Cure and hygienists of high repute almost unanimously advise their patients and students to "flush out" their systems with large quantities of water. They advise their followers to drink glasses, quarts—yes—gallons of water, whether they feel the need of it or not.

It seems so easy and sounds so plausible to "flush out" everything that does not belong in our systems—one can do it with a sewer, why not with a body? The difference, however, lies in this: Flushing out a sewer is a mechanical process, while cleaning out a human body is a chemical process.

The cleansing of the human organism depends upon the **concentration** of vital fluids and secretions, not on their dilution with large quantities of water.

Blood, lymph, saliva, gastric juice, bile, pancreatic juice and all other fluids and secretions of the body are chemical solutions, and chemical solutions do not become stronger by adding to it two or three cups of water. Neither will the fluids of the body become more effective in their work by continuous water flooding.

Modern blood analysis demonstrates the fact that human blood is too thin already; almost every sample which comes in for analysis to the laboratory contains too many fluids in proportion to solids. If the blood does not carry enough iron, sodium, calcium, silicon, etc., to satisfy the demands of cells and tissues, there is bound to be abnormal function or disease.

Anaemia, for instance, is a misnomer, for it is not due, as the name would indicate, to a lack of blood, but to a lack in the blood of mineral elements, especially of iron, sodium and calcium. There is no lack of quantity, but a lack of quality due to abnormal composition of constituent elements. To such abnormal conditions of the blood Dr. Lahmann has applied the better name of dysaemia, which we shall adopt from now on.

We have learned before that uric acid diseases are due to a lack of sodium, whose office it is to neutralize uric acid, sulphuric acid and carbonic acid and to carry these waste products out of the system through the various channels of elimination. Bone diseases are due to lack of calcium and phosphates. In similar manner all other diseases are caused or accompanied by a deficiency of organic salts in blood and tissues.

The introduction of more water into the blood through mouth or rectum reduces still further the proportion of organic salts to fluids; in other words, the blood becomes more watery than ever, it carries less of the mineral elements for purposes of oxygenation, purification and for the generation of electro-magnetic currents. We therefore recommend drinking only when Nature calls for it by the sign of thirst.

People often remark, "Flushing makes the bowels lazy; after awhile they will not act at all."

There is a good deal of truth in this, for the following reasons: The free and natural action of the bowels depends on copious secretions from the mucous membranes of the intestinal tract. These secretions are incited by dryness of the tract. This sensation of dryness is telegraphed to headquarters in the brain and from thence in response to the call, the command comes back to the cells of the mucous membrane in the intestinal tract "to furnish secretions."

When the bowels are constantly flooded with fluids by water drinking and flushing, dryness, the incentive to secretion, is missing, there is no demand for fluids telegraphed to the brain and from the brain no impulse to secretion is returned. In other words, the bowels, being artificially flooded with water, become inactive and lazy, because dryness, the natural stimulus to secretion, is lacking.

For these and other reasons before mentioned a purely milk diet, is persisted in for any length of time, always tends to biliousness, constipations, and to unhealthy fat formation. A watery condition of the blood and other vital fluids and a corresponding deficiency of organic salts produce sluggish digestion and only partial reduction of food materials and tissues. Instead of reducing proteids and carbohydrates into heat and energy and into protoplasmic cell material, the transformation of food remains incomplete and stops at the formation of fat. This process is very similar to the production of fat on pigs and cattle by feeding them with salted food and giving them large quantities of water. Salt creates thirst, water causes dysaemia, and watery dysaemia makes unhealthy adipose tissue.

It is this apparent gain in weight and fat which attracts people to water flushing and milk diet. The majority of people and many doctors as well, gauge health by bulk and weight and are therefore deceived by the artificial gain under the milk cure regime. But their exultation over the acquisition of a few pounds of flesh is usually of short duration, for sooner or later the reaction comes and the abnormal gain is lost even more rapidly than it was acquired. We have witnessed many such a collapse after the "wonderful" milk cures.

Many of our readers, however, will tell us after reading this article of the undeniable benefits which they themselves or their friends have at times experienced under the milk treatment. We do not deny that this is true. We know that under certain circumstances the milk diet is, temporarily at least, very beneficial.

A glance at our tables of food analyses in former numbers of this Magazine will disclose the reason why this must be so.

On examining the milk analysis we are struck by the very low percentage of proteid constituents, despite the fact that milk is Nature's perfect food for the growing animal, which naturally demands much more proteid material for the building of new tissues than the full grown organism. What an argument this presents against our cereal, peanut and bean-eating vegetarians, or against the meat and egg-stuffing regulars.

When the system is carbonic acid or uric acid poisoned by a one-sided cereal or meat diet, the change to a straight milk diet with its very low percentage of carbohydrate, hydrocarbon and proteid materials is certainly of immense benefit. It puts the system, so to speak, on a temporary proteid fast and gives it a chance to eliminate the poisons accumulated in the excessive consumption of uric acid producing food elements. In buttermilk the proportion of organic salts to fats and proteid is still greater than in milk, and it is therefore in many forms of systemic poisoning more cooling and eliminating than full milk.

If, however, the milk diet is persisted in the deleterious effects above described will soon manifest in the forms of fermentation, gas formation, biliousness, constipation and occasional collapse.

If the flushing theory were correct it should be especially advisable in cases of chronic constipation on account of the heated and dry condition of the bowels. I admit that in such cases "flushing" is greatly to be preferred to the old barbaric system of purging by means of calomel (mercury) and salts. We sometimes use the syringe for temporary relief, but if persisted in, excessive water drinking and flushing, for reasons before stated, will have a tendency to aggravate disease conditions in general and to make the bowels more inactive than ever.

We ourselves invariably put all cases of chronic constipation on a dry diet; that is, we instruct our patients to drink moderately when thirst compels them, and so far we have rarely failed to perfect a cure, no matter how old and stubborn the condition. Some of these patients assured us that they had not had a single natural movement of the bowels without recourse to drugs or injections in five, ten or even twenty years, but even then, two or three months of natural diet, water cure, osteopathy, massage of the bowels and moderate water drinking have always sufficed to produce free and natural action.

The only exceptions to this rule as far as we can remember were a few cases of chronic constipation in which the bowels were completely burned out and atrophied by long continued use of calomel and salts, and a few others due to "successful" operations for appendicitis.

Thus has practical experience in hundreds of cases convinced us that the secretions of the digestive organs, as well as all other vital fluids, are more effective when concentrated than when diluted with large quantities of water.

A rational vegetarian diet properly combined, consisting of dairy products, the positive vegetables, and the medium positive fruits with just enough of starchy and proteid foods to supply the needs of the body for tissue building and fuel material, will be found to be an ideal diet for human beings fully sufficient to keep them in health and strength under the most trying circumstances.

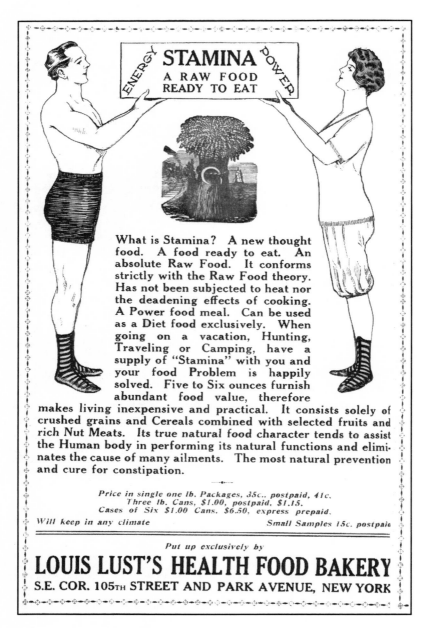

Louis Lust, Benedict's brother, produced innovative raw food products
such as an energy powder called Stamina.

OVEREATING

by Henry Lindlahr, M.D.

The Naturopath and Herald of Health, XV(10), 611-612. (1910)

The most wholesome foods become injurious when taken in excessive quantities. Whatever we cannot properly digest and assimilate, ferments and decays, filling the system with waste matter and poisons. Many persons squander their vitality in eliminating noxious food ballast, and wonder why they are so weak *in spite of a good appetite and rich foods.* When the organs of digestion are continually overworked, they weaken and are unable to convert the over-supply of food into the proper constituents for healthy blood and lymph; waste matter accumulates, creating noxious gases and systematic poisons. Poisonous miasms thus contaminate the vital fluid, causing corruption and obstruction in organs and tissues, furnishing a luxurious soil for all kinds of parasites, germs and bacteria.

This is so evident that we cannot comprehend why the "regular" profession persists in stuffing the weak bodies of consumptives and other invalids with enormous quantities of food, under the impression that the patients are thus strengthened and restored. The profession does not realize that the stomach and bowels of these poor sufferers are feeble, and as incapable of exertion as their arms and legs.

Suppose that one of these patients, hardly able to walk, complained of extreme weakness and was told by his physician to go home and chop a cord of wood daily; the patient would be of the opinion that there was a "loose screw" somewhere in the thinking apparatus of the food doctor. But when the latter tells him to go home and load his stomach every hour or two with eggs, meats, soups, beer, tonics, brandy and other solids and liquids, he goes home, does as advised, praises the wisdom of his doctor— and peacefully gives up the ghost.

The good minister attributes his death to the inscrutable will of Providence. We suspect that he succumbed to an overdose of professional ignorance. The health and strength of the body do not depend upon the quantity eaten, but upon the quantity properly digested and assimilated. When will doctors learn that digestion and exertion are in themselves a great strain on vitality? Have they never experienced that "lazy feeling" after a heavy metal?

In severe diseases and states of nervous and physical prostration, the ordinary functions are at a standstill—as is apparent from the extreme weakness and helplessness of the patient. Much less food is required than in times of healthy activity. Does not Nature herself, in acute diseases, protest against eating, by loss of appetite, nausea and vomiting? Nevertheless, although the patient himself objects to the enforced feeding, and his whole organism revolts against it, the wise doctor still insists that he "must eat to keep up strength," so-called "sedatives" are given to paralyze the stomach into insensibility and down go chicken soup, eggs and beef tea!

In acute febrile disease, feeding is not only useless but actually harmful, because in such conditions, which we recognize as Nature's healing and cleansing efforts, the normal activities of the organism, including the processes of digestion and assimilation, are at a standstill. All efforts are concentrated on elimination; the stomach and bowels are also called upon to assist in the general house cleaning. Instead of assimilating, they too are eliminating noxious poisons, which produce nausea, vomiting, diarrhoeas and catarrhal excretions. The digestive organs normally acting like a sponge, but now the process is reversed, the sponge is being squeezed. It is giving off old, filthy accumulations, thus aiding the "cleansing crisis." As soon as food is given, this beneficial elimination through stomach and bowels is hindered and interrupted; as a consequence, the temperature immediately rises and is followed by an aggravation of all symptoms.

The danger lies not so much in under-feeding, as in over-feeding. To one who dies from lack of food, thousands die from over-eating. If the truth were known, we should be surprised at the small amount of food required to keep the body in perfect condition.

Cornaro, an Italian nobleman, when forty years of age, was declared by his doctors to be dying from the effects of dissipation. Instead of resigning himself to this fate, he determined to enter upon a little experiment of his own. He cut his food supply down to a few ounces a day and, before long, regained health and strength. At a hundred years of age, he wrote a book recounting his experiments and the wonderful effects of temperate living.

The only safe guide in eating is "hunger, not appetite;" this Nature's sign that more food is needed, and that the organism is in a condition to take care of it.

If the doctors and friends of patients better understood and applied this principle, many who are now carried to the grave would remain with us and enjoy life a little longer.

1911

Drink At Meals
J. H. Neff

Care And Feeding Of Infants
Otto Carqué

EAT and be HEALTHY !

Why fast every once in a while, or go on some rigid diet,

when, if you knew how, you could just as well **Eat and be Healthy?** **Fasting,** like medicine, **merely removes effects, not causes.** How absurd to have to be fasting for illnesses, mere effects caused by wrong eating!

Eat right and you will never need to fast!

How?—"Eat and be Healthy," unquestionably the simplest and yet the most comprehensive and scientific book on the diet question ever written, tells you. **If you want to know the very heart of the diet question, read this book!** Send $2.50 for your copy now!

DR. VIRGIL MacMICKLE
807 Dekum Bldg., Portland, Oregon

Dr. MacMickle, a Naturopath from Oregon, placed this ad in 1919.

Drink At Meals

by J. H. Neff

The Naturopath and Herald of Health, XVI(6), 381. (1911)

Never, no, never drink a drop of any liquid at meals. If you do, it will be decidedly injurious; for no amount of liquid at meals can aid or help one iota in digesting your food. It only prevents digestion and causes ill-health.

The Creator knew far better what was needed for mankind's best health, than knows disobedient man. He gave man teeth to first chew his food to a pulp, that it might be thoroughly saturated with nature's liquid, the only liquid needed—the saliva, which forms the first part of digestion.

When the food is thus completely masticated to a pulp, then it is ready and easy to be sent down the narrow way to the chemical laboratory—the stomach—for the gastric fluid to further complete the second part of digestion, and so on to the end of the elementary thoroughfare of nature's operation.

When you drink at meals, you wash the food down long before it is chewed finely enough, or before it has received half of the saliva needed to prepare the food for the gastric operation. Hence fermentation sets in, accompanied by stomach troubles and other evils.

If one ounce of gastric fluid will digest half a pound of solid food at meals in two hours' time, how long will the same amount take to digest the same quantity of food when diluted with 40 to 60 times its amount of some other liquid? And when thus gorged three times a day with such destructive methods, can you not see the evil of such inhuman practice and also the suffering that will follow?

Drinking at meals is one of the worst acts of gluttony mankind can be guilty of.

What can be more gluttonous than not to chew the food half, and then wash it down with some liquid. Some are so greedy or gluttonous that they put a pile of cow grease (butter) on certain foods or pitchers of chalk-water (milk), etc., so they can gulp it down without taking time to chew the food as nature demands—thus eating by wholesale, nay, not eating, only scooping it down in a thunderstorm flood-like manner—no matter how or what may follow.

Thus they scoop or pitch what they got into their hopper for their wet grist to be ground as fast as their ability can exercise their gluttonous operation.

Is it any wonder people suffer with all kinds of stomach troubles, etc.? Why, the animals have better sense than that. They never drink when they eat, and yet, how well and chaste they are, as compared to disobedient man. When will mankind get sense or wisdom enough to eat when hungry, drink when thirsty, but never at meals, and stop this gluttony of drinking at meal times?!

Never, no, never drink a drop of any liquid at meals.

If one ounce of gastric fluid will digest half a pound of solid food at meals in two hours' time, how long will the same amount take to digest the same quantity of food when diluted with 40 to 60 times its amount of some other liquid?

Drinking at meals is one of the worst acts of gluttony mankind can be guilty of.

Care And Feeding Of Infants

by Otto Carqué

The Naturopath and Herald of Health, XVI(11), 788-790. (1911)

The question of diet in infancy and childhood is most important, because during especially the first year of life, improper feeding causes nearly all the so-called children's diseases. The period of early childhood is decisive for the rest of our life and the amount of vitality to resist injurious influences, aside from heredity, largely depends on the quality of nourishment we receive in the first year of our existence. "The child is the father of the man," and as the formation of the healthy and strong body is necessary for the development of the healthy mind, the importance of a sound foundation of the growing organism cannot be too strongly emphasized.

Reason and common sense tell us that mother's milk is the best form of nourishment during the early months of life, and that every mother who is physically able shall nurse their baby. It is a deplorable fact that less than one-third of mothers in so-called civilized countries are unable to perform this function. Many mothers do not nurse their infants because of ignorance. They do not know what it means to the child's future. Any mother who does not nurse her child because it is not convenient, because she does not wish to be tied down to her child during the first few months of its life, is committing a crime and is not fit to be a mother.

Statistics show that infants fed on the breast milk of a healthy woman are stronger and better able to resist disease. While it is true that babies may be reared on artificial food and remain apparently healthy, the percentage of robust bottle-fed babies is much smaller than that of healthy breast-fed children. The injurious effects of improper feeding are not always immediately noted, and often a food may temporarily show no ill effects, but does much harm when used permanently. It is often the case that a child will became fat on some particular form of food, but if there is an absence from the food of one necessary element, it may be months before the lack of this element is noticed. Scrofulosis, scurvy, rickets, chronic indigestion and many acute diseases are caused by improper feeding.

Infant mortality remains one of the biggest problems that confront society. For years it has been the object of serious concern to governments and municipalities, not only in this country, but also in France, Germany and England. In spite of everything that has been done, however, the total number of deaths among infants has not appreciably decreased. During 1907 in New York City the number of deaths of infants under one year of age was 17,437. In other words, about 150 babies out of every thousand born died before they reached the first year of age, from causes which were largely preventable. Considering the poor population during the hot weather alone, the rate in congested quarters was from 200 to 400 deaths per thousand births.

Cow's milk, which is used in most instances as a substitute for mother's milk, is most readily affected, not only by the food of the animals, but also by the conditions and environments in which it is living. Even if produced under ideal conditions and taken in its natural state, without boiling or pasteurizing, cow's milk is physiologically unsuitable for infant feeding.

It must be remembered that however carefully a milk mixture may be made and however closely it resembles human milk in composition, such mixture can only be regarded as a poor substitute for mother's milk, which is the best of all foods for infants. So-called modified milk may appear to the analytical chemist a good imitation of human milk because its proportions of proteids, fats and carbohydrates are about right, but actually the discrepancy is very great when studied from the standpoint of physiological chemistry.

The digestion and growth of a calf are quite different from those of and infant. The chief characteristic of cow casein is its ready coagulation into large indigestible masses, rich in fat, while human casein coagulates into fine soft flocks containing much less fat, easily acted upon by the gastric juice. The stomach contents of a child after a meal of cow's milk at the end of 45 minutes show casein clots still undigested; furthermore, the mineral elements of organic salts of cow's milk, chiefly lime, are not well assimilated, fully one-third being lost in the bowel discharges. The mineral salts of cow's milk which are of importance are those of sodium, calcium, potassium and magnesium chloride, and they are more than twice as abundant as in human milk. In contradistinction to the organic salts in human milk, they frequently act as an irritant, even when artificially reduced to the same or lower percentage found in breast milk.

Pasteurization or sterilization, which is still advocated by some physicians in order to destroy germs and bacteria is a delusion. Dr. E. M. Hill, New York, writes: "It has been my fortune for a number of years to oversee the feeding of many hundred babies, and after numerous and careful experiments with feeding babies on pasteurized milk, I am forced to believe that it, in the vast majority of cases, produces rickets and scurvy or scurvy rickets and kindred diseases, if given continuously, these diseases being cured by the use of raw milk with no other treatment. Several years ago when there was so much talk of the virtues of pasteurized milk for babies, I examined several hundred babies so fed and found that 97 per cent of them showed signs of rickets, scurvy and scrofulosis, and it was only after these careful observations that the fallacy of heated milk in infant feeding was made clear to me."

Pasteurization of milk so changes its organic ingredients that it is no longer food fit for the proper nourishment of an infant. That commercially pasteurized milk is more unsafe and less to be trusted than ordinary milk is abundantly proven by the investigation of Pennington and McClintock of Philadelphia, and is also true of other cities. Experiments on the germicidal action of cow's milk have shown that the relative increase of bacteria in milk is more pronounced if heated to 75 degrees C. or 100 degrees C. (167 degrees F. to 210 degrees F.) than in raw milk or milk heated to 56 degrees C. (132 degrees F.), proving that the heating of milk destroys or greatly impairs its germicidal action.

Animal milk, used as an exclusive infant's food, should not be heated above blood heat, as a temperature above that disorganizes the albumenoids and mineral constituents, on which the development and growth of the child depends. To be sure, uncontaminated milk is necessary for successful infant feeding, but contaminated milk, no matter how carefully pasteurized, will cause disordered digestion, improper assimilation and consequently disease. Pasteurization does by no means destroy the impurities, and heating inferior, unclean milk that is full of bacteria does not improve the health of children. Raw milk should always be preferred, even if it's not so pure and free from bacteria as we wish.

Some people have an idea that it matters not how filthy a cow's milk is, or how many germs it may contain, if it be pasteurized or sterilized it then becomes a fit food for children. This is not true, because in the first place, even prolonged boiling does not kill the spores of all bacteria; and, in the second place, the chemical poisons produced by certain germs are not altered by the temperature of boiling milk.

The first effect of using sterilized milk is that the child will be constipated. It is for this reason decidedly objectionable. The same refers to condensed milk, which probably does more harm than any other of the infants' foods, because it contains a large amount of refined sugar. If cow's milk is used at all, it should come from clean and healthy animals, living out of doors. It should be handled in scrupulously clean vessels and used as soon as possible.

A diet of fresh cow's milk is best modified by small quantities of fresh fruit juice; for example, orange juice, apple juice. The general opinion is that children should not be given fruit until they have well passed the period of infancy. This may be true of fruits in general, but the giving of the strained juices of certain fruits is not only conducive, but is actually essential to the baby's health. A teaspoonful of orange juice three times a day has been found very beneficial, especially in cases of rickets and other disorders of nutrition. In giving fruit juices to infants, several points have to be observed. The juices must be made from perfectly ripe fruit and must always be carefully strained. They should be given about two hours after milk feeding and at least half an hour before the next milk feeding.

In nearly all cases the infants enjoy this pleasant modification of their diet. Since mother's milk is free from the objections made to all artificial foods, it is not necessary to give fruit juices to breast-fed infants; nevertheless, it will be always advantageous to do so. Fresh fruit juices are the best preventatives of infantile diarrhea, as their mild acids and alkaline salts are natural disinfectants of the alimentary canal.

One of the most frequent mistakes in the feeding of infants is the tendency to overfeed. Nearly all cases of colic and diarrhea in babies are due to this cause. A large number of infantile diseases can be overcome by regulating the hours of feeding. The child is not always hungry when it cries, and a few sips of water, especially during the night, will produce better sleep and give the little stomach a much needed rest.

Infants, as well as children, should not be given refined sugar in any form. The extensive use of artificial sweets is responsible for a large number of diseases of the digestive organs. Not enough can be said in warning against the prevalent use of refined sugar in the various forms of pastry and confectionary. That the general public is not aware of the injurious effect of artificial sweets seems to be indicated by the rapid increase of the manufacture and consumption of sugar. Statistics show that the average American consumes half of his own weight, or over 82 pounds of sugar, every year.

The use of artificial sweets in connection with white flour products is one of the most pernicious customs of the day, causing defective development of the skeleton of the infantile body and in later years a morbid softening of the bones, making dentistry one of the most lucrative professions of this country. Of 1,500 children examined carefully by the Bureau of Municipal Research of New York, 75 per cent were found to need dental treatment.

The taste of sweets is natural and indicates a physiological demand. This demand, however, can only be met without injury by the natural sweets existing principally in sweet fruits. Like all other acquired tastes, the sugar-eating habit is hard to give up, but numerous tests have shown that the habit is once broken the natural taste of food appears more pleasant than when it is disguised by manufactured sugar.

The feeding of growing children with an excess of bread, breakfast foods, ice cream, confectionary, meat and eggs furnishes too much nitrogen and phosphoric acid and not enough of the alkaline salts to the system, causing anemic and scrofulous conditions. At the same time these foods favor a morbid overgrowth of the tissues, as enlarged glands, adenoids and a catarrhal condition of all the mucous membranes. To relieve these conditions by surgical operations betrays very little knowledge of the physiological functions of the human body. Such illogical treatment is the outcome of the ruling medical system which constantly confounds cause and effect. Children as well as adults cannot keep in the best of health without an adequate supply of fruits during all seasons of the year.

Any mother who does not nurse her child because it is not convenient, because she does not wish to be tied down to her child during the first few months of its life, is committing a crime and is not fit to be a mother.

Even if produced under ideal conditions and taken in its natural state, without boiling or pasteurizing, cow's milk is physiologically unsuitable for infant feeding.

The chief characteristic of cow casein is its ready coagulation into large indigestible masses, rich in fat, while human casein coagulates into fine soft flocks containing much less fat, easily acted upon by the gastric juice.

Several years ago when there was so much talk of the virtues of pasteurized milk for babies, I examined several hundred babies so fed and found that 97 per cent of them showed signs of rickets, scurvy and scrofulosis, and it was only after these careful observations that the fallacy of heated milk in infant feeding was made clear to me.

Pasteurization of milk so changes its organic ingredients that it is no longer food fit for the proper nourishment of an infant.

A teaspoonful of orange juice three times a day has been found very beneficial, especially in cases of rickets and other disorders of nutrition. In giving fruit juices to infants, several points have to be observed.

Statistics show that the average American consumes half of his own weight, or over 82 pounds of sugar, every year.

The Food We Eat And The Food We Should Eat
Eugene Christian, F. S.

To Salt Or Not To Salt
Henry Lindlahr, M. D.

California "LikeFresh" Fruits,
Their Nutritive And Hygienic Value
Otto Carqué

A NEW BOOK

ON

Curative Diet

Called

"250 Meatless Menus"

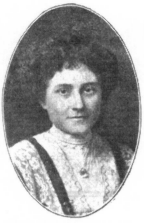

Here are some of the Chapters:

Dietetic Do's and Don'ts

Diet for School Children

Feeding the Pregnant and Nursing Mother

Over=eating

Feminine Freedom and Feminine Beauty.

Balanced Menus for the Sedentary Worker.

Balanced Menus for the Manual Laborer.

Balanced Menus for the 4 Seasons of the Year

Refrigerator and Kitchen Hygiene.

THE PURPOSE OF THIS BOOK IS:

To make the food the Family Doctor.
To increase the pleasure of eating and decrease the expense account.
It is beautifully illustrated and bound in vellum and gold. Price $1.00, postpaid.
P. S.—Read this book—if you are not satisfied, return it and I will refund your money.

VIENO BRAN

An infallible food cure for constipation. **Six recipes** and twenty health rules in each box. **Agents wanted** everywhere. Send 25c. for full size package, by mail.

ADDRESS

MOLLIE GRISWOLD CHRISTIAN

42 Seventh Avenue, Brooklyn, N. Y.

Mollie Christian shared her husband's zeal for vegetarianism.

The Food We Eat And The Food We Should Eat

by Eugene Christian, F. S.

The Naturopath and Herald of Health, XVII(1), 6-7. (1912)

[This interesting article is the second of a series to be published in The Natur-opath on the very important question of man's health and the food he eats. These articles will be written by Mr. Eugene Christian, who as an authority on matters of diet should prove of great interest to our readers. The first article was published in the December issue. Editor, B. Lust]

Under present economic conditions, the amount of food necessary to sustain life is a perplexing problem with many people, but if ideal socialistic conditions were to prevail, and the supply of food to every person was unlimited, the most important phase of the food question would still be unsolved, viz., to determine what is food and what is not food. To determine how to select our food so as to give to the body all the elements of nourishment it needs under the varying conditions of age, climate and work, and how to combine our food so as to make chemically harmonious when taken into the body.

About 90 per cent of all human disease originates in the stomach, caused by errors in eating. If the highest earning power of each individual could be realized and our luxuries and leisure's vastly increased, the abuses of eating would be correspondingly multiplied and human ills would increase at the same ratio.

Recognition of these facts very naturally introduces the question of scientific feeding, as a method of removing the causes of and curing diseases, in opposition to the time honored practice of healing with drugs and medicines, for in order to cure disease we must remove its causes. The majority of causes being the wrong or unnatural use of food, preventative methods or preventative medicine flows back to the food question as surely as all water flows back to the sea.

All disease is merely an expression of violated natural law. Diseases caused by violating the laws of nutrition can only be cured by obeying these laws, in other words, standing out of Nature's way and giving her the material to work with and she will do the curing.

Two million Christian Scientists, one million mental scientists, or so-called New Thought people, the various accepted schools of drugless healing, such as Hydrotherapy, Electrotherapy, Osteopathy, Mechano-Therapy, Naturopathy, Autology, and the new theory of Food Science, all point with much emphasis to the fact that there is something radically wrong with the old school of medicine, i. e., treating disease with drugs.

The best posted physicians in the country admit that there are twenty million people in the United States who do not believe in drugs, and who, therefore, advocate some form of drugless healing. This is authentic evidence that there is room for a new school of healing, but a new school could not survive without followers and it will not have followers unless it gives results.

If 90 per cent or even 50 per cent of human disease is caused by incorrect eating, then the food question, not the supply of food but the use of food, becomes the most important problem before civilization, for it matters not how plentiful food might become under ideal co-operative or social conditions. Human disease and suffering could not be decreased unless we know something about the Science of Human Nutrition—unless we know how to make food give natural result, which is health.

The way to destroy an effect is to remove its cause. Disease is an abnormal condition of the human body caused by congestion or the retention of poisons, which the body is unable to throw off. Nearly all of these poisons are caused from food taken in wrong selections, proportions and combinations. Therefore, the natural way to cure a disease is to remove its cause, by eating foods in such combinations as will give the body every element of nourishment it requires in the right proportions. This is standing out of Nature's way.

Man is physically what he eats. What we take into our stomachs either nourishes and gives us strength and health, or poisons and produces disease.

When one speaks of poison we are apt to think of strychnine or carbolic acid, but these are not the kind of poisons that cause most suffering and deaths. Meat from diseased animals, ptomains in decayed food, formaldehyde in preserved milk, and other poisons used by criminal manufacturers to preserve or color food, and the decay or undigested or unused food in the body, cause more deaths that strychnine, arsenic or acid. The United States Government, recognizing this fact, established the pure food law to purify as much as possible our National food supply and prevent this needless waste of human life.

The pure food law was modified, however, to suit the "interests," it is imperfect, and full of "holes," but it is a little step in the right direction.

When a man has taken arsenic or eaten embalmed beef, and is sick, we say he is poisoned, but what of the man who has dyspepsia, rheumatism, intestinal gas, constipation or nervousness? He is just as truly poisoned.

Science has given us the chemical composition of every article of food it requires. It should therefore, be a very easy matter to unite these two things (the food and the body) so as to produce a perfectly natural result, which would be health.

Knowing the chemistry of the body and the chemistry of our food,

Health is your Birthright

Some men sell their Birthright of Health and Happiness for a Mess of Pottage. Some sell it for a Plate of Homemade Doughnuts. And some sell it for a Midnight Snpper.

But the final accounting discloses the fact that the Price paid in each instance is the same. Poor Digestion! No Appetite! Insomnia! Loss of Health!

If your food has made you ill, if you have stomach trouble, if you are obese or emaciated, if you are full of aches and pains or are nervous and brain fagged,

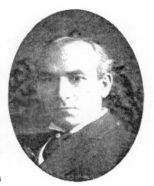

Send for my book and learn

"HOW FOODS CURE"

Read these letters from those who have learned

February 17th, 1909.
Mr. Eugene Christian, 7 East 41st St., N. Y.
My Dear Sir: I beg to acknowledge receipt of your favor of the 10 inst., and replying to the last paragraph of same, beg to say that I am entirely pleased with your dietetic treatment, and I thank the day that I first saw your advertisement, as at that time I was suffering everything possible from indigestion, constipation, etc., etc. I was suffering with pains of all kinds at first, then my condition changed to being unable to keep anything on my stomach—not even the lightest foods, and I felt as if I did not care to live any longer. Upon taking your treatment I gradually was able to retain some food, until at the present time I am able to eat almost anything, and with great relish.
Thanking you for your kindness to me in bringing me back to my former health, and wishing you all the luck in the world, I remain,
Yours very sincerely,
T. T. BANKERD.

La Cross, Wis., October 5th, 1908.
Dear Mr. Christian:
I am immensely pleased with the contents of your letter as it is a pleasure to know that you are grateful for my appreciation of what you have done and are doing for me. My main regret is that I cannot express what I feel. You have rescued me from a quicksand of disease and improper living. You have lifted a loan of dread from my heart and are put-

ting in its place, hope, health, energy, ambition and restored ability to carry on my work in life.. I would indeed be an ingrate were I not willing to give you credit and to try to spread your theories for the benefit of others. After all, life, in the broad sense, is valuable only as we improve it to benefit mankind. That is why I feel sure you find so much gratification in your work, even though you must fairly fight to get people's permission to help them. Many, I fear, have taken so much medicine they eye the word "cure" with suspicion. I feel certain that among the hundreds of people you have helped there are many who have appreciation in their hearts, but like the "cub" reporter cannot transfer it to paper.
Very truly yours,
W. V. KIDDER.

1412 Hyperwin Ave., Los Angeles, Cal., Sept. 28, 1909.
My Dear Mr. Christian: This is my final report and I am happy to say a very satisfactory one. The three months have passed very swiftly and I can testify to your being the best "doctor" I ever knew in all my long life. Your prescriptions are not only the most sensible, but all so delightful, so dainty, so æsthetic, that I am a complete captive to your theories, and shall never go back to the troublesome old ways of cooked foods. There is also a marked improvement in the family menus, for they are not going to let "Grand'ma" have all the good things.
Yours sincerely,
FRANCIS M. RICHARDS.

You may not be "under the doctor's care"; but if you don't feel **all right all the time**, you can read my book with profit to yourself. Write right now! It is sent Free.

Eugene Christian, FOOD SCIENTIST
7 East 41st St., Suite 60, New York City

Eugene Christian, an advocate of the vegetarian lifestyle, authored *How Foods Cure* (1911) and *Uncooked Foods and How to Use Them* (1924).

we could very easily learn the laws of chemical harmony, and we should be able thereby to produce many special results by special or scientific feeding.

If we know we are to be exposed to zero weather, we should be able to select such food and proportion it so as to keep up the bodily warmth to meet this emergency.

We should know how to select and combine our food during extremely hot weather so as to keep up the maximum of vitality and the minimum of heat. If this was done there would be no such thing as sun strokes or heat prostrations.

We should know how to select food that would remove causes of indigestion, constipation, rheumatism, gout, Bright's disease, obesity and nearly all abnormal conditions we call disease.

In our food we can find every chemical element of which the body is composed, therefore, eating can be made both remedial and curative. To do this only requires some knowledge of the chemical requirements of the body and the different foods that will supply these under different conditions, such as age, temperature of the atmosphere, whether winter or summer, and the kind of labor engaged in.

Household food science is therefore most useful of all reforms because it builds a foundation for the nation's greatest asset, which is health.

About 90 per cent of all human disease originates in the stomach, caused by errors in eating.

The majority of causes being the wrong or unnatural use of food, preventative methods or preventative medicine flows back to the food question as surely as all water flows back to the sea.

Science has given us the chemical composition of every article of food it requires. It should therefore, be a very easy matter to unite these two things (the food and the body) so as to produce a perfectly natural result, which would be health.

To Salt Or Not To Salt

by H. Lindlahr, M.D., Chicago

The Naturopath and Herald of Health, XVII(4), 218-220. (1912)

Like Barquo's ghost this question will not down. Pro or con it has been discussed by every diet specialist and food reformer. Vegetarians say, "Don't;" meat eaters say, "Do." Both may be right. How can that be?

Common inorganic table salt is chemically composed of sodium and chlorin. This and all other minerals we call organic, when they enter into chemical combinations with carbon in the living cells of plants and animals.

In our article on "Natural Dietetics," we have learned that proteids, starches, fats and sugars, in the process of digestion, form large amounts of carbonic, uric, sulphuric, hippuric acids and various poisonous alkaloids, such as xantin, creatin[e] and ptomaines, which become, when not rapidly and thoroughly eliminated, the most fruitful source of disease.

The neutralization and elimination of these food poisons depend largely upon sodium. The ordinary American diet, consisting of meats, peas, beans, potatoes, white bread, pastry, coffee and sugar, contains an excessive amount of the poison-producing food elements and only very small amounts of the eliminating sodium. Fruits and vegetables, however, are very rich in organic sodium as well as all other "organic salts." Keeping in mind these premises, we shall see how both vegetarian and meat eater may be right in their stand on the salt question.

The vegetarian whose daily dietary contains a liberal amount of uncooked fruits and vegetables and only moderate amounts of proteids and starches, has no need and no desire for inorganic table salt. His demands for sodium are fully satisfied *in a natural way by the organic sodium* contained in the raw foods.

On the other hand, people whose dietary consists largely of meats, potatoes, peas, beans, cereal foods, white flour bread and pastry, coffee, tea and refined sugar, must have table salt (sodium chlorin*) therefore they crave it.

The foods above mentioned, as we have learned, produce large amounts of poisonous acids and alkaloids, and unless these are promptly neutralized and eliminated by sodium, disease and death would be the inevitable results. Since the above described standard American dietary is deficient in the organic salts of fruits and vegetables, inorganic table salt (sodium chlorin) must serve as a poor substitute, but it is far better for the system to have the inorganic substitute than no salt at all.

---

*Henry Lindlahr's spelling, 'sodiam chlorin,' is understood to mean 'sodium chloride' today. *Ed.*

The fact that many people have lived almost entirely on meats or cereal foods with table salt as seasoning and have reached a ripe old age, indicates that the organism *can* use the inorganic salt as a substitute for the organic.

We have learned that many elements, though congenial to the body, when taken in the inorganic form show in the iris, but table salt even when habitually taken in large quantities does not show, indicating that we cannot class it among the poison foods. It is congenial to the system, being naturally present in the blood, in organic combinations, in large quantities. Like uric acid, caffeine, theine, alcohol and nicotine, which also do not show in the iris by distinct signs, it becomes poisonous to the system only when taken habitually in large quantities.

Table salt, however, should be used very moderately even by meat eaters. Its excessive use easily becomes a habit. Its elimination greatly irritates the kidneys and withdraws from the blood large quantities of serum. This creates great thirst, which necessitates the drinking of much water. This in turn dilutes the blood and other secretions of the organism, causing a watery dysaemia (anemia), watery blood makes fat. Thus salt is turned into fat.

Inorganic salt, when absorbed in large quantities, pickles the tissues. It destroys albuminous compounds and causes their excessive secretion in the urine, albuminuria. Therefore, it leeches the protoplasm of the cells, weakening their resistance and breaking down their normal structures.

This is shown clearly in scurvy, which is caused by excessive use of salt meats and lack of fresh vegetables (organic salts). This disease, which is characterized by decay and bleeding of the gums, proves that Nature limits the substitution of inorganic salt for the organic, and it strongly indicates that the latter is the most desirable form.

As soon as scurvy patients are put on a fruit and vegetable diet, the destruction of tissues, the bleeding resulting from it and other symptoms promptly abate.

Another indication that inorganic sodium-chlorid is not congenial to the system is indicated by the fact that considerable amounts of the organic salt contained in fruits and vegetables or in their extracts do not create thirst, while comparatively small amounts of the inorganic table salt cause irritation of the kidneys, great thirst, overwork, albuminuria, and weakening of the cell structure. These influences undoubtedly favor the development of kidney diseases.

When the dietary contains liberal amounts of uncooked fruits and vegetables, very little or no salt will be needed. The addition of salt is advantageous to vegetarian foods which contain large amounts of proteids, fats and starches, such as eggs, butter, peas, beans, lentils, potatoes, cereals, rice etc.

Vegetables when properly steamed in their own juices, so that none of their mineral constituents are wasted, do not need additional condiments, their own salts are the best flavoring.

Patients and visitors often think that our vegetable soups are over-salted. This is due to the fact that through the cooking process the salts are precipitated in the inorganic form, and act as such on the system. This is one of the reasons why we use vegetable soups sparingly.

In conclusion, we must remember that fruits and vegetables often do not contain the normal amounts of organic salts, because for ages the soil on which they grow has been robbed of its mineral constituents.

It is this deficiency in mineral elements which lowers the resistance of vegetable grains, and fruits, impairs their development, causes decay and facilitates the work of destructive worms, insects and germs, just as low-ered resistance favors the development of germs and bacteria in human bodies.

Nitrogenous fertilizers have been provided plentifully, but the neces-sity of mineral fertilizers was never thought of until Julius Hensel, the German food chemist, called attention to the fact.

The soil and its products, therefore, as well as human beings, suffer from mineral starvation. African explorers state that in certain parts of Africa the soil and its products are lacking in sodium chlorin, and that in these sections animals and human beings suffer from salt starvation, which expresses itself in many curious ways.

The following clipping from a daily paper is of interest in this con-nection.

REGION OF SALT FAMINE

All living creatures in this region are crazy for salt, just like oxen on a 'sour' veldt. Salt is far the best coinage you can take among the Chi-bokwe. I do not mean our white table salt. They reject that with scorn, thinking it is sugar or something equally useless, but for the coarse and dirty 'bay salt' they will sell almost anything, and a pinch of it is a greater treat to a child than a whole bride cake would be in England.

I have tested it especially with the bees that swarm in these forests and produce most of the beeswax that goes to Europe. I first noticed their love of salt when I salted some water one afternoon in the vain hope of curing the poisoned sores on my feet. In half an hour the swarms of bees had driven me from my tent. I was stung ten times and had to wait about in the forest till the sun set, when the bees vanished as if by signal.

Another afternoon I tested them by putting a heap of sugar, a paper smeared with condensed milk and a bag of salt tightly wrapped up in tar-paper side by side on the ground. I gave them twenty minutes, and then I found nothing on the sugar, five flies on the milk, and the tar-paper so densely covered with bees that they overlapped each other as when they swarm. For want of anything better, they will fight over a sweaty shirt in the same way; and once, but the banks of a stream, they sent all my carriers howling along the path by creeping up under their loin-cloths. The butterflies seek salt also. If you spread out a damp rag anywhere in tropical Africa, you will soon have brilliant butterflies on it. But if you add a little salt in the Hungry Country the rag will be a blaze of colors, unless the bees come and drive the butterflies off.

BURN GRASS FOR SUBSTITUTE

As I said, the natives feel the longing, too. Among the Chibokwe the women burn a marsh grass into a potash powder as a substitute; and if a native squats down in front of you, puts out a long pink tongue and strokes it appealingly with his finger you may know it is salt he wants.

The addition of small quantities of table salt to a vegetarian diet is, therefore, not to be condemned, but its use should be confined to butter, eggs and such cooked foods as we have mentioned.

Do not use it at the table, except on eggs. It is barbaric to kill with salt and pepper the delicate flavors of fruits and vegetables. But, says our friend, the meat eater, I have to add condiments and spices, or I cannot taste anything.

No wonder, when the bulbs in the tongue are paralyzed by salt, pepper, nicotine and alcohol. Return to a natural diet and your nerves of taste will soon regain their normal sensitiveness. Then you will enjoy the beautiful flavors of fruits and vegetables and things will taste as good as when mother made them.

In summing up and comparing our evidence, we come to the conclusion that here, as elsewhere, it is not well to run into extremes. As usual, the middle, common-sense way is the safest way.

> *The vegetarian whose daily dietary contains a liberal amount of uncooked fruits and vegetables and only moderate amounts of proteids and starches, has no need and no desire for inorganic table salt. His demands for sodium are fully satisfied in a natural way by the organic sodium contained in the raw foods.*
>
> *[Salt's] elimination greatly irritates the kidneys and withdraws from the blood large quantities of serum.*

California "Likefresh" Fruit, Their Nutritive And Hygienic Value

by Otto Carqué, Food Expert

The Naturopath and Herald of Health, XVII(12), 730-735. (1912)

No other State in the Union has gained so much fame and prominence all over the world as California. The early pioneers in their hunt for gold hardly realized the wonderful and inexhaustible treasures which lay hidden besides the yellow metal in the fertile hills and valleys. It is California's excellent fruit crop, the result of soil, sunshine, and an abundant water supply from the eternal snows of the high Sierras which will insure forever her unique position among her sister States. Scenery and climate are certainly two great assets of the Golden State, but the greatest of all is her ever-increasing harvest of delicious fruits, which are now sent to all parts of the world, bringing California sunshine in a condensed form to those who live in less favored states and countries.

Unfortunately, the value of fresh and dried fruits is still very much underestimated by the majority of people. They realize but slowly the fact that it is easier to prevent sickness than to cure it, and that fruits, if used judiciously possess all the curative properties required by the systems. A glance into our newspapers and magazines will convince us that at least half of the American people are suffering from one physical ailment or another. Otherwise the numerous manufacturers of patent medicines could not spend millions of dollars every year for advertisements in order to unload their abominable nostrums upon a credulous public, which is still foolish enough to believe that health can be bought in the forms of pills, powders, and portions. No chemist, however clever, can imitate the highly organized food principles which Nature has stored up so wonderfully in her luscious gifts for the health and delight of man.

Statistics show that of the total amount of money spent for food in the United States only 5 per cent is expended for fruit, while flesh foods, dairy products and cereals predominate in the average dietary. The great hygienic value, of fruits in general is not yet realized; on the contrary, many persons frequently avoid fruits as the cause of more or less painful disturbances in the digestive organs. Fermentation and other disagreeable symptoms in the stomach and in the intestinal canal are in most instances produced by artificially prepared foods eaten in connection with fruits rather than by fruits alone. Especially starchy foods in the form of pies, pudding and pastry sweetened with manufactured sugar, considerably retard the processes of digestion and assimilation and give rise to fermentation in the alimentary canal. Moreover, fruits are frequently eaten on top of a heavy meal. Their beneficial effect upon the system is thereby entirely lost and they become the source of much distress, as in the case of the farmer who ate a few apples after a hearty meal of pork and pastry. Being tortured by severe pains during the following night, he condemned the apples as the cause of his pitiable condition and decided to carefully exclude them from his dietary in the future.

Fruit Sugar Versus Refined Sugar

Modern physiology shows that there are two important factors in sustaining the health and vigor of the body—first, adequate nutrition, and second the conservation of vital force. Fruits which we receive direct from the hands of nature contain the necessary elements for our body in the highest form of organization and in about the right proportion; they will therefore insure perfect nutrition. In the process of digestion fresh, ripe fruits, if eaten by themselves, require only a small expenditure of nerve force; they are superior to starchy foods, which draw more heavily upon nerve force, overtaxing and gradually weakening the organs of digestion and elimination.

In the carbohydrates of plant foods nature has organized those elements which give heat, energy and endurance to the body. The heat-giving elements, carbon and hydrogen, exist in different forms, principally as starch and sugar. In fruits we find these elements in the form of fruit sugar (levulose) or grape sugar (glucose) already prepared for immediate assimilation. Here the rays of sun have practically performed the work of the cook by bringing the carbohydrates into the most perfect and soluble form. That sugar is the most economical source of animal heat and energy has been proven by many scientific experiments, but we must always discriminate between the sugar as it exists in fruits or succulent plants, and the refined sugar of commerce, although their chemical composition is similar. The former is intimately associated with other elements, making a complete food, while the latter is a chemically isolated food principle which cannot maintain health and vitality, except for a very brief period. Experiments prove that the regular use of refined sugar, whether in the form of candy, syrup or diluted in water, in time produces catarrh of the stomach and induces various disorders of the digestive organs.

Refined Sugar, A Starvation Food

The reason for the injurious effects of manufactured sugar and glucose is that they are artificially extracted from those organic combinations which are necessary for building of tissues and bones, for the proper functioning of the nervous system, and the purification of the blood.

Refined sugar consists only of three elements: oxygen, hydrogen, and carbon, while the human body is composed of fifteen elements, all of which are important for the formation of healthy and firm tissues and in the performance of the various physiological functions of the organism. These elements can only be assimilated by our system in an organized form, as they are contained in natural foods, such as fruits, nuts, whole cereals, and vegetables. Life and health cannot be maintained by proximate food principles such as refined sugar, starch, gluten obtained by mechanical or chemical processes. A German scientist who has made a large number of experiments, found that animals if fed on pure gluten and sugar, died sooner than those not fed at all. Mineral waters and preparations which contain iron, sulphur, lime, magnesia, etc., in their inorganic state, are of no value for our nutrition. On the contrary, they impair and obstruct vital action.

In selecting and preparing our food we should always bear in mind that we cannot improve on nature, and that any food we can relish in its natural state is best adapted for the proper nourishment of the body.

Not enough can be said in warning against the prevalent and extensive use of refined sugar in the various forms of pastry and confectionary. That the general public is not aware of the injurious effect of artificial sweets seems to be indicated by the rapid increase of the manufacture and consumption of sugar. Statistics show that the average American consumes half its own weight, or over 82 pounds of sugar every year. The total consumption of sugar in the United States in 1907 amounted to over 7000 million pounds. Calculating this enormous total at the average retail price of 51-2 cents per pound, we get a total of 385 million dollars to the consumer, or more than one million dollars for every day in the year. Whatever interest these figures may possess from a commercial standpoint, considered from a hygienic point of view, they are deplorable. Indeed, the use of artificial sweets is one of the most pernicious customs of the day, causing defective development of the skeleton on the infantile body, and in later years a morbid softening of the bones, making dentistry one of the most lucrative professions in this country.

The extensive use of artificial sweets, especially in connection with white flour products, is responsible for a large number of diseases of the digestive organs. The liver and kidneys are severely affected by the increased formation of toxic substances and the consequent accumulation of acids in the blood causes a catarrhal condition of all the mucous membranes.

Organic Salts In Fruits

There prevails a mistaken idea that the mineral elements are present in all our foods in superabundant measure, and that therefore the study of this matter is not of importance. If it were ever true that in our natural choice of foods we could not fail to get an adequate supply of these elements, this condition has been entirely changed with the advent of modern milling processes, with the establishment of sugar and starch factories and the irrational preparation of foodstuffs for the table of the average household to-day.

The importance of the organic salts in the vital processes of the cell lies almost entirely in their physical and chemical properties. The chemical reactions in the body which constitute the physical basis of life take place between substances in solution, and it is by means of the electrical charges carried by the particles in solution that reactions are possible. Through their peculiar electro-chemical attributes the organic salts maintain, therefore, a very important relation to practically all of the vital processes and they enter into the composition of every tissue and fluid of the body.

Calcium, phosphorus, sulphur and iron are used in the formation of the essential structures of the body. Without a constant renewal of the elements of iron and sodium, the blood cannot take up sufficient oxygen and the products of combustion (carbon dioxide, uric acid, etc.) cannot be neutralized and eliminated. As proteid substances are used up in the life processes of the cells of the body, the phosphorus and the sulphur contained therein give rise to the formation of sulphuric and phosphoric acids. These and certain other acids must be neutralized in order to preserve the alkalinity of the blood and tissues. The normal alkalinity of the blood rests chiefly on the sodium ions and is essential to the physiologic oxidation of the nutritive cell contents of the tissues. This alkalinity is increased by fruit and greenleaf vegetables and lessened by meats, broths and cereals.

If there is a deficiency of alkaline salts in the food, ammonia, for a time, will be split off from the proteids of the body, but entire absence of alkaline salts from the food for even a brief period will cause death from autointoxication.

The alkaline salts of fruits and vegetables act as natural laxatives by promoting the action of the secreting glands; they also assist in the preservation of normal physical conditions within the cells. The chlorides furnish the chlorine of the hydrochloric acid in the gastric juice, pepsin being inactive except in the presence of hydrochloric acid. In the small intestine the alkaline salts assist in the digestion of fats.

To enjoy permanent health and immunity from disease, our blood must contain all the necessary elements in the right proportions and combinations, because it is the blood which carries them to the different parts of the body, nourishing and cleansing the tissues, creating animal heat, magnetism and electricity. As long as the importance of the organic salts in our system is not recognized and understood, so long must there exist a deplorable guesswork, both in regard to diagnosis and the treatment of disease.

Diabetes, kidney and bladder diseases, calculus, stones and gravel are caused by insufficient oxidation and consequent acidity of the blood, due to an excess of meat, sweets, starches, table salt and frequent indulgence in alcoholic beverages. Phosphate of potash is almost the only mineral basis present in meat and cereals, while only small quantities of other salts are present. Bladder stones consist chiefly of phosphates and oxalates of lime and compounds of urea. Only when the alkaline elements are introduced in the right proportions can the acid reaction of the blood be brought back to its normal alkaline state and the solid concretion dissolved and eliminated.

The feeding of growing children with an excess of bread, breakfast foods, refined sugar, meat and eggs furnished too much nitrogen and phosphate potash and too little sodium to the system, causing anemic and scrofulous condition. At the same time these foods favor a morbid overgrowth of the tissues, as enlarged glands, adenoids, and as already stated, a catarrhal condition of all the numerous membranes. To relieve these conditions by surgical operations betrays very little knowledge of the physiological functions of the human body. Such illogical treatment is the outcome of the ruling medical system which constantly confounds cause and effect. Children as well as adults cannot keep in the best of health without an adequate supply of fruits during all seasons of the year. *The fact that man is by nature frugivorous cannot be successfully refuted, and the nearer one is able to live to this ideal the better it will be for one's health and power to resist disease.*

SULPHURED FRUITS INJURIOUS TO HEALTH

The season for fresh fruits in less favored countries than California is comparatively short and to supply the demand for fruit, a large part of California's annual fruit crop is now canned and dried. Special care should be taken, however, by the consumer in the selection of his dried fruits, as in most instances chemical processes are employed during the preparation, which detract considerably from the hygienic value of the fruit. In the drying process sulphurous acid is chiefly employed in the form of the fumes of burning sulphur, applied either to the food products themselves in the course of manufacture, or to the containers in which the food products are held. Desiccated fruits, pared or unpared, are subjected after the removal of the pit or core, to the fumes of burning sulphur in what is known as a "sulphur box." Following reasons are given for the practice of sulphuring:

1. To produce as clear and intense a yellow color as possible.

2. To conceal decayed portions of the fruit.

3. To prevent fermentation and decay during the drying of the fruit.

4. To protect the fruit during drying from flies and other insects, the larvae of which would otherwise develop after the fruit was stored.

5. To kill the cells of the fruit and thus make the texture more porous, which expedites drying.

Numerous experiments carried on by Dr. H. Wiley, former chief chemist of the United States Department of Agriculture, have shown that the use of sulphurous acid in foods is deleterious, that it never adds anything to the flavor or quality of a food, but renders it both less palatable and less healthful. Sulphurous acid retards the assimilation of food material and overworks the kidneys, which have to remove the added sulphur from the body. Another effect which the administration of sulphur produces and one of a more serious character still, is formed by the impoverishment of the blood in respect of the number of red and white corpuscles therein. Sulphur, like all other preservatives, as benzoic acid, saccharin, etc., is purely a drug, devoid of food value, and exerting deleterious and harmful effects. The addition of any form of sulphurous acid to products intended for human food should therefore be avoided.

Dr. Wiley says in part, after his extended investigations:

> From a careful consideration of the data in the individual cases and the summaries of the results, it appears that the administration of sulphurous acid in the food, either in the form of sulphurous acid gas in solution, or in the form of sulphites, is objectionable and produces serious disturbances of the metabolic functions, and injury to health and digestion.

> The experiments show what an immense burden has been added to the already over-worked kidneys, which are called upon in this case to remove nearly all, if not quite all, of the added sulphur from the body, previously converted, in great part, to sulphuric acid. It is not possible that placing upon the kidneys this increased work of excreting sulphur can result in anything but injury.

> The further observation that there is a marked tendency to the production of albuminaria, although of an incipient character, is an indication of the unfavorable results of the administration of the sulphurous acid. It is therefore evident that by increasing the burden upon the excretory organs, the administration of sulphur in the form mentioned is highly detrimental to health.

> The conclusion, therefore, is inevitable that, as a whole, the changes produced in the metabolic activity by the administration of sulphur in the forms noted above in the comparatively short time covered by the experiments, are decidedly injurious.

> The verdict which must be pronounced in this case is decidedly unfavorable to the use of this preservative in any quantity, or for any period of

time, and shows the desirability of avoiding the addition of any form of sulphurous acid to products intended for human food.

Several years ago, Germany, which has an old-fashioned idea that the health of its people is of more importance than the wealth of its manufacturers, forbade the admission of California dried fruits unless they contained only a very small amount of sulphur.

Whenever the sulphuring of dried fruit has been criticized or threatened by law, the California fruit packers have claimed that to forbid this practice would ruin a great California industry. This would certainly be a bad thing, although not so bad as the injuring of the health of hundreds of thousands of people. Such a calamity need not, however, now follow the non-sulphuring of fruits.

The demand for dried fruits and vegetables that will meet the requirements of the pure food laws has been a question of vital interest to the fruit and vegetable grower for several years. What is desired more than anything else is a dried fruit free from sulphur or other chemicals. This can be secured by using the "LIKEFRESH" SYSTEM OF FRUIT PRESERVATION invented by William H. Swett, now of Berkeley, Cal. The process is called "Likefreshing" because the article preserved in this manner regains its original color and flavor when placed in water or cooked in the ordinary way.

The "Likefresh" system, which is based on scientific principles hitherto entirely overlooked will revolutionize the dried fruit industry of the Pacific Coast, besides doing away with the objectionable sulphuring of fruit in order to preserve its color at the cost of its natural flavor.

The ideas of the inventor are incorporated in an evaporating apparatus which dries almost any food product perfectly and completely within twenty-four hours, without deterioration of color, flavor or nutritive value.

Heat energy, if properly applied, has no power to change chemically the quality of any organic material, but improperly applied it causes the deterioration through a geometrical arrangement of the molecules of the cell structure, thus permitting the admixture of the oxygen of the air with the constituent parts any material being dried, producing by the combination a deleterious effect and until investigators familiarize themselves with heat energy effects, they will not be able to perfect a drying apparatus that will dry fruits or vegetables and retain their nutritive elements without impairment.

This system is meeting the indorsement of scientific men and creating intense interest not alone among fruit growers and truck farmers, but packers, canners and consuming public as well. The soil and the climatic conditions necessary to grow fine fruit are not found in every locality, and the idea of a system that will allow the less favored localities the

TREE-RIPENED FLORIDA

ORANGES
GRAPEFRUIT
TANGERINES

Direct From TREE to Your TABLE

We are sure you will be highly pleased with a box of our very best fruit. Being tree ripened, the quality and flavor is not to be compared with what you buy in stores. Send us your check today and we will ship you by express either of the following, f. o. b. Zellwood, Tangerine, Fla.

No. 1, Full Box Tree-Ripened, Best Quality Oranges, per box, **$5.00; $8.00** from N. Y. Depot.
No. 2, Full Box Tree-Ripened, Best Quality Grapefruit, per box, **$6.00; $9.00** from N. Y. Depot.
No. 3, Full Box Tree-Ripened, Best Quality, Assorted—Half Oranges, Half Grapefruit, per box, **$5.50; $8.50** from N. Y. Depot.
No. 4, Full Box Tree-Ripened, Best Quality, Assorted — Half Tangerines, Half Grapefruit, per box, **$7.00; $10.00** from N. Y. Depot.

This fruit is picked, packed and shipped same day order is received. We use Standard Packing Box, holding 1 3-5 bushels. If fruit is to be prepaid add $2 for express charges.

Adress all orders to

DR. B. LUST, Tangerine, Florida

N. Y. City Office and Depot:
Dr. B. LUST, 110 E. 41st. Street

Benedict Lust established a second Yungborn sanatorium in Tangerine, Florida.

luxury of fresh sanitary fruit and a fruit that is almost as good as the fresh article, appeals to the public mind and demands attention. Pies made from "Likefreshed" apples, peaches, apricots or pumpkin are as good as though made from the fresh article and have been accepted by connoisseurs as fresh product. This is impossible with the ordinary dried fruits. Dried peaches or apricots can be soaked in water for a few hours and served with cream and sugar as fresh fruits.

The inventor has worked many years to perfect a machine, simple and complete, yet economical in its operation and capable of drying fruit and vegetables in commercial quantities. The result of his work is the "LIKE-FRESH EVAPORATOR."

The process is a radical departure from the old lines in which the moisture is driven out by overheated air, which destroys the cell structure. Our drying is by evaporation which does not change the cell structure nor cause waste by dripping and leaves the fruit in its original condition with the water extracted.

The Carqué Pure Food Co., 1607 Magnolia Av., Los Angeles, Cal., has undertaken to introduce the "Likefresh" Fruits and is in the position to offer a limited amount of the 1912 crop of "Likefresh" fruits, such as figs, peaches, pears, prunes, apples, etc., and will furnish samples and prices on application, also give further information about the "Likefresh" Evaporators.

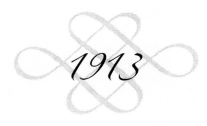

1913

THE NATUROPATH AND HERALD OF HEALTH'S

Apyrotropher

Section

DEVOTED TO

**APYROTROPHY—the Science, Art and Practice of Living
on the Moral Unfired Diet for the Perpetuation
of Perfect Health and Cure of Disease.**

It is also the organ of the Apyrotropher (*Unfired-fooder*) Society.

Address all communications for this department to its editor,

GEORGE J. DREWS, AL.D., 3220 Thomas Street, CHICAGO, ILLINOIS

JANUARY, 1913

The masthead for the first issue of the Apyrotrophy section in *The Naturopath and Herald of Health,* January, 1913

A Plea For An Apyrotropher Society

by Mrs. Helen Sherry, Associate Editor, Alamogordo, N.M.

The Naturopath and Herald of Health, XVIII(1), 50-52. (1913)

This is an age of organization. Whenever a group of men find that they have united under the canopy of a single important idea they seem to recall the maxim, that "in union there is strength" and at once issue a call for the clans of the idea to come together. Having foregathered they lose no time giving themselves a local habitation and a name.

As there are now scattered over the world, in two hemispheres, thousands of men and women who are deeply convinced that a diet of unfired foods is the only one which is absolutely correct, health-giving and founded on scientific research of the most painstaking and authentic character, it now behooves them to effect such a union of forces as will materially increase their numbers and help promulgate the dietary doctrines dear to them.

When you approach a man with a view of gaining his assent to a new doctrine he usually asks you what you can offer him as a compensation for abandoning rooted beliefs and cherished practices. To such inquiries we would reply: The advantages of Apyrotrophy fall naturally into three divisions, physical, metaphysical and economic. That is to say, the feeding on unfired foods affects a man's body, his mind, his soul and his material conditions.

When we consider its effect upon his body we are at once reminded of the poet's happy thought,

"We are what suns and skies

And winds and waters make us."

Without launching into a long series of proofs of this fact we may briefly refer to the Georgia clay-eaters, the cretinism of certain Alpine regions and the leprosy of the Orient as illustrations of what the physical conditions surrounding man can do to modify his bodily frame.

If the elements which merely surround man have so much influence on his being, how much more must those elements which he takes into his body, and which go to the building up and repair of tissue, help to make or mar his life!

But a prospective proselyte in a mood of resistance, may here object: "You preach the eating of fruits and vegetable and all the natural products of the soil, in preference to meats which are always likely to prove injurious. Behold! I am already a vegetarian, and by seeking to indoctrinate me you are but carrying coals to Newcastle."

"Nay, nay, friend, we answer, we are not satisfied with eating the products of the soil; we must have them in their natural condition, not sodden or cremated. We must have all the organic salts which they contain in their *unfired state*. The action of heat, as a rule, utterly destroys all the organic salts. It is not enough for us to eat the *right things*; we must eat them in the *right way*, while they are yet in their right form, that is, a form in which their contents are capable of subserving in the highest degree the nutrition of the tissues. The vegetarian of the old school acquiesces, like the cooked-meat-eater, in the destruction of the nutritive value of his food before he ingests it. The *new vegetarian* wants his food with all its nutritive value to the system, that is to say, he wants it uncooked, or unfired, and for that he calls himself an Unfired Fooder, or, in Greek, an Apyrotropher.

The old style vegetarianism has, indeed, done some good in its day by banishing from the dietary that mass of cooked and toughened animal fibre with which the advocate of cooked meats fills his digestive tract. This was, and is still, fertile in rheumatism, fibrous and malignant tumors and many other diseases. It, however, leaves so much to be desired as a sound dietary that there are no words for it. The next great step which vegetarianism needed to take has now been taken by the inventors of the unfired food system. Let us fall in and keep step with them. Their efforts, so valuable to the race, deserves this at our hands.

But food ingested into the body of man reacts not only upon his body but upon his mind and soul as well. To those who might be inclined to deny the effect of a system of feeding upon man's faculties and his intellectual career we ask leave to submit a few facts. Let us begin our observations on her who prepares the food for us—the too little known and appreciated housewife. We hear much from a class of not unduly ambitious women of the too absorbing duties of the household. The appalling drudgery of cooking, added to the care which the cleanliness of a house requires and aggravated by the rapidly intermittent periods of illness which are apt to swoop without warning, on the average home, making the care of a house a horror instead of pleasure. The unremitting cry goes up from thousands of overburdened and sorrowing mothers (for many of them must yet bury their dead ones) that there is no time left for education or culture.

If, then, this is true, and no genuine observer of things human will call into question, who can measure the good that would accrue to humanity from a system of diet that would have—even as a sole advantage over a previous one—that of being prepared in but half the time and with much greater ease? This alone would enable the housewife to cultivate her mind in a manner befitting the dignity of her position. This precious opportunity Apyrotrophy would most surely secure for her.

Not the mother alone but other members of the family are as likely to share in the cultural disasters which too often attend a vicious system of diet. The too frequent tale of men and women is that premature illness and death on the part of mother or father—brought about by malnutrition—had forced them to suspend their scarcely-begun education and go to work just at the moment when formal instruction would have been of most avail. Would not, then, any system of diet be a blessing which would make all men and women strong and sound and able to bear all the burdens of parenthood, and continue bearing them until such time as the children, which they have taken the responsibility of bringing into the world, have been properly equipped to face, in their turn, the battle of life; not thrust, feeble and unprepared, unto that grueling struggle to which, even under the best conditions, far too many succumb before the allotted time? Would it not be a grand cause to fight for, that which should give all men the only foundation possible for an effective career?

What this wrecking of careers has meant to the race in the higher and finer walks of life we all too well know. Indeed, it needs no argument to show that the purest and loftiest plans for the improvement of mankind are all houses built on sand when not accompanied by bodily health sufficient to secure the energetically laboring faculties against the misfortune of suddenly tottering and falling, never to rise again. How often do we read that men and women, nobly exerting themselves for the good of the race, have fallen by the wayside from premature exhaustion, with nobody to take their empty places in the human ranks, mankind mourning the while the irretrievable loss of its workers and friends!

In spite of the many proofs that the Anglo-Saxon race has given of its sharing the universal fallibility of mankind, it yet remains true that they are conspicuously a moral people, that is to say, the moral pre-occupation is always at hand in their consideration of any proposition presented to them. Indeed, it is in the name of the moral effects attending them that so many metaphysical sects have recently made their way with them, even to the superseding of ancient and deep-rooted religions. In their eyes, therefore, it will add to the value of this movement (for a more rational and sane dietary) that it penetrates the soul with that religious feeling which attends all work of self-denial, for the man who can and will forswear ancient practices, sanctioned by time and the most tender associations, is a man in whom the moral fibre is exceedingly strong—a man against whose firm stand against time-honored evil the very gates of hell shall not prevail! And such self-denial is required by the complete revolution which the new diet entails, that highest order of self-denial which is at the root of all true religion. Besides other advantages of more material character, therefore, an apyrothroper has the satisfaction of feeling that he has added immeasurably to his moral stature. He is a better, healthier and, mentally, a saner man than he ever was before.

If further points were required to this argument we might call attention to the results of investigation in that department of psychology which treats of the origin of the criminal instincts. The criminologist tells us to-day, in accents that grow deeper and more authoritative as time passes, that the bad man is a sick man, and jurisprudence, following suit, now treats him at the hospital and no longer by means of scourges and dungeons.

Truth to tell, the moral point of view has more angels than we can well take account of within our limits. Let us, however, consider this one: Is not embezzlement of mere money, which but deprives a man of material goods, regarded as a vastly immoral act? But how can it compare with that more tragic form of the crime which consists in the wanton waste by a parent of the bodily vigor which it is his most sacred duty to transmit intact to his offspring; for it is the only physical capital which they have to build their own lives upon, and if, by vicious diet, the parent has vitiated and rotted his tissues what hope can there be for the innocent and helpless victims of such spoliation? Here, again, Apyrotrophy comes to the rescue. It will strengthen the parent so that he will transmit a pure blood stream and strong nerves and muscles to his offspring, and the same diet followed in their turn by the children will maintain the physical advantages bestowed by the parent, thus forming an enormous capital of bodily energy to hand down to the third generation.

In these days of burning economic questions it will surely not be amiss to add to our list another point of merit to the system advocated here, and call attention to the fact that Apyrotrophy will greatly lessen the cost of living. For the burden of the buyer's bill of charge lies not in the real necessities of life, but rather in the injurious luxuries of the table—hot bread, rich sauces, fritters, puddings, pies, cakes and the liver racking candy confections that greet us every where, to say nothing of the market-meats, most of which are either poisoned by disease, cold storage or the injection of harmful antiseptics. If Apyrotrophy did but make living cheaper it would certainly confer an inestimable boon upon society as now constituted and burdened.

If, then, to summarize, we have shown that, besides adding to the normal nature and intellectual opportunities of man, the unfired diet is both easier and prompter of preparation, healthier and more economical than its predecessor in popular favor, it must be allowed that we have justified our propaganda.

Let us, then, all join hands together in the new generous emulation for the building up of a finer and stronger race, let us erect, as a temple to our endeavor and our cause this Society of Apyrotrophers and make our bedside book of this little magazine, which shall be the medium for communicating thought and sentiment, fresh visions and discoveries along new lines of feeding advocated in its pages. Let it be to us the sacred tie that binds!

Do You "Troph"?

by Mrs. Helen Sherry

The Naturopath and Herald of Health, XVII(2), 124-126. (1913)

"Do you 'troph'?" was the heading of an article published by the *Chicago World*, the *Los Angeles Record* and a number of other papers.

The reporter of one of these papers paid us a visit one fine day last summer, took a few snapshots and wrote the article from which we will here quote a portion.

"It's the way to health. The eating plan of Dr. Drews: Raise vegetables in your little back yard, turn your kitchen into a 'trophery,' eat your garden stuff unfired, and laugh at the doctors and the food trust."

Dr. Drews has the sovereign remedy for the high cost of living. "Trophing," he calls it.

Vulgarly speaking, the remedy is "greens." They must be eaten green, though. That's half the secret. Greens eaten green turn the trick.

A plot of ground twelve feet square will produce all the green vegetables that two people can eat in eight months of the year, says Dr. Drews.

He has proved it. Also, he has proved to his own satisfaction, at least, that cooked foods aren't fit for human beings to eat. His clear eye and healthy skin back up his words.

In his back yard he grows three times as much green stuff as the whole household can eat.

The doctor will show you his twenty-five by forty-foot garden. It's a most astonishing garden. It's pretty safe to say that there isn't another just like it in the world.

Here are rows upon rows of green stuff, scores of different kinds of vegetables and synede (salad) plants, some familiar, some that you have heard of, but have never seen before, and some you never even heard of.

Here a row of endive, there a row of sorrel; here a row of upland cress, there one of nasturtiums; here a row of ice plants, there one of corn salad; here a bed of dandelions, there a vigorous row of white mustard—a botanical garden—but it's really a severely practical trophery (none-firing kitchen) garden with a view to furnishing a regular procession of synede (salad) leaves and green vegetables from April till frost.

With these green things for "roughage" and tonic elements, nuts for protein, unfired nut and cereal bread, (which he calls "artos"), fruits, honey instead of sugar, and some olive oil, Dr. Drews makes up his "natural" diet.

He holds that cooked food is unnatural, that the chemical make-up of the food is perverted by cooking, that the organic salts have been freed, mineralized and neutralized, and that cooked food is thus disposed to fermentation and further decay in the stomach and intestines; thus being the cause of auto-intoxication.

As for meat, he holds that it is only for hyenas to eat, since it is necessarily charged with animal refuse and with injurious acids and alkaloids—in other words, is at best, but a form of carrion.

The basis of his "piece de resistance" dishes is a meal of four courses consisting of an eupos (health drink), a synede (saltless salad), a relish and a meliart (unfired bread).

THE TROPHERY GARDEN

Now is the time when all nature-loving people of the Northern Hemisphere should commence to plan their trophery (kitchen) garden. Seed catalogues should be sent for and a list of vegetable seeds should be made from them.

The proposed garden plot should be measured and a plan be drawn for the early sowing. No matter how small the piece of ground is that you can spare for vegetables; it can always be made a source of health preserving food.

Those who have the experience know that vegetables absolutely fresh from the trophery garden have a flavor far superior and more delicate than any that can be produced in the market. Last spring we had crisp and sweet cultivated dandelions, under glass protection, twelve inches tall of the first of March. On the fifteenth of April we had white mustard four inches tall, ready to be cut for synede (salad) greens; while all the other vegetables sown at the same time were less than one inch and a half. The reason for this early crop of white mustard, is because this vegetable grows three times as fast as any other cultivated vegetable. This is the sweetest and mildest of all the mustards grown for greens and it does not develop any stringy fibre until the seed commences to develop.

If you do not wish the weeds to grow ahead of the vegetables, then sow early, say, between April the first and fifth and between the fifteenth and nineteenth. If you sow between first and the fifth of May the soil must not be spaded, plowed and raked longer than a day or two before the sowing or the weed will get ahead of the vegetables.

The reason for sowing between the above-mentioned dates is that a rain generally follows these periods to help the vegetables to sprout before the weeks; whereas, if you sow before these dates the weeds sprout before the vegetables.

The lots in the larger cities are generally so small that there is very little room for the cultivation of synede herbs and roots. Every family in the city should cultivate at least two hundred square feet of fertile soil for food of a plot ten by twenty feet. Such an area judiciously cultivated and arranged can produce all the synede greens and roots an average

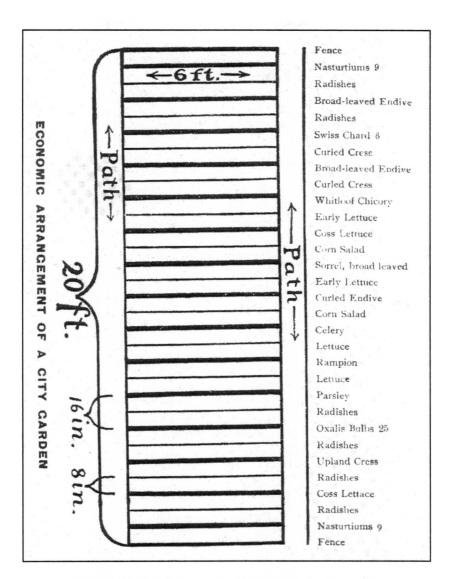

Diagram showing the economic arrangement of a city garden.

family may require, for their health, throughout the spring, summer and autumn.

Study the following diagram and note how the late vegetables are alternated with the early ones to make a perpetual garden. In place of the rampion and corn salad sow white mustard and take notice how much faster it grows than the other vegetables; but be sure to have it cut and eaten before it is twelve inches tall.

Take notice that every other row is lettuce, radishes, curled cress, or white mustard. These rows should be used up before they crowd the later and larger herbs. The nasturtiums, Swiss chard, Whiloof chicory, sorrel, celery and parsley are late herbs and require the space of the other three rows after the early vegetables are out. Sow the chicory, sorrel, celery, parsley, cress and white mustard closely in a drill, traced with the finger. Plant two seeds of nasturtium every six or eight inches. Plant four Swiss chard seed every ten inches and when the plants are six inches high cut the three smallest ones away and leave the largest ones grow until the mature leaves can be broken from the side. The oxalis bulbs should be planted two or three inches apart. The radishes should be sown in the drill so that the seeds come about a half to an inch apart. The lettuce must be sown dense enough that the sparrows can take a few sprouts also. Do not cut the celery and parsley off like chives, but break away the mature and drooping leaves from the side of the rows as they grow. The young leaves should not be picked or cut off the plant unless you wish to kill it or retard its later growth.

If the troph (food-preparer) will practice a little economy there will be no old leaves to waste, because she will have used them before they are old. If the garden is large enough it is advisable to cultivate a bed of dandelions and sour dock for early spring synedes to be grown under glass from the first of February till the night frosts are over.

Carrots, turnips, kohl-rabi, salsify (oyster plant) and parsnips should not be forgotten in a larger garden. Jerusalem artichokes may grow in a waste corner of the garden. Tomatoes, cucumbers, and sweet potatoes need more space than the city garden can afford. If there is room for these last then do not forget dahlias for their delicious tubers. The dahlia tuber for food will have to be introduced by the apyrotrophers (unfired fooders) because this tuber is delicious only in the unfired state.

For a closer description and preparation of the above mentioned vegetables see *Unfired Food.*

A plot of ground twelve feel square will produce all the green vegetables that two people can eat in eight months of the year, says Dr. Drews.

The Cruciferae

by George J. Drews

The Naturopath and Herald of Health, XVIII(3), 201-204. (1913)

The Cruciferae or cross-bearing vegetables and flowers are a family of plants which have four petals arranged like the arms of a cross. This family of plants presents itself in greater variety of form than any other family known. It is practically the largest edible family of plants which supplies man with more variety of food than any other family of plants and of which every variety is wholesome.

All the following vegetables and flowers are Cruciferae, i.e., the cresses, the mustards, the cabbages, the kales, the radishes, the turnips, the kohlrabis, the cauliflowers and many ornamental plants of which, later, both the leaves and especially the flowers may be used as food.

The water cress is such a well-known plant that a description of its uses is almost superfluous. The Paris market is always abundantly supplied with it. Apyrotrophers (unfired-fooders) use it, chopped, as an ingredient of aesthetic synedes (ornamental salads) or as the foundation of nut synedes. For the preparation of aesthetic synedes see *Unfired Food* page 142. The nut and cress synede is composed of four ounces of chopped cress and two ounces of finely ground unroasted peanuts or other nuts, and the cress, mixed with the nuts or separate, may be dressed with either honey, lemon juice or oil or a combination of these according to taste.

The Upland or Belle Isle cress resembles water cress in both the shape of its leaves and its flavor. This cress can be cultivated in any trophery (kitchen) garden. It is used in synedes just like water cress.

Curled garden cress, common garden cress, broad-leaved cress and golden garden cress differ in the shape and color of their leaves, but they have the same pungent flavor as the water cress and are used just like it. These may be sown broadcast or in drills, and will thrive in any trophery garden.

There are five or more varieties of rock cresses, cultivated for ornamental purposes, but the apyrotropher uses its tender fleshy leaves and also its flowers for synedes.

Scurvy grass is well known as an anti-scorbutic plant, but it is no less wholesome for all. The leaves of this plant resemble those of water cress and are equally useful for synedes.

Let us say right here that the whole family of Cruciferae has anti-scorbutic properties when eaten unfired in synedes.

Rocket salad has leaves which resemble those of radishes, but are more fleshy and pungent.

The leaves of Turkish rocket resemble those of horse radish, but are

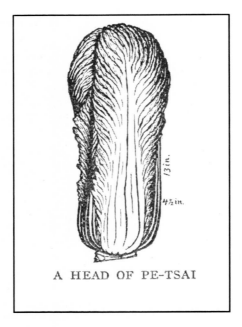

A HEAD OF PE-TSAI

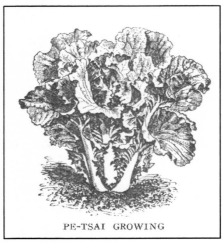

PE-TSAI GROWING

A head of Pe-tsai and its growing.

more tender. This plant is highly spoken of as a trophery garden plant, because it is a hardy perennial and commences to grow very early in spring, where other fresh green vegetables are scarce, resisting both cold weather and drought. This plant is as easily grown as chicory.

The blanched leaf stalks of sea kale make good synedes, but this plant should be only cultivated by truck farmers.

Sea rocket grows wild on northern lake shores. The tender and fleshy leaflets and tops may be gathered for synedes and prepared like water cress which it resembles in flavor.

The black and brown seeded mustards, the Chinese cabbage-leafed mustard and Chinese curled mustard make wholesome synede material, but for trophery gardens we prefer to advise the cultivation of white mustard, which is milder and more tender than the other varieties of mustard. Provided that all vegetables are sown on the same day, the white mustard will have grown three inches when other vegetables have only grown one inch at most. It never develops fibre in its stem until it goes to seed; therefore, the stems of white mustard are as desirable for synede material as the leaves.

There is a Chinese tuberous-rooted mustard of which the leaves and the radish-like roots are equally desirable for synede material.

In 1904 there were 64 varieties of radishes cultivated in France with as many descriptions. It is unnecessary to say anything about the use of radishes except that the extremest pungency of the hottest radish is reduced to a pleasant warmth by eating it, together with whole or ground unfired peanuts. The leaves of radishes may also be used for greens.

There are also about 64 varieties of turnips. These very few people know how to use uncooked except the apyrotrophers who shred then on a fluted grater for their synedes. When the turnips are not yet fully developed their leaves make good synede material.

There are also eight varieties of turnip-rooted cabbages which develop large roots instead of heads.

More than seventy varieties of smooth-leaved cabbages and seventeen varieties of crimped cabbages are cultivated. You do not deserve to be called, much less eutroph (unfired food artist) if you could not prepare a tasty and tempting synede of a scant cupful of chopped cabbage, a heaping spoonful of chopped onion, to fill the cup, one-half of a lemon which contains a spoonful of peanut oil or olive oil, as much ground caraway seed as will lay on a five-cent piece, a pinch of curry powder and two spoonfuls of water if the combination is too dry. This quantity is a full portion for one person.

There are three varieties of Chinese cabbage of which the "Improved Heading Chinese (or Pe-tsai) Cabbage" is the best for vigorous and rapid growth. It can be recommended as a winter vegetable for mild climates.

The leaves are large, light green, and curved at the edge; the rib is broad and white, only slightly bare at the base. The first leaves are spreading and curved outwards, the later ones cover one another like those of Cos lettuce, and form a fine, tall head, weighing easily four pounds and over. It should be sown during summer for use in the autumn and winter. This cabbage is milder and more crisp than other cabbages.

The editor prepared pe-tsai as given above for cabbage and was delighted with it. Pe-tsai was sent to Chicago from California during December and January. Those retailers who called it "celery-cabbage" and "French lettuce" sold it at 15 cents per pound, but the Bosto store called it Chinese cabbage and sold it at 5 cents per pound. We will send enough seed of this cabbage to the readers of this magazine, to try it out on receipt of 15 cents in stamps.

The twenty-five varieties of kale; dwarf, tall, curled, smooth, and ornamental; develop their best flavor after they have received frost. On account of their hardiness and compactness of leaf tissue they make a very substantial food, much relished by apyrotrophers.

Brussels sprouts are only another form of cabbage which develops many small heads at the axils of the leaves instead of one large head.

In the approximately forty-eight varieties of cabbage known as cauliflowers and broccoli, it is the flower stems which have been artificially modified in the course of cultivation. The flowers have almost been rendered abortive, and the bractlets, which bear them, have gained in thickness what they have lost in length, form a regular solid corymb, which is seldom interrupted by small leaves growing through it. The thick and tender floral bractlets form the generally known edible part, but we wish to say that the leaf stems also make a desirable food as they are sweeter than the corymb. The corymb, for synedes, may be shredded on a fluted grater and the leaf stems may be sliced or chopped across the grain.

The flowers and leaves of sweet alyssum, candytuft and sweet rocket, cultivated only for ornaments, are perfectly wholesome, but they are, rather, too pungent for most people.

The wall flower is also a Cruciferae.

The last but not less important for food are all the varieties of stocks, also called gilliflowers. The leaves of these plants are no more pungent than water cress, but a little more substantial and when prepared like water cress with ground peanuts, a trace of lemon juice and oil make a perfectly delicious synede. The double flowers of these plants we cannot speak of too highly, as they are tender, slightly sweet and have only a desirable trace of pungency which can hardly be detected when combined with ground nuts. These flowers, of any color, when chopped, may be used as an ingredient of the aesthetic synede, referred to above, or they may be used whole as an edible garish, planted artistically over the synede.

Many people think that it is a sin to eat beautiful and delicate flowers, but they forget that this sin cannot be compared with the taking of sentient life, nor can the partaking of dead food be compared with it; for even the Bible says "he that partaketh of death shall surely die."

The Cruciferae or cross-bearing vegetables and flowers are a family of plants which have four petals arranged like the arms of a cross. This family of plants presents itself in greater variety of form than any other family known. It is practically the largest edible family of plants which supplies man with more variety of food than any other family of plants and of which every variety is wholesome.

All the following vegetables and flowers are Cruciferae, i.e., the cresses, the mustards, the cabbages, the kales, the radishes, the turnips, the kohlrabis, the cauliflowers and many ornamental plants of which, later, both the leaves and especially the flowers may be used as food.

In 1904 there were 64 varieties of radishes cultivated in France with as many descriptions.

More than seventy varieties of smooth-leaved cabbages and seventeen varieties of crimped cabbages are cultivated.

CURLED DOCK

by George J. Drews

The Naturopath and Herald of Health, XVIII(4), 266. (1913)

From the standpoint of diet the apyrotrophers are the most economical people known, for they know how to use to best advantage every fruit, every wholesome wild and cultivated vegetable, the nuts and even the flowers of wholesome plants.

Nearly everywhere in the northern states, next to the dandelion, in the woods, in the meadows, in the waste fields, in the waste lots of cities, in the back yards, in the hedges and by the roadside grows the curled or yellow dock.

This dock comes to usefulness about the same time as the dandelion and like the last, it is an excellent spring tonic food. It is, like spinach, rich in all the essential organic salts for toning the blood and for aiding the kidneys and the other glands in eliminating from the blood and tissues accumulated impurities, wastes and irritants.

The leaves of this dock are from 6 inches to 12 inches long, tapering towards both ends and about one and one-half inches wide. The surface and the edges of the leaves are sometimes slightly crimpt and this is all the reason why it is called curled dock. The flavor of the leaves is acid at first taste, but the acidity quickly leaves when the leaf is properly masticated and then changes into a pleasant bread-like flavor.

Bitter dock looks like curled dock in every respect except that its leaves are twice as wide and has no acid flavor.

The curled dock plant can be forced to furnish tender leaves during summer and fall when prevented from running to seed. When you must go far to get curled dock then gather enough for a few days and on arriving home place the leaves, stem end down, into a bucket containing about two or three inches of water and let it stand in a cool place.

There is nothing in dock roots that is superior tonic food than what the system can get from the leaves.

[Curled Dock] is, like spinach, rich in all the essential organic salts for toning the blood and for aiding the kidneys and the other glands in eliminating from the blood and tissues accumulated impurities, wastes and irritants.

Building Brain By Diet

by Dortch Campbell

The Naturopath and Herald of Health, XVIII(11), 727-728. (1913)

To me this is one of the most fascinating studies in the realms of heal-ing—the construction of mental power through the judicious use of foods, for I believe that it is pregnant with great possibilities for the happi-ness of mankind. During the last ten or fifteen years I have made a sincere investigation of this subject and my efforts have been amply rewarded, yet I have been shown that the field is practically without any limit.

Many people ridicule the idea that there is such a thing as "brain food," that is, that certain kinds of foods nourish the brain. This belief is, moreover, not confined to the average layman. Some well-known inves-tigators say there is no such thing as "brain food," neither flesh nor fowl, yet admitting, for the most part, that brawn-food exists. Of course, we are all aware of the ancient superstition of the value of fish for brain nour-ishment. As a matter of fact, the idea is not entirely without foundation, being founded, perhaps, on a physiological idea of the phorphorus in fish as well as in brain-substance.

As for those who ridicule the statement of "brain food," I, for one, know that they have been somewhat premature, inasmuch as my inves-tigations have shown me that there is nourishment for brain as well as body, that certain elements build up gray-matter equally as well as other elements bring about muscular activity.

Even the tyro in health theories knows that a man can not be muscu-larly strong on fruit of the juicy kind and green vegetables, such as lettuce, onions, etc., or bread by itself. This being so—and none deny it—can not it be true also that certain foods build up the mental machinery of a person?

I am not arguing for Sophie Leppel dietary, although I have the great-est respect for this former English food scientist, who taught the necessity of so called "brain-foods." I simply state as a fact that there are: Foods—for fat, energy, heat, muscular activity, brain-power, elimination.

Apparently, however, there has been a grievous mistake in the advo-cacy of a "brainy diet" so-called. Having proved that there are special foods that nourish the brain, advocates of this dietary have swung the pendulum to the extreme and have concluded, therefore, that mentality—brain-power—depends entirely on brain foods.

Brain integrity depends on foods that nourish, or build up the brain; depends on those elements in the vegetable world that nourish the body.

As for mental endurance and intelligence—which for a good many persons is the all-important thing—this depends primarily, or, at least, partly, on other factors of living, such, for instance, as sleep and rest, the process of recuperation.

Still one can not build up the mental machinery for enduring work without foods that properly nourish the brain. Oftentimes, moreover, the lack of mind endurance—the power to work with the brain—is due to an absence of the "soluble phosphates" that nourish the gray-matter "inside the head" and along the spinal way. It behooves us, therefore, to thoroughly understand the science of "selection, combination and pro-portioning" of foods, through which one may learn the process of brain as well as body building.

There are good and bad brain foods, as well as weak and strong. Good, because they nourish the mental apparatus without wasting the energy of the brain; bad, because they dissipate mind strength. Foods that build the brain are: Lean meats, fish, milk, eggs, cheese, beans, peas, len-tils, nuts, and, in the highest, most psychic sense, certain kinds of fruits.

Nuts are the best brain foods. To get full benefit, however, they should be properly combined with other foods, eaten at meal time only, taken in average quantities and thoroughly masticated. One can rarely learn to eat for brain nourishment—in the very highest, or the most perfect, sense—without a competent instructor.

Generally, the persons who know that special kinds of foods nourish the brain think that meat is the best food for that purpose. This error is unwarranted and grows out of the fact that flesh foods are most easily digested by the present stomach, which is abnormal. The average diges-tive apparatus has fallen away from its original strength. The average individual, therefore, can not digest nuts until he has developed a normal stomach.

I can recommend lean, tender flesh foods to persons whose vitality is greatly lowered and to the aged and infirm, but not as an ideal brain-food. Why flesh foods are not suitable for man's use have been so thoroughly explained in this publication that I see no need of further elucidating this point.

One often finds when illness is extreme that flesh foods must be con-tinued; that nuts can not be digested. This is not to the discredit of nuts as an ideal brain-food, rather it is to the discredit of the average man's digestive machinery. In other words, the abnormal stomach can best, in illness, at least, handle that to which it has been accustomed, an abnormal brain-food, but train the stomach to normal strength and it will spurn flesh-foods, digesting readily the various kinds of real nut brain-foods.

As for peas, beans, cheese, lentils, etc., they are even inferior to flesh-foods as brain-builders. This class of brain-builders is very difficult to digest, even by the normal stomach, and, therefore, should not be used.

Milk is a delightful and nourishing food and is, moreover, of benefit in a mono-diet. It is not the best, however, for brain-workers, as it is "weak" for that purpose, being more suitable for infant brains.

Eggs are strong as brain nourishment, but the yolk seems to have an aging effect when used constantly, hence eggs are excluded somewhat from our dietary.

That leaves us, therefore, for the very best brain foods—pecans, filberts, walnuts, almonds, butternuts, pine-nuts, etc., etc.

Fruits such as pears, apricots, grapes, apples, etc., are more like psychic food than brain-builders and, therefore, can not be used for our purpose—the construction of the animal brain. They help to develop our higher powers and natures when not used as anti-toxic, purifying and eliminating foods.

There are good and bad brain foods, as well as weak and strong. Good, because they nourish the mental apparatus without wasting the energy of the brain; bad, because they dissipate mind strength. Foods that build the brain are: Lean meats, fish, milk, eggs, cheese, beans, peas, lentils, nuts, and, in the highest, most psychic sense, certain kinds of fruits.

The very best brain foods—pecans, filberts, walnuts, almonds, butternuts, pine-nuts, etc., etc.

1914

EUGENE CHRISTIAN—THE FOOD SCIENCE DOCTOR
VALDEMAR BLAD

EDIBLE THISTLES
GEORGE J. DREWS

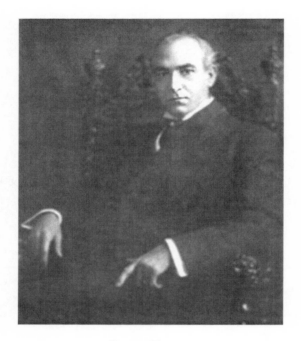

Eugene Christian.

Eugene Christian—The Food Science Doctor

by Valdemar Blad

The Naturopath and Herald of Health, XIX(9), 605-606. (1914)

We live in an age of specialists. Scattered throughout the country, each in his own workshop and with a definite plan of his special task fixed in his mind, are thousands of sincere, tireless men (women too), engaged in forming and perfecting the parts which in due course are to be fitted into each other as a new social structure.

Clumsy, obsolete and unsatisfactory, diseased and impotent, dusty, wrinkles, pathetic, all forlorn, the old system lies at the mercy of the scrutinizing gaze of the advanced modern thinker who, with Edison, has succeeded in penetrating beneath the surface of things, watching with amazement the hidden clockwork of human and universal life as it has wound and unwound from the beginning of time.

Edison as the wizard of electricity has shown that we stand on the threshold of discoveries which will show that human life, thoughts, emotions, passions, impulses, actions, health and diseases in their every manifestation are and have always been controlled and operated by the natural laws of the universe.

Eugene Christian, for twenty years in modest seclusion, has faithfully devoted his life to the mission of discovering the chemistry of the human body, the chemistry of food and the method of uniting these two branches of science. His work has been directed toward ascertaining how to select, combine and proportion food so as to build up both the mental and physical vitality to the highest degree of energy the body is capable of taking; in other words, to produce a condition in which all the functions of the body would work harmoniously together and produce that joyous, luxurious state known as youth and health—the capacity for thinking and doing—the mastering of self and problems.

There are many other forces in Nature which Dr. Christian recognizes as important factors in removing the causes of disease and producing health, but food he claims is one of the most important.

Food supplies the raw material from which the body is constructed. After life is created it must depend for its growth and development upon nutrition. This is one subject that up to date scientists and the world in general have given very little attention.

Men, more than all other animals, have eaten at random and have therefore built up their bodies entirely by guess work. Dr. Christian's work has been directed wholly toward ascertaining what food is and its true purpose, how to select it, how to combine it and how to proportion it so as to make it produce specific results when taken into the body.

Dr. Christian has shown that when food is properly selected and administered, and eaten according to one's age, occupation and the time of the year, it will, in the great majority of cases, produce a perfectly normal result; that is, all the organs of digestion and assimilation as well as those of elimination will work in harmony and automatically. He has further shown that when they work automatically or without expression it is evidence of health, but that the moment there is any evidence of disturbance certain changes should be made so as to prevent that abnormal condition called disease.

Dr. Christian in his various works has also shown that food has a most direct effect and influence upon the morals. He has shown that the history of primitive man was mostly a history of strife and bloodshed. Wars of conquest and cruelty were the most important events in his national life. Up to a few centuries ago man with a few exceptions was a fighting animal. He knew of no way to enforce his opinions, to secure his desires or distinguish himself except by the sword, but the human mind has undergone and is still undergoing a great change and within a few years from today internecine wars such as are now appalling the civilized world will be a thing of the past and the instruments with which he kills his fellow creatures will in the coming true civilization be exhibited as relics of barbarism.

It is well known among dog breeders and trainers that a flesh diet will cause these docile animals to become vicious and will generally tend toward the development of the fighting instinct; likewise with people whose diet is largely composed of the flesh of other animals (which must be obtained by killing). They are not shocked by killing and after a while they will naturally take on the instincts of the carnivora which is to kill and subsist and prey upon other forms of life.

War has changed the map of various countries and the government of people. It has extended the dominion of rulers and made nations appear great from the standpoint of primitive fighting man, but true greatness lies in producing the most learned, the most just and the most merciful people, therefore Dr. Christian claims with good reason that the highest civilization cannot be attained unless the diet is perfected, unless people subsist upon true food which must be obtained from the vegetable world.

Dr. Christian has in all probability made of the food question the most profound study of any living man and under conditions that have given him real knowledge instead of theory. Most writers first draw their conclusions from theory—what seems to be true—then various tests are made with various acid solvents on food in glass test tubes. From this purely laboratory work new theories go forth about foods and feeding which have not been proved by experiments in the human body, but with Dr. Christian's work it is different.

After recovering his health he came to New York and began to practice Scientific Dietetics. The human stomach was his crucible; the intestinal tract was his test tube; the gastric juices, bile and pancreatic fluids were his chemicals, and natural food was the thing to be tested and studied while the human body was the delicate machine, the thermometer, as it were, that told accurately the results of every change, every different combination, every different proportion that went into it.

Dr. Christian has compiled and correlated his knowledge and experience in five splendid volumes, constituting the compendium of all his study during his twenty years of actual practice and experience. Two decades of practice as a food specialist and a year spent abroad under the greatest scientists in Europe gave him the opportunity to build up, as it were, this set of books out of proven facts that could never have been secured in any other way.

Encyclopedia of Diet, therefore, comes to the public from the actual field of experience. It is a contribution to the world from that only source which produces great books, namely experience.

Earnest, sincere and unpretentious in his style, Dr. Christian should be read by all students, sick or well, who recognize the supreme importance of food in the economic system of man. His is a great and good life-work, which will lighten the burdens and light a new path for many perplexed minds.

Eugene Christian, for twenty years in modest seclusion, has faithfully devoted his life to the mission of discovering the chemistry of the human body, the chemistry of food and the method of uniting these two branches of science.

The human stomach was his crucible; the intestinal tract was his test tube; the gastric juices, bile and pancreatic fluids were his chemicals, and natural food was the thing to be tested and studied while the human body was the delicate machine, the thermometer, as it were, that told accurately the results of every change, every different combination, every different proportion that went into it.

Dr. Christian has compiled and correlated his knowledge and experience in five splendid volumes, constituting the compendium of all his study during his twenty years of actual practice and experience.

EDIBLE THISTLES

by George J. Drews

The Naturopath and Herald of Health, XIX(12), 832-833. (1914)

From the fifteenth of June until July the common large thistle (Bull T., *Cnicus lanceolatus*) has attained a height of four to six feet and commences to bloom. The base of the stem is about one and a half inches and more in diameter. Such a stem has an edible pith which is about as hard as a young carrot and taste like sweet lettuce. In order to get to the pith the plant is bent to the earth with a stick and then the stem is cut with a sharp knife at the base. The leaves are then sliced from the stem with an upward stroke to prevent being stung by the pricks. The prickless stem is then carefully picked up and the fibrous rind is carefully shelled from the pith to be eaten.

The pith of a large Burdock plant has practically the same sweet flavor as that of the thistle, except that the fibrous rind must be more carefully shelled because it is bitter but not disagreeably so.

In Spain, France, Italy, and Holland a very prickly thistle is cultivated for its lettuce-flavored root which is about one inch thick and ten to twelve inches long. The flavor of this root reminds one of that of sweet milk and in this respect the root is sweeter than the pith of the bull-thistle. It is known as Golden Thistle (*Scolymus hispanicus*). Golden—because of its golden yellow flower.

The first of May we sowed a fifteen foot row of this thistle for an experiment. The first of July we pulled the sturdiest plant which had a root three-fourths of an inch thick and fifteen inches long. The root was tender and could not be described better than has been done above. Since that time we have pulled a plant once a week with roots not quite an inch thick.

In those countries where the ground does not freeze more than an inch the roots can be gathered all winter. This plant is a biennial and the roots can be left in the frozen ground like parsnips and gathered in the early spring until it commences to produce a stem, when the root becomes fibrous. Some of the plants produce a flowering stem the first year. Such plants must be pulled before the stem is six inches tall, because the pith of the root develops woody fibre as the plant grows taller.

One who has never seen nor tasted the root of the Golden Thistle could never rationally expect to find such a delicious root under such cruelly thorny leaves. Those, however, who are experienced in handling the plant, though they have tender hands, can pull it barehanded without being pricked.

They say that this root tastes like oister plant when cooked; but we find it much more delicious in its natural state after it is scrubbed in clean water. The clean roots can be shredded or coarsely grated or thinly sliced and combined in a synede (salad) with lettuce or endive like carrots or parsnips. See *Unfired Food** page 142 for the preparation of an aesthetic synede.

To those whose alimentary canal is not in a perfectly healthy state this root has a mild laxative property; because many essential organic salts are then still in the milky juice from which they can be easily absorbed into the blood stream.

The "vitamines" or "activators" of this plant cannot bear the boiling temperature without being destroyed.

> *One who has never seen nor tasted the root of the Golden Thistle could never rationally expect to find such a delicious root under such cruelly thorny leaves.*

Unfired Food was written and published by George J. Drews in 1912. *Ed.*

Unfired Food and Trophotherapy—By Drews

A Text Book for Nurses, Physicians, Students and Mothers. A book embracing five volumes in one. Contains 325 pages, bound in black cloth and stamped in white foil. Illustrated with 30 halftones and numerous etchings. It takes in the whole field of the Unfired Diet.   **Price $5.15**

The Improved Mono Diet—By Drews

Is based on a one course per meal, so arranged, that it is most valuable for Nature Cure doctors, to give to their patients, and those who want to insure continued health.   **Price, cloth bound, $1.15**

DR. BENEDICT LUST
110 East 41st St., New York, N. Y.

Ad for *Unfired Food and Tropotherapy* and *The Improved Mono Diet* by Drews.

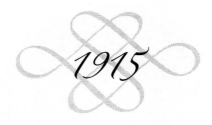

1915

HOW TO EAT DAHLIA TUBERS
GEORGE J. DREWS

LIFE AND DEATH IN DIET
AXIL EMIL GIBSON

SCIENTIFIC DIETETICS—FASTING
R. MOERSHELL

THE DASHEEN
GEORGE J. DREWS, AI.D., D.C.

DULSE AS FOOD
GEORGE J. DREWS, AI.D.

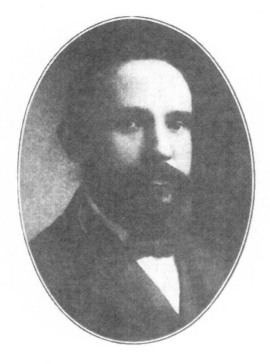

George J. Drews, author of *Unfired Foods* and *Tropho-Therapy* (1912).

How To Eat Dahlia Tubers

by George J. Drews

The Naturopath and Herald of Health, XX(2), 69-70. (1915)

The Dahlia is a genus of plants native to Mexico and Central America, of the order Compositae, of which the fascicled tuberous roots are edible and wholesome.

The plant is named after the Swedish botanist Andrew Dahl, a contemporary with Linnaeus. Dahl introduced this ornamental as well as useful plant as an addition to the common potato.

The following is a quotation from *Unfired Food*, page 292: "The tuberous roots of the dahlia make a most delicious and wholesome food. They are as crisp as the finest young radishes. They have a warm spicy flavor which is at once relished and craved. The tubers may be peeled and cut into sections and served like radishes, or they may be chopped and combined with other vegetables and nuts to form salads. Hereafter that variety which is productive or the finest, the largest and the roundest tubers will be selected and cultivated for food. The most perfect tubers are now found among the red and yellow varieties. In good soil they are as productive as the sweet potato. They will be in great demand when their value is known."

Last spring we had four fascicles of these tubers. We broke each fascicle into three parts by forcing a pointed knife into the hollow of the parental stem and thereby forcing the fascicle into two unequal parts, then we cut the largest part through the stem in two; thus making three or four plants out of each. Then we cut the largest tubers off from each section for food, leaving only one or two small tubers to nourish the young shoots. We planted these sections two feet apart each way. Now in November after the first heavy frost we harvested two bushels of the finest and most shapely dahlia tubers that you ever laid eyes on. The weight of these tubers ranged from four ounces to a pound. We put the tubers into the cellar and covered them with slightly moist sand.

At this point we were interrupted by a call for dinner and we have just enjoyed a large dahlia-buttermilk synede (salad) and it was so satisfactory that we ate nothing else. Last week at this time we enjoyed a synede composed of chopped celery, chopped cabbage, shredded dahlia tuber and flaked peanuts, dressed with a little honey. Yesterday we ate two peeled tubers at noon in place of apples, each weighing about four ounces. Two days ago we had a dahlia supawn introduced by a dahlia posset. The supawn was made as follows: A six ounce dahlia tuber was peeled and grated on a fine grater and four ounces of the juice was strained from this pulp for the posset. This pulp was then combined with two ounces of grated celeriac root, one ounce of cubed banana and an ounce and a half of flaked peanuts and all stirred together and served. To the four ounces of dahlia juice was added a pinch of ground fennel seed and a half teaspoon of honey, stirred and served as posset. This posset would make a very good tonic drink for invalids and those whose stomach needs a rest

Eat the dahlia tuber as you would eat radishes. The majority of people will enjoy the eating of the dahlia tuber most when they will learn to eat it like radishes.

There is hardly any wholesome herb, root, fruit or even nut that someone does not dislike, or that does not give someone distress; but that has nothing to do with the fact that the majority of people may like it and enjoy it with benefit. We have, furthermore, proven that herbs, roots or fruits that cause distress or aversion through idiosyncrasy, inherited characteristics or evil memory of the stomach may be made enjoyable by proper combination to the majority of such cases. The dahlia tuber, in our experience, meets with the same likes and dislikes that other natural edibles are subject to; and we know of a few people who dislike radishes very much, but who enjoy extreme pleasure in eating of this tuber.

The reason why the dahlia tuber has not come into general favor as a wholesome food is because of the inculcated habit and desire to cook everything that grows underground, and since this tuber after being cooked is not a success, it is passed as unfit for food. To a great extent the desire to cook is influenced by the misinformation that uncooked roots are indigestible or unwholesome. Another less effective reason is that some people attach an inexplicable sacredness to plants that are grown as flowers to the extent that they dread to use them as food. We have often come in personal contact with this sacred dread to eat flowers when demonstrating and explaining the palatability and usefulness of the stock and dandelion flowers.

We advise all apyrtrophers who have some cultivatable soil to plant some dahlias for food next spring.* They are easy to cultivate, for they only need a little weeding and howing before they are one foot tall and after that they take care of themselves and besides become quite ornamental with their beautiful flowers before the tubers are ripe. Different from the murphy there is no bug or worm that feeds on the leaves or tubers of the dahlia, hence needs no care or watching after the plant is established.

> *The tuberous roots of the dahlia make a most delicious and wholesome food. They are as crisp as the finest young radishes. They have a warm spicy flavor which is at once relished and craved.*

---

*George Drews adopted another spelling for Apyrotrophers—Apyrtrophers. *Ed.*

Life And Death In Diet

by Axel Emil Gibson, Los Angeles, Cal.

The Naturopath and Herald of Health. XX(2), 99. (1915)

Starvation By Overfeeding

When the famous English suffragette, Emily Pankhurst, introduced fasting as a means of frightening her jailers into submission, she little dreamed that the road to self-destruction leads almost as quickly to the goal by feasting as by fasting. And though we may not realize it, yet so common is suicide by overfeeding, that for each death caused by actual starvation, hundreds are caused by overeating or wrong eating.

A man may so over-indulge in food that it brings about his starvation. Hence not infrequently we starve in the midst of plenty. A dinner made up by incongruous and disharmonious food elements may be so indigestible that the vital expense involved in its digestion overbalances the vital income arising from its assimilation. Hence, so far from food always being a source of health, strength and beauty, it may become a positive cause to sickness, feebleness and ugliness.

But starvation from food is only one of the dangers that arise from indulgence in ill-balanced food mixtures—poisoning, auto-intoxication, is another. For man is what he eats: his blood, his muscles, his several organs, are fundamentally and absolutely at the mercy of the food he puts into his stomach. And if the foods turn into decomposition in place of digestion, corrupting in place of nourishing the body, the nerves, sustained on the poisoned blood, lose their power to safely and sanely conduct the vital force-currents, on which life depends, for its orderly and organized expression. Next thing, we have the system speedily turned into a breeding place and playground for the alien micro-organisms, ever ready to invade a body, whose physiological balance, by unwise modes of living has been broken.

Whether operating inside or outside the body, the laws of chemistry cannot be broken, without subsequent suffering and restitution of the culprit. Certain foods, no matter how healthy in themselves, when indulged at the same meal will generate certain fermentative processes in the stomach. It is from fermentation that those gases are evolved—the alcohol, ammonia, uric, carbonic, oxalic and other toxic acids—which gradually but surely poison the system, and bring about those degenerative changes, known and suffered as catarrh, asthma, bronchitis, rheumatism and neuralgia, with its various forms of nerve racking headaches.

Crazed by repeated poisoning, the nerves gradually lose control, both over themselves and over the physiological processes they are superintending. Digestion is turned into decomposition, assimilation into malnutrition;—in the place of living, healthy tissue, lining the alimentary track, we see the growth of devitalized and devitalizing tissues;—a vicious fungoid or catarrhal covering, spreading like a noxious weed from orifice to orifice, upwards and downward, until every vessel and passage of the body, including the entire alimentary tract, stomach, kidneys, bladder, liver, lungs, pharynx, ear, eye and nose, are all in the grip of this deadly tissue, which like an impenetrable barrier interrupts the vital exchanges between the circulating fluids of nutrition and their absorption. This of course means starvation of the tissues and their eventual breakdown, into established chronic disorders.

NINETY PER CENT OF THE WORLD'S DISEASE ARE DUE TO OVEREATING

It is safe to say that out of the world's diseases ninety per cent are due to errors in diet. For, remember, that every time the stomach is disturbed with gas after eating, processes of fermentation are at work, turning out the fatal death poisons into the system. Remember further that premature weakness and frailty, accompanying an entirely too early old age, is due to the wholesale expenditure of vitality, required by the system in its life-and-death struggle in holding its own, over and against the swarms of bacteria, envading the devitalized and anemic tissues—an expenditure, which normally directed, would bring us easily within the century mark, or higher, in our career of health, power and joyful usefulness.

Diseases are cumulative; they grow silently and unnoticed. The promiscuous eater may yet triumph for a season, and gloat in his conceit of having cheated nature of her dues; but an expert accountant is busy in the function of every cell keeping an account of every item in the income and expense of man's vital economy. And though the transgressor may lull himself into the false hope of having escaped the pending installments,— the final payment, the ultimate adjustment between man and nature, is inevitable. Recurring diseases and suffering marks the jagged course in the enforced payment of human delinquency, as nature relentlessly presses him onward in the process of restoring the broken harmony in his relation to the laws of life.

We starve in the midst of plenty. Meal after meal may pass down the "via dolorosa" of man's subverted digestion, carrying the seed of corruption in the incongruous, law-defying nature of the food mixtures. In place of bringing health and strength to man, such eating injects into the very cell-life of his system the death-poisons of decomposition.

This gives a logical and scientific explanation to the fact that an individual may gain in weight while fasting. The poisons constantly generated from the fermentation of foods in the stomach, discontinued by fasting, enables the system, through the vitally constructive processes of oxygenation, to assimilate the unused proteids, already present in the circulation, and thus actually give rise to new, organized, concrete tissue.

Sooner or later, however, the effect of our dietetic transgressions will come into evidence. In place of rising from the table with a feeling of buoyancy, energy and optimism, we experience dullness and dizziness in the head, accompanied by sour stomach and general discomfort. These symptoms are warning-signals of nature, indicating that dangers are ahead, and that the individual would do best in changing his course of living.

The Appeal To The Drug And Its Response

In our predicament we take recourse to the apothecary's bottle which frequently is followed by temporary relief. Any betterment, however, not due to a more rational mode of living, is a mere whip on the nervous system, bringing out and exhausting the protective reserve forces of a vitally insolvent organism, and thus leaving the individual in a more helpless state then ever; as it is only a question of time when the worn out functions will fail to respond, even to this last scourge of artificial animation. Drug treatment, in chronic cases, is the proverbial whip on the lame, used-up horse dragging a load up hill, while straining every muscle in the climb to the point of bursting. For there is no more reasonableness in giving credit to medicine, as a source of vitality, then to give credit to the whip as a source of strength to a horse. In either case the system has to cover its own expense,—unrecompensated and unreplenished.

What Vegetarianism Can Do For Us

Nothing but food can help us; good, dietetically balanced food, and so combined, that its ingredients cannot give rise to fermentation in the stomach. But the mere absence of meat in a dietary does not change the chemical principles of food. Meat or no meat, any preparation of food which admits a mixture of acids, starches, "sweets", fruits, salads, milk, and any form of pastry, at the same meal, undermines the constitution of the eater, by using up his vital forces in neutralizing and subduing the inevitable fermentation and decomposition, arising from the incongruous mixtures. And it can be stated without risk of scientific contradiction that the unwise mixtures of sweets, starches and acids, in the ordinary vegetarian menu, has caused more indigestion and catarrh than any other violation of dietetic principles. It is not the purity of the food that is questioned, nor the efficiency of the cook, but the bringing together in the stomach of food stuffs that defy the action of every law and principle of physiological chemistry.

INDIVIDUALITY AND DIET

Yet even if the general rules of diet are complied with, and the patient is careful in his indulgence both as to quality and quantity of diet, there still remains the question of individuality. The statement that one man's meat is another man's poison, like so many other popular adages, has its basis and significance in the very root and center of human nature, in the temperament and atmosphere of man's mental life. Thus a diet which prescribes the same elements and combinations of foods for the nervous and highstrung, as for the lymphatic and sluggish, may not only be useless but positively harmful. The foods that stimulate the latter into a quicker momentum of energy, would become a lash of consuming irritation on the quivering sensibility of the nervous.

For each individual is a world in himself—distinct and unique; while back of every predisposition and aptitude of his physiological nature is found a corresponding disposition and attitude of his mind. And as every article of diet, especially fruits and vegetables, stand for definite and unchangeable principles, with definite reactions on the mind, as transmitted through the circuit of the nervous system, so in the proper knowledge of the principles and virtues, inherent in food selection, a combination of diet may be effected, capable of restoring fundamentally and permanently the balance of health, strength and beauty, which man in his ignorance or wickedness has caused to be broken. It is thus by a close observation of himself in his relation to food, as means and ends in his daily routine existence, that the individual will succeed in solving the perplexing question of life and death, as influenced by a right or wrong system of diet.

THE RACE OF LIFE AND HOW WE LOSE IT

Our limitation with regard to the power of deeper diagnosis often deceives us with regards to our actual position in relation to health. We often hear people boast over their powers of digestion, defying with impunity every rule and principle of diet. Those people, however, are short-sighted. They have subverted, not converted nature, and their escapes are only temporary. The race of life does not commence before sixty. At this age man feels his great change of life—his climectory; when suspended in the balance of life, his vital records are thrown into the scale with him. It will then be seen whether in the financing of his vital business of life and health, he has laid up sufficient funds to carry him through his critical period, and land him in safety and triumph of graceful old age; or if wantonly, in senseless gluttony, he has used up the birthright-promise of a long, happy and useful existence.

Mother Nature, thankful and proficient in her care and sustenance of her creatures, has equipped each individual with a vital "old age pension" on which to rely for support when his self-generative powers are waning. Normally, this biological reserve should complete a century of unimpaired virility and usefulness of the human life-cycle; but in the overwhelming majority of cases, at the time when man arrives at the end of his first division and applies for his vital allowance, he finds his account overdrawn, his checks turned down, and himself a biologic vagrant, bankrupt, insolvent, used up—a staggering, decrepit and worthless wreck, broken on the wheels of his own transgressions, and ready to be buried in a grave dug by his own teeth.

[But] starvation from food is only one of the dangers that arise from indulgence in ill-balanced food mixtures—poisoning, auto-intoxication, is another.

Digestion is turned into decomposition, assimilation into malnutrition;—in the place of living, healthy tissue, lining the alimentary track, we see the growth of devitalized and devitalizing tissues;—a vicious fungoid or catarrhal covering, spreading like a noxious weed from orifice to orifice, upwards and downward, until every vessel and passage of the body, including the entire alimentary tract, stomach, kidneys, bladder, liver, lungs, pharynx, ear, eye and nose, are all in the grip of this deadly tissue, which like an impenetrable barrier interrupts the vital exchanges between the circulating fluids of nutrition and their absorption.

It is safe to say that out of the world's diseases ninety per cent are due to errors in diet.

Diseases are cumulative; they grow silently and unnoticed.

SCIENTIFIC DIETETICS—FASTING

by Dr. R. Moershell

The Naturopath and Herald of Health, XX(2), 104-106. (1915)

Fasting means the abstention from all food, liquid or solid, water only being permissible. Fasting is a means to rid the body of accumulated poisons, waste material and worn out tissues. During the period of abstention the body has the opportunity to eliminate all debris, thus laying a foundation for the rebuilding of new tissue, new blood which presages perfect health.

While fasting all the organs of elimination are working to assist this process of blood purification, but the brunt of it all is upon the **mucus membranes**. The mucus surfaces of the body eliminate most of the effete material: too little attention is given to the amount of work that is done by the mucus cells, for they are of the utmost importance, even more so, while fasting, than the skin. While the skin is of great importance, I have been forced to the conclusion that the mucus surfaces of the body eliminate most of the poisons.

Since the greater amount of excretory material is deposited by the mucus cells, special effort should be made to clear these surfaces from time to time and the one way to remove the accumulations is by the drinking of **hot water**. Drink at least from three to five cupfuls during the day. Hot water dilutes and dissolves all the excretions, stimulates the circulation, in fact, [hot] water flushes the entire body, stimulating every organ of elimination to increased activity.

The skin being one of the important avenues of elimination, all means to aid its function should therefore be used. The various natural methods, such as all hydrotherapeutic, mechanical and thermal treatments should be used and among these I consider the sun bath par excellence as a stimulant to the capillary circulation of the skin. The lungs are assisted by having free supply of fresh air, with moderate exercise. The more oxygen that is absorbed and the greater the activity of the lungs, the more waste material will there be burned and a larger amount of carbon dioxide will be thrown off.

The bowels, liver and kidneys are stimulated by the use of the enema and the drinking of hot water combined with the various exercises for the abdominal and lower spinal muscles.

Now as to the mental attitude, I caution you never to fast if you are afraid. If benefit is to be received fear must be eliminated, for men have actually "starved to death," better to say that they were frightened to death within a few days from fear of starvation: therefore never fast unless you free yourself from all fear regarding it. Worry is another enemy as is also anger. These mental enemies actually cause poisons to be thrown into the circulation, this has been proved many times; so if you expect the beneficial results that are anticipated see that the mind is free from these conditions. An optimistic, cheerful and care-free attitude will do a great deal to instill success, and too much stress cannot be laid upon these factors.

The enema, uses of hot water, symptoms observed during the fast, and methods for alleviation, milk diet, raw food diet with various food used in youth and old age, etc., will be taken up later.

These various subjects will be thoroughly dealt with and any question that puzzles you will be gladly answered in this column.

Symptoms And Other Manifestations

Allow me to state that it is not needed for you to become anxious or alarmed about the various symptoms that usually occur, for there is absolutely no danger, as sane fasting is productive of good results only and no injury whatever can result from a short fast. Right here I wish to warn you against long fasts, fasting until the return of natural hunger or what is sometimes termed "fasting to a finish," for rest assured "finish" it may be. A fast of over three or four days should never be undertaken by the novice. It is sheer insanity to even attempt a longer fast when you know little or nothing regarding this form of treatment. If you wish to fast until there is no vestige of poisonous material left, make it a series of short fasts, each fast being of two or three days duration. You will then avoid all possible danger.

Many persons have actually caused their death and many have ruined their constitutions by following the advice of some **idiotic advocate of the long fast.** It fairly makes my blood boil to think of some who have simply wrecked their lives by listening to these imbeciles. Please understand that I am not criticizing some of our modern writers who have penned their personal experiences with the long fast; in studying their articles you will find that they, as a rule, do not advocate this kind of fast to a beginner, unless he is in a sanatorium where fasts of this kind are conducted, or is under the personal supervision of one who has thoroughly studied this treatment and is capable of handling such cases. Furthermore, cases that require such a strenuous regime are few in number, such fasts are unnatural, extreme, and are too much of a shock to the system. Better results will be obtained without the attending danger, by the series of short fasts. I never have been partial to the long fast except in very exceptional cases.

Weakness

The first and most noticeable symptom is that of **weakness**, better to say **a feeling of weakness.** Really you are **not weak**, the fact is that the body is storing energy during this period of rest. It is impossible for

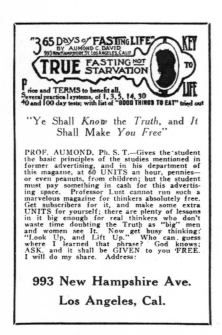

"365 Days of FASTING LIFE"
BY AUMOND C. DAVID
993 New Hampshire St. Los Angeles, Calif.
TRUE FASTING NOT STARVATION
KEY TO LIFE
Price and TERMS to benefit all.
Several practical systems, of 1, 3, 5, 14, 30
40 and 100 day tests; with list of "GOOD THINGS TO EAT" tried out

"Ye Shall *Know* the *Truth*, and *It*
Shall Make *You Free*"

PROF. AUMOND, Ph. S. T.—Gives the student
the basic principles of the studies mentioned in
former advertising, and in his department of
this magazine, at 60 UNITS an hour, pennies—
or even peanuts, from children; but the student
must pay something in cash for this advertising space. Professor Lust cannot run such a
marvelous magazine for thinkers absolutely free.
Get subscribers for it, and make some extra
UNITS for yourself; there are plenty of lessons
in it big enough for real thinkers who don't
waste time doubting the Truth as "big" men
and women see It. Now get busy thinking:
"Look Up, and Lift Up." Who can guess
where I learned that phrase? God knows;
ASK, and it shall be GIVEN to you 'FREE.
I will do my share. Address:

**993 New Hampshire Ave.
Los Angeles, Cal.**

Ad for "Key To True Fasting Not Starvation".

a short fast to cause real weakness, unless the vitality is unusually low. This deceptive feeling of weakness is due to the sudden withdrawal of food, the withdrawal of a stimulant, in other words, you are suffering from the lack of food stimulation. All food, regardless of its nature, or the way in which it is prepared, stimulates. You will feel strong and full of energy after a meal, yet the food has not even been digested and assimilated, hence the fact that you feel stronger after partaking of food is merely due to stimulation, not from nourishment. Let the inebriate cease to imbibe alcoholic drinks, he will feel weak and irritable; the same may be said of the user of tobacco or of any other form of stimulation. Thus the nerves, having been accustomed to the oft repeated food stimulation naturally rebel when all food is withheld.

COATED TONGUE

Were you able to see the entire surface of the alimentary canal, you would find a coating similar to that on the tongue. This symptom indicates the vast quantities of foul matter or reeking filth that is being eliminated by way of the mucus cells, thus we can see that these cells serve as a sort of filter and are unusually active during the fast. The importance at this time cannot be overestimated.

FOUL BREATH

This symptom is indicative of the activity of the lungs in helping the system to rid itself of poisonous matter; a free supply of fresh air is indispensable to assist the lungs in this great putrifying process. The oxygen of the air is absorbed into the blood stream where it unites with the iron of these cells and is carried to the tissues of the body to burn waste matter. A chemical change takes place resulting in the formation of carbon dioxide and water; the carbon dioxide is then carried back to the lungs to be thrown off. Since the more oxygen that is absorbed the greater the amount of waste material will there be consumed.

INCREASED ACTIVITY OF THE GLANDS OF THE SKIN

The sudoriferous and sebaceous glands of the skin are especially active as is noted by the tendency to perspire upon the least exertion: of course there is a continual excretion (perspiration) which is not detected because of the rapid evaporation that is continually taking place. The oily skin denotes the activity of the sebaceous glands, the watery matter being taken care of by the sudoriferous glands.

THE SALIVA

The salivary secretion becomes thick and quite pasty indicating that the function of these glands has been changed to that of elimination of poison; so it is with every cell and organ, their normal function is at once changed to that of a purifying nature.

SYMPTOMS OF IRRITATION

The symptoms of irritation are as follows: Headache, dizziness and spots before the eyes upon suddenly arising from the sitting position, palpitation of the heart, mental irritability, fatigue or general aching sensations over the body, sometimes a sudden sharp pain will be experienced in a certain part caused by a temporary, but severe congestion. The various symptoms mentioned are due to the poisons floating in the blood stream, that have been thrown out by the various cells and tissues, these poisons acting as an irritant to the nerve centers.

THE ACCUMULATION OF GAS IN THE LARGE BOWEL

The gas will sometimes accumulate in large quantities, thus causing a great deal of distress. The cause of this manifestation is due to the lamentation and decomposition of remaining particles of food and tough cellulose tissue that have not been excreted, hence nature strives to rid the system of the debris by resolving this material into its native elements. Sometimes large amounts of gas form in the stomach and palpitations of the heart results, either by direct pressure of by reflex irritation: while direct pressure may occasionally be the cause of the rapid heart. I think that in the majority of cases the irritation is reflected over the sympathetic nervous system: it is the sympathetic nerves that accelerate the heart. All natural methods used to rid the alimentary canal of this gas can always be relied upon.

> *There is absolutely no danger, as sane fasting is productive of good results only and no injury whatever can result from a short fast.*

THE DASHEEN

by George J. Drews, Al.D.

The Naturopath and Herald of Health, XX(6), 399-400. (1915)

The Dasheen is a tuber or corm of a variety of the *Caladium esculentum*, commonly known as elephants ear and its corm differs from that of the latter in being less fiberous in texture and lighter in color.

We saw them for the first time in the Chicago market in February of this year, when we procured a corm to experiment with for the apyrtropher diet, and find it perfectly wholesome to be eaten in the unfired state.* Of all the tubers we have tasted it is the blandest and is practically devoid of flavor. For those who dislike the natural flavor of the common Irish potato the dasheen is ideal and yet some have objected to its having no flavor and called it insipid.

In firmness it resembles that of the sweet-potato. It makes an excellent admixture for the vegetable synede when shredded on a "shoestring grater," and for the toothless it can be grated on a common grater without becoming soggy. We have not yet found in the dasheen any special medicinal properties, with the exception that it contains an etheric substance which slightly touches the nerves of the lungs, the solar plexus and the small intestines perceptible only the first time by highly sensitive people. Its prophylactic properties are like those of the Irish potato and the artichoke when eaten unfired. In the cooked form it is just as immoral for health as any of the other tubers, and even more so as it has a tendency to remain soggy after the most careful draining and steaming.

In the dasheen Nature has provided a delectable tuber for some of those with whom the other tubers do not go well and an additional chance for variety for those who want variety.

The dasheen will be enjoyed most by the majority of apyrtrophers when combined with some vegetable that has a strong flavor of its own. It may be used as a substitute for one of the ingredients in the aesthetic synede prescribed on page 142 of our book *Unfired Food and Trophotherapy*.

For those who have not got our book we propose the following recipe:

---

*George Drews adopted another spelling for Apyrotrophers—Apyrtrophers. *Ed.*

Dasheen Synede

1. One fourth cup of chopped water cress,
2. One fourth cup of shredded dasheen,
3. One fourth cup of chopped tomato,
4. One fourth cup of ground peanuts and
5. One small teaspoon full of honey for dressing. Mix all together and serve.

Nasturtium leaves or flowers, garden cress, white mustard leaves, sorrel, French dock, curled dock, dandelions or chicory may be substituted for number one. Cubed banana or cucumber may be substituted for number three. Ground almonds or pignolias may be substituted for number four. Olive oil or lemon juice or a combination of these may be substituted for number five.

By means of these substitutes the troph can prepare an almost endless variety of synedes and still use dasheen for the second ingredient or, if so desired, other tubers may be substituted for the dasheen.

The Dasheen is a tuber or corm of a variety of the caladium esculentum, commonly known as elephants ear and its corm differs from that of the latter in being less fiberous in texture and lighter in color.

DULSE AS FOOD

by George J. Drews, Al.D.

The Naturopath and Herald of Health, XX(11), 714. (1915)

Several algae or cryptogamic seaplants known under the commercial term Dulse are useful as food, even for apyrtrophers. Webster says "Dulse, a seaweed of a reddish brown color, which is sometimes eaten, as in Scotland. The true dulse is *Sarcophylis edulis*; the common is **Rhodymenia**."

Rand-McNally in his Encyclopedia says "Dulse (**Rhodymenia palmata**), a seaweed, one of the **Ceramiaceae**, growing on rocks in the sea, and used as food by the poor on the coasts, occasionally also as a luxury by some of the wealthier classes who have acquired a taste for it."

Commercial dulse is taken from the sea and dried in the sun with the natural sea-salt adhering to it, and is thus packed for the market. The sea-salt is very soluble in fresh water and is therefore easily rinsed off in the short time of one minute when it is not stuck together in hard lumps. The rinsed dulse is perfectly bland as to flavor and will be liked by all who are not slaves to the use of condiments. If, however, any flavoring must be used then ground bayleaf, ground turmeric or ginger can be used. Dulse can be procured in most of the larger department stores.

From the standpoint of trophotherapy dulse is rich in organic iodine which has none of the harmful after-effects that are known to follow the use of the unorganized and concentrated iodine prescribed by the M. Ds.

We have tried and from our experience can see no reason why it should not be used occasionally for variety in diet and with benefit.

Sea-lettuce (Ulva), which is also used as food, is different from dulse in that it is green instead of red.

We do not recommend the eating of dulse with the salt in it. Rinsed dulse can be eaten alone or as admixture with greens and nuts in the form of a synede (salad).

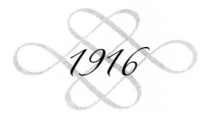

MILK FOR APYRTROPHERS

GEORGE J. DREWS, AI.D.

SPRING SUGGESTIONS

GEORGE J. DREWS, AI.D.

THE MILK CURE

By Philip Karell, M. D.

AMID the allurements of a thousand remedies (so-called) for disease, the milk cure takes high rank as a source of nutrition where the system refuses to assimilate any other form of diet. Dr. Karell in this pamphlet assures us that by means of an exclusive milk regimen, he has had the most gratifying success. He describes in full his method of treatment in many well-defined diseases.

He analyses milk, showing its composition of water, fat, albumen, sugar and mineral salts, making it a perfect food. By reason of the fact that digested milk leaves little residue, and contains little fat, it produces constipation in many people, which is corrected by swallowing a few tablespoonfuls of bran saturated in milk per day and eating boiled prunes and apples, with, or without, the assistance of an enema.

Dr. Karell has studied the milk cure from the standpoint of scientific feeding and tells us that milk is both diuretic and sudorific and therefore hastens to remove the fluids of the body, since poisons are secreted by the urine and in perspiration this effect is anti-poisonous. These poisons are mostly acids and the great efficacy of milk in general, results from its being an alkaline fluid of strong anti-acid power. Another fact is that milk renders the blood more alkaline, and the more free from acid the blood becomes, the more the body becomes resistant to the inroads of disease.

He points out that great care must be exercised to obtain milk from cows living in the open and not in stables, so that their milk will not sour readily. Good milk is neutral and does not react to testing, that is, it will neither redden blue litmus paper, nor make the red one blue. If milk reddens blue litmus paper it reacts sour, and therefore cannot be anti-acid, diuretic and sudorific, and anti-poisonous.

This is a most important analysis of the milk cure.

Price in paper, prepaid, 50 cents.

The Nature Cure Publishing Co.
Butler, N. J.

The milk cure was a popular dietary system for some Naturopaths.

Milk For Apyrtrophers

by George J. Drews, Al.D.

Herald of Health and Naturopath, XXI(2), 119-120. (1916)

Many people who now count their seventy summers will live the time when pasteurizing and sterilizing will be a thing of the past. For example, in Chicago there are enough people, especially mothers, who realize that pasteurized and sterilized milk is unwholesome for them and more so for their children, that it has become a good business for specializing dairies who advertise unpasteurized milk, infant milk or milk for children, and milk for invalids, charging double price for same.

Just before this bug killing craze will receive its fatal blow it may become profitable to advertise apyrotropher milk.

Those who live in large cities and wish to procure natural milk that comes from healthy cows must inquire for certified milk.

Apyrtrophers do not use much milk because the foods they select are mostly so rich that milk becomes superfluous, but when they do use milk they want it unfired like all their other foods, i. e., natural as it comes from a clean and healthy cow. They want its chemistry absolutely unchanged. They want no dead food of any kind that is fit for incubating scavengers, the bacilli and cocci. Warm dead milk is just the stuff that the tubercle bacilli like to feed on; for they do not on feed on living tissue until it is dead.

We hear someone say "tubercle bacilli are found in living lung, muscle and bone tissue." Yes that is true; but they can do no harm until they find cooked stuff or tissue waste to scavenge on and from this they produce their own more poisonous, dreadfully poisonous, waste which then irritates, paralyzes, and kills the surrounding tissue.

All living disease scavengers are perfectly harmless until they find something dead to eat and dead milk, at the proper temperature, is good incubating material.

Some M.Ds. are conscious of the fact that they would go to starvation if the people did not eat cooked food and partake of pasteurized milk.

We read somewhere, of a doctor in Europe, who, just before the war, proved that pasteurized milk from healthy cows was productive of tuberculosis and that fresh (unpasteurized) milk from consumptive cows did not produce tuberculosis; that the doctor himself partook of milk from consumptive cows without fear of contracting the disease; but he would not use pasteurized milk.

Here is what Dr. Brook in *Brain and Brawn* says on the subject:

> Skimmed milk is a good food, and much neglected. The only difference between milk and whole milk is that skimmed milk contains four per cent less of fat.

Pasteurized milk is devitalized milk. Sterilized milk still more so, because it is subjected to greater heat. If you eat other foods, it does so much difference, but pasteurized milk, fed exclusively to infants, will produce rickets, constipation, and finally, consumption.

Sterilizing—and in a less degree pasteurizing—of milk not only causes it to putrify easily, but coagulates the albumin, making it difficult of digestion, and also radically changes the organic salts. For this reason pasteurized or sterilized milk is a starvation food, and should never be fed exclusively to infants. Get as pure milk as you can from pure cows in a clean dairy. Do not let the fear of "bugs" lead you to starve your infant.

Buttermilk is a food that can be used by many who cannot tolerate sweet milk. Not a beverage, mind you. Like all other foods, it must be 'chewed', or it will disagree. It is hard for city dwellers to get pure, fresh buttermilk 'like mother used to make'.

Desiring to learn something about buttermilk, as sold in Los Angeles, I addressed a letter of inquiry to the local inspector of food and drugs for the California State Board of Health. In his reply he said: 'Most of the alleged buttermilk for sale in drug stores and saloons in Los Angeles is artificial buttermilk, the ingredients used being desiccated buttermilk, or desiccated skimmed milk, to which a small amount of fresh milks and plenty of water are added, together with a composition known as Bacillus Bulgaricus. The compound is then submitted to a certain treatment, where after it is put on the market as buttermilk without any qualification.'

The late Dr. C. S. Carr said on the subject:

It is a great mistake to suppose old sour buttermilk is poison. It is a very natural mistake to make, however. Lactic fermentation of milk is wholesome, no matter how far it may be advanced, but at the same time, milk is exposed to the lactic ferment germs, it is also exposed to the putrefactic germs, but the germs of putrefaction have no chance to get in their work so long as the germs of lactic fermentation are at work. They are the stronger and they destroy the putrefactic germs, or at least prevent them from getting a foothold.

Natural milk allowed to sour will not putrefy, but if the milk has been pasteurized, or sterilized the germs of fermentation have been destroyed, which gives the germs of putrefaction a chance. Such milk will not sour in a natural way, but will putrefy and is poisonous.

We would rather say that the natural food for the lactic acid germ is destroyed by the pasteurization and the food for the putrefactive germ has been increased.

Beware of milk that has been pasteurized and sterilized. It can not sour, it can only putrefy. If drunk immediately after pasteurization or sterilization it is not poisonous but very unwholesome. The milk's nutritive qualities have been greatly impaired and its use induces severe constipation. But if pasteurized or sterilized milk is allowed to stand, except on ice, it will very soon putrefy and become poisonous.

Pasteurized milk is devitalized milk. Sterilized milk still more so, because it is subjected to greater heat.

Sterilizing—and in a less degree pasteurizing—of milk not only causes it to putrify easily, but coagulates the albumin, making it difficult of digestion, and also radically changes the organic salts.

Lactic fermentation of milk is wholesome, no matter how far it may be advanced, but at the same time, milk is exposed to the lactic ferment germs, it is also exposed to the putrefactic germs, but the germs of putrefaction have no chance to get in their work so long as the germs of lactic fermentation are at work.

SPRING SUGGESTIONS

by George J. Drews, Al.D.

Herald of Health and Naturopath, XXI(6), 403. (1916)

These suggestions have been delayed because our department was omit-ted in the March issue for want of space, so we have discarded much that would have been useful a month earlier.

We would like to remind all apyrtrophers who have any available garden space, and others, not to forget to plant dahlias and Jerusalem artichokes for next winter's use in synedes.

In selecting dahlias for food-crops it is best to choose the red and pink varieties. The red variety, however, in our experience, produces the largest tubers. If any reader does not know what these dahlia tubers taste like we would advise him to go to his neighbor and ask him for a sample tuber. The first expense for plants is somewhat forbidding; but after that they can be produced as cheaply as those of sweet potatoes and in a simi-lar way. To those who have learned to like the dahlia tuber, any price is insignificant to the pleasure of eating them.

Our government went to much expense to introduce the dasheen (the tuber of a variety of the cala or elephant's ear), and yet this tuber has noth-ing in flavor, consistency or wholesomeness to be recommended.

The juice of the dahlia tuber (in our experience), lends strength to the muscles of the intestinal peristalsis and courage to the nerves that control them. With this we do not mean to say that it acts like laxatives. It would by truly consistent to advise the eating of these tubers as an early spring tonic, on account of the tonic salts they contain.

Do not worry about the soil in which to plant dahlias for they will grow in any soil which you can cultivate, provided they get a reasonable amount of sunshine.

The artichoke likes a richer soil; but a poor soil will not prevent it from growing and producing good tubers. Any unsightly corner of the garden or yard is the best place to plant artichokes.

Vaughn's Seed House, of Chicago and New York, advertises a French novelty artichoke of a rose color, which they say is more smooth and more productive than the common variety. We have procured some of these rose artichokes to try them in our garden this summer. They look as beautiful as the rose murphies; but cannot be compared with them as to flavor.

Another suggestion is about dandelion flowers. Take every oppor-tunity this spring to eat the flowers of the dandelion. In order to get the sweetest flowers it is essential to get out early and beat the bee. The flow-ers that unfold for the first time in the morning are tender and sweet.

The full grown buds before they are unfolded together with their stems are best to be chopped up for synede material; because they are then not so dry.

It is a good idea to have some dandelions growing in the garden in order that absolutely fresh flowers can be had at any time for synede garnish.

Of all edible flowers the stock is the queen; because we know of no one that was not delighted with their flavor and crispness. If you wish to give somebody pleasure some time, then sow some stocks now.

Another suggestion is about dandelion flowers. Take every opportunity this spring to eat the flowers of the dandelion. In order to get the sweetest flowers it is essential to get out early and beat the bee.

MY DIET OF HEALING
ARNOLD EHRET, DIETIST

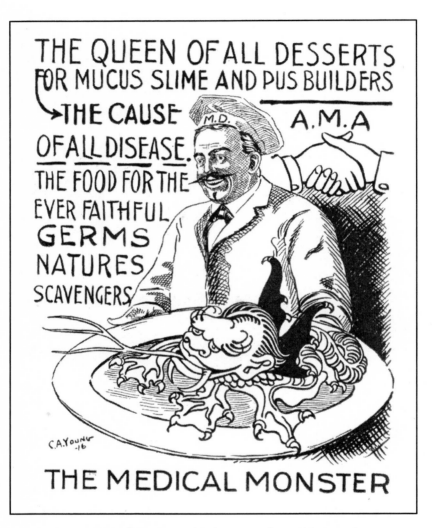

A cartoon that appeared in the September 1923 issue of
Herald of Health and Naturopath.

My Diet Of Healing

by Arnold Ehret, Dietist, W. Alhambra, California

Herald of Health and Naturopath, XXII(5), 257-260. (1917)

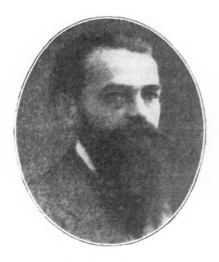

Professor Arnold Ehret

At present, there is no want of dietetic systems in Naturopathy. What we shall eat is a question of the highest importance, just as it has become vitally important at present in Europe. Physiological Naturopathy owes more and more its success to radical diet. To fast and drink water only will help in most diseases, if everything else fails. In the most severe cases, nature heals by refusing to eat; hence the logical conclusion that a sick person cannot eat too little. "The more you nourish the sick, the more you harm him," says Hippocrates, the greatest physician and dietist. In cases of acute sickness, the patient instinctively obeys the natural antagonism to food; his appetite is simply taken away. He who dies today of an acute disease is the victim of the modern insistence for forced nourishment.

The success of the fasting cure has banished more and more the spectre of starving to death, and that of under-nourishment. Every Naturopathic patient knows that he must observe restriction of diet in order that the supplementary physical administrations may be successful. The so-called scientific nourishment of allopathy has received its death blow by the present war situation in Europe. A German lady who is a follower of my method wrote to her son in the United States during the first year of the war, "Everything that Ehret rejects as unhealthful eating is extremely expensive at present."

In Germany, the greatest enemy of health, French pastry, was utterly exterminated by the first order of the department of provisions. The Ehretists do not feel sorry, and no one scoffs at the name of "Ehret." The thundering of the cannon had to come to establish his doctrine. One believes again in strict moderation in eating in all methods of healing. Abstinence from meat, alcohol, tobacco, coffee and tea is not enough with regard to diet. The discoveries and methods of the pioneers, Schroth, Priessnitz,

Kuhne, Kneipp, Lahmann, Just, Engelhardt and others, are based more or less on restricted diet. Heretofore the desire of sick humanity was to eat, and the medical profession's false doctrine of nourishment had diminished the importance of low diet.

Although the minimum requirement of food for the sick, as well as the healthy, is not yet fully established, every follower of Naturopathy knows that all maladies are caused, more or less, not by too little nourishment, but by overfeeding. What else charges the body with poisonous, contagious matter, and causes more and more deterioration of the blood, the principal source of all disease, but the undigested nutriment which will in time saturate the entire system with its poison, and give rise to any kind of disorder. This effete matter manifests itself by various secretions, notably mucus, and these secretions are the breeding grounds for all kinds of germs, which, as Béchamp has shown, are simply the evolution of the microenzymes that are the basis of all organic life.

Mucus is so much superfluous matter, which, being decomposed by fermentation and putrefaction, becomes mucus (see my book *Rational Fasting*, published by B. Lust, Butler, N. J.). All maladies, sickness and disease are nothing more than internal uncleanliness. The human body is healthy only as long as it is able to eliminate such poisons by virtue of vital power and good hygienic conditions.

This definition gives us the answer why a drunkard can reach a high age, but not a glutton. A few years ago, I improved this fundamental dietetical perception of Graham, with the sentence: We have centenarians that smoke, ninety-year-old coffee drinkers, and eighty-year old drunkards, but we have no gluttons that reach old age. Nobody can show me a man possessing an obese corporation who is ninety years old, because such a person does not exist.

Do not the poorest countries produce the maximum of centenarians?

Where everything else has failed, one can gain results by eating less and eating not so often. This is slower but more convenient than fasting. It is the natural and is, therefore, the unfailing measure against overeating and thereby becoming sick. Altogether, the progressive moderation of taking food results in many cases in regaining health without abjuring any kind of food, or even the so-called poisons of civilization.

Of course, the absolute fast, graded in severity according to the powers of reaction in a given individual, is the most potent and rapid method of restoring the digestive functions to their normal condition, but short of an actual fast, frugality in eating is and always will remain the open secret for attaining a happy and healthful old age.

A systematic program with regard to frugality, number and regularity of meals is in most cases a successful remedy for those patients which for some reason cannot waive the tid bits of civilization.

The quality of the diet of healing must also be considered. What shall we eat to become and remain healthy, if gluttony and wrong eating are the principal causes of sickness? Our investigation discloses a chaos of theories and systems, all of which will find approval by some, but which are condemned by others, a confusion that runs riot even in the camp of Naturopathy. My investigations have disclosed the profound truth that the straight road to health consists in **Fasting and the Fruit Diet,** as I have shown in my booklet *Rational Fasting.*

Fasting is the only genuine and unfailing power to heal sick humanity. It alone can unmucusize the human race. It is a practice that has existed in the animal kingdom in all ages. As to food, there is no reason why fruit should not be to-day, as heretofore, the most perfect nourishment, and therefore the healing food of the human race. It was the food of the first man before he learned to use the spear and fire, and thus established a form of civilization whose blessings have yet to be discovered.

It is pure legend to speak of the first man as a cave dweller, as science to-day pretends. He only became such after he was forced to leave the shelter of his cocoanut and date palms by reason of his disobedience in eating of forbidden food. It is not too late to again believe in biblical health and eat of the fruit of the God-made gardens of earth. But the road thither leads through the purgatory of fasting and a fruit diet.

The failure of all the experiments of so-called fasting and fruit-diet experts does not contradict the truth.

Fruit as the best factor in the healing diet is continually doubted and discredited because most of the adherents of such a diet suffer shipwreck for want of experience and proper management. Even experts explain the preliminary critical state of weakness as undernourishment, while in reality it is caused by the excretions of poisons, the very same thing that happens in fasting.

No other form of treatment needs to be so carefully watched, or so highly individualized and directed with such progressive zeal as the diet of healing. The layman thinks the more drastic the treatment, the better. He wants to fast to an extreme extent once he gets enthused with fasting, and seeks in matters of diet to transform himself overnight from an epicure to a radical fruit eater. The change is too sudden, and he partakes of the most senseless combination of food only to become the possessor of a mass of effete matter. In most cases, he has the naïve superstition that for every special case of sickness there is a specific dietetic prescription.

A fast, or a healing diet, or both combined, are not to be prescribed for certain diseases, but are to be determined with regard to general conditions, age, sex, and profession of the sick person.

My system distinguishes itself by being based upon the following considerations. First, the quality and quantity of the mucus diet. Secondly, the quality and quantity of the non-mucus diet. Thirdly, the composition of the absolutely frugivorous diet.

The meager of mucus diet consists essentially of fruits, vegetables, and vegetable salads. Meat, eggs, milk, and all kinds of starchy foods are not included, for technical reasons of nourishment, being held in reserve to moderate too radical fruitarian aliment.

In my investigation with a strictly fruitarian diet, I have evolved various menus that are well adapted for the treatment of specific physical temperaments. These I call systems of cure, and they are very efficient agents of regeneration.

SYSTEM 1.

This is adapted for heavily afflicted elderly persons. Here are the right combinations of foods—the most intricate having to be prescribed individually.

SYSTEM 2.

This consists of fruit, vegetables and vegetable salads only, with fats of vegetable origin. It is the continuation of System 1, and can be applied direct to younger people, who are affected with minor ailments.

SYSTEM 3.

This is the absolute fruit diet which was the paradisiacal food of primitive man. To achieve a permanent form of nourishment with fruits is most difficult, because the fruit eater does not regain his maximum of energy until the last trace of morbid matter rooted in his tissues is eliminated. His whole system must undergo purification and then physical regeneration is accomplished.

This, of course, takes time and painstaking observation, as critical conditions of secretion return continually, and right here is the obstacle met by most. This is the reason why to-day not a dozen individuals are fully convinced of the nourishing power of fruit. Other difficulties in the way of the fruit diet are social conditions. Whoever antagonizes these, knows what it is to do so by experience.

My healing diet pursues the principle to successively withdraw all contaminating mucus-forming food, which consists of meat, eggs, milk and its products, bread, potatoes, and all carbohydrates, in order to create blood from grape sugar. Why should not the sugar be taken direct from the grape? Besides this, I employ vegetable and lettuce salads as purifying mucus-cleansers to augment the aperient, cleansing effect of fruit, with due regard to choice and combination. Further, I adjust the activity of the healing process to the condition and occupation of the patient, and choose and prepare the meals in such a way that no privation exists, but to the end that the healing diet becomes a greater attraction than all the dainties of modern cooking.

"Your food will be remedies and your remedies shall be food," said Hippocrates, the first and greatest physician and dietist.

The utterance of a German poet concerning diet is apropos of my theme: "Not until the last cook-book is hung up with the last cook's gut, shall suffering humanity be liberated." In this sentence is the historical misery of mankind revealed.

The natural healing method does not accomplish its mission if merely limited to the healing of patients spoiled by medicine. The healing diet that I advocate has a greater mission to fulfill, and that is, to create a new god-like being, a veritable superman, to fill the ranks of a new evolution of humanity. The chosen ones are those who are willing to pass through the most intense putrifying fire of tropical fruits, and receive as their reward the key to the lost paradise, and so to speak live without sorrow or sickness under its palms in absolute happiness.

I do not, like most reformers, desire to alter the entire customs of mankind by theories alone, but as a finale to my mission to create a new blood nobility, a crimson-blooded race, regenerated by the healing qualities of the purest and most nutritious food.

A frugivorous diet will nourish humanity in absolute health, which will then contain the potency of the superman. The garden of wedlock will thus not merely propagate in kind but will lift posterity to a higher plane of existence, by a new and wonderful thoroughbred of the human race.

This I understand not in a figurative, but in a very real and practical sense. We have already the germinating life, and all we now require is the fecund soil.

The cradle of mankind was situated in a tropical garden where the sunshine from a cloudless sky ripened a variety of succulent fruits sufficient to sustain man in health and happiness. Not far away, the uplands ripened the fruits of the temperate clime also.

My method of healing, then, leads mankind back to the menu chosen by God in His infinite wisdom as that form of food which will produce the highest earthly felicity, and when God had spread the banquet amid the vineyards of Mesopotamia for beings destined for immortality, He sat down amid the glowing oranges, the dates, bananas, grapes, apples, figs, pears and pomegranates of paradise, and, blessing these alimentary delights as necessary rudiments for the health and life of mankind, declared that all His work was good.

My healing diet pursues the principle to successively with-draw all contaminating mucus-forming food, which consists of meat, eggs, milk and its products, bread, potatoes, and all carbohydrates.

Rational Fasting

Regeneration Diet and Natural Cure for all Diseases

By ARNOLD EHRET

Synopsis of contents:

I. **The common fundamental cause of diseases.**

II. **Remedies for the removal of the common fundamental cause of disease and the prevention of their reoccurrence.**

III. **The fundamental cause of grow= ing old and ugly, of the falling out and getting gray of the hair.**

IV. **Death.**

THIS is a severely scientific treatise on the rationale of fasting. The argument goes directly to the point and shows how the chronic stuffing of th body mucus-generating foods is the prime cause of disease, premature old age, and death.

Our author declares that disease is nothing else but a clogging-up of the smaller blood vessels, the arterioles and capillaries by mucus, by effete food-products. This clogging up leads to decomposition, to fermentation of the dead matter, that is nature's effort to rid the system of wholly offensive and boiled-dead food products. These decay partially in the living body, causing abscesses, cancer, tuberculosis, syphilis, lupus, etc. The decomposed material gives birth to microbes that are not the cause but the product of decomposition. They are only discernable in an advanced stage of the disease, and by their excretions, called toxins, they also poison surrounding tissues. The prescribed remedy for this state of things is to fast entirely from food, for a long or short period, according to the vitality of the faster.

The energy of the system when not engaged in digesting food attacks the decomposing mucus, slime, or paste, that over-indulgence in food stores up in the system, and cleanses the body from the offensive material.

Mr. Ehret declares war not merely on meat and alcohol, but on cereal and white flour products, being a fruitarian. Walnuts, figs, dates, oranges, bananas, do not generate in the system floral and faunal fermentive slimes and pastes that so readily decompose and produce death dealing diseases. Nobody who values health can afford to overlook this splendid pamphlet that discloses the natural cure for all diseases.

Price, postpaid, $1.00

The Nature Cure Publishing Co.
Butler, N. J.

An ad for *Rational Fasting*, one of the several books written by Arnold Ehret.

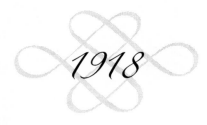

1918

The New Science Of Healing
Louis Kuhne

—·—

Cocoa Bread
Translated From The German by David Ammann

—·—

Kitchen And Table, Menus For Purification
Mrs. Louise Lust

—·—

A Nut And Fruit Dietary For Brain Workers
Sophie Leppel

—·—

Healthful Eating
E. Howard Tunison

NEO-NATUROPATHY
THE NEW SCIENCE OF HEALING
By LOUIS KUHNE

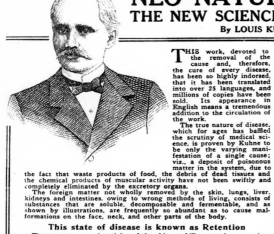

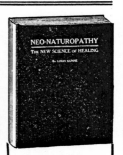

THIS work, devoted to the removal of the cause and, therefore, the cure of every disease, has been so highly indorsed, that it has been translated into over 25 languages, and millions of copies have been sold. Its appearance in English means a tremendous addition to the circulation of the work.

The true nature of disease, which for ages has baffled the scrutiny of medical science, is proven by Kuhne to be only the varying manifestation of a single cause; viz., a deposit of poisonous matter in the system, due to the fact that waste products of food, the debris of dead tissues and the chemical products of muscular activity have not been swiftly and completely eliminated by the excretory organs.

The foreign matter not wholly removed by the skin, lungs, liver, kidneys and intestines, owing to wrong methods of living, consists of substances that are soluble, decomposable and fermentable, and as shown by illustrations, are frequently so abundant as to cause malformations on the face, neck, and other parts of the body.

This state of disease is known as Retention

The symptoms are inactivity of the skin, a chilly sensation, sneezing, great nervous tension, a dread of cold air, an excited pulse owing to capillary obstruction, coated tongue, hyperacidity of the stomach, soreness of the muscles, perversion of taste, loss of smell, catarrh, etc.

These conditions cause acute or chronic Enervation

The symptoms of Enervation are low vitality, lack of metabolism, emaciation, a weak heart, neurasthenia, sleepiness by day and sleeplessness at night, great weakness of the sympathetic system, owing to which the cells refuse the natural nutrients in the blood. Retention and Enervation together furnish the conditions for the development of the various micro-organisms that produce the various infections and contagious diseases that afflict mankind, thereby hindering progress.

Such condition is known as Invasion

as medical science supposes that disease is caused by an invasion of microbes from without, a wholly false conception in the great majority of cases.

There is only one disease and, as regards essentials, only one method of treatment is actually necessary

Now comes the immense value of this great work. Kuhne, the master of disease, rejects drugs in toto and employs Natural Methods of healing, describing the same so fully, so clearly and so simply that nobody needs any more to visit a drugging doctor, as he or she can be cured at home by employing the methods of healing recommended in the book.

His remedial agents include the use of steam baths, sun baths, followed by the cooling and friction sitz-baths, and other treatments supplemented by a system of vegetation diet that raises the vitality of the body. The sympathetic nervous system is in particular the object of his keen regard, as it is the citadel of strength and power in the body.

Kuhne shows how his remedial treatments can be most successfully practiced at home. He devotes fifty pages of the work to the testimonials of those who have cured themselves of every conceivable disease by following his wise and benign advice.

To an ailing man, this book is worth a thousand dollars. Price, only $3.00

SEND FOR IT TODAY

START YOUR CURE WITHOUT DELAY

DR. BENEDICT LUST
110 East 41st Street   **New York City**

NEO-NATUROPATHY
The New Science of Healing
By LOUIS KUHNE
Cloth Bound, 300 pages, $3.00

SYNOPSIS

Part I

What led me to the discovery of The New Science of Healing—How does disease arise—The nature and cure of children's diseases — measles, scarlet fever, diphtheria, etc — Disease a transmission of morbid matter — Rheumatism and gout; their cause and cure—Cold hands and feet; their cause and cure—The science of facial expression—My remedial agents—What shall we eat? What shall we drink? Indigestibility of denatured food—A rational, natural system of diet—Man a frugivorous animal—Beneficial value of vegetable diet—Simple home recipes.

Part II

Nervous and mental diseases—Pulmonary affections—Cause and cure of nodules—Tuberculin inoculation condemned—Sexual diseases—curative crises—Diseases of the bladder and kidneys—Heart disease—Poverty of the blood—Epileptic fits—Diseases of the eye and ear—Diseases of the teeth—Diseases of the throat—Headache — Inflammation of the brain—Typhus—Dysentery—Cholera and Diarrhea—Climatic and tropical fevers—Leprosy—Scabies; parasites—Hernia—Cancer — Proud flesh.

Part III

Treatment and cure of wounds, without drugs and operations—Diseases of women —How to bring about safe and easy parturition—Conduct after birth—The bringing up of children.

Part IV

Reports of cures and of appreciation (fifty pages)—Illustrating the science of facial expression—Child inoculated with tuberculin forty-five times, and the results.

Benedict Lust translated Louis Kuhne's book, *The New Science of Healing,* in 1917 and renamed the book, *Neo-Naturopathy, the New Science of Healing.*

THE NEW SCIENCE OF HEALING

by Louis Kuhne

Herald of Health, XXIII(1), 42-55. (1918)

WHAT SHALL WE EAT? WHAT SHALL WE DRINK? THE DIGESTIVE PROCESS

From the explanation given about the friction sitz-bath and human vitality, we have seen that disease can only arise as a consequence of wrong food. It is only through bad digestion that foreign matter can form and disease develop in the body. Thus the questions: "What shall we eat? —What shall we drink?" are of the greatest importance for us.

As is well known, in order to produce electric power, or a constant electric current, certain definite elements are necessary. It is only with the aid of an acid that we are able through the decomposition or transformation of the zinc and carbon plates, to set free the power which formerly was required to retain the plates in their original structure. This power is then conducted as positive and negative current through wires, to be used as electricity. If, however, in place of these elements (zinc and carbon), we were to substitute others, which resemble them—or consist of similar constituents, or even of the same materials (zinc and carbon), but in another form, for instance, pulverized—we should soon notice a difference. We should, then, either get no generation of electric power at all, or it would be essentially changed, diminished, in spite of the fact that the conditions may otherwise be exactly the same as in the case of the zinc and carbon plates. It is similar with the generation of vital power in the human body. Here, also, the development of more or less vital power, depends upon the right choice of elements, in this instance, of food. This is most clearly to be seen in the case of atmospheric air, our chief food. We have only to take a person for some minutes away from his normal air, and put him into another gaseous atmosphere, and we shall see at once how he dies in a few minutes, the new element not enabling him to maintain his vital power.

The injurious effects of a wrong diet are slower and less striking. The boundary between natural food and deadly poison is very wide. The step from the natural to the unnatural is often so small as to be at first scarcely perceptible. But as we know that foreign matter only forms as the result of wrong food, that is, can only arise in the body as the result of bad digestion, it must be our task to avoid such wrong foods and such bad digestion.

In order to make clear this matter of wrong food and bad digestion, I will here cite a few instances which occur in daily life. We meet stout, corpulent people, who assure us that they eat and drink very little, but

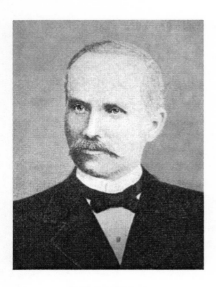

Dr. Louis Kuhne.

complain that they nevertheless are always growing stouter and stouter. Such persons suffer from over-nutrition. Others are scraggy, lean, emaciated, although they are consuming unusually freely what, in their opinion, are the most nutritious foods and drinks. Judging by the quantity consumed, such persons should be in quite another condition. The food passes through the body, but the latter is unable to benefit by it. A large part of the food passes away unused, or at all events insufficiently utilized. This proves that the mere fact of foods and drinks passing through the body, is no proof at all of a normal digestion, as many people, unfortunately, seem to think.

We thus have two opposite classes of people. The one demonstrates to us how, by eating and drinking little, one becomes stouter, the other, how by eating and drinking much, one becomes thinner. In spite of apparent contradiction, the reason for the ailment is in both cases the same; that is, bad digestion and wrong feeding. This premised, and we can readily understand how, for instance a consumptive person can eat what he considers the most strengthening, nutritious food without his body benefiting at all; whilst, on the other hand, we shall no longer wonder about the want of appetite on the part of apparently strong, but nervous people.

After these explanations, and remembering the remarks upon vital power in the last chapter, it is not difficult for us to find the way to avoid over-nutrition. The reflective reader will no doubt already have come to the conviction, that the most nourishing and suitable foods and beverages are not flesh-meat, eggs, extracts, wine, beer, cocoa, coffee, tea, etc., but only such foods as can be quickly and easily digested. The more rapidly our body can digest the food presented to it, the more it will be able to utilize such, and therefore the more vital power it will be able to generate. The degree of vitality depends, therefore, upon the digestibility of foods consumed.

The more difficult of digestion a food is, the longer the time required by the body to perform the work of digestion. If we consume such foods, then we must at any rate, if we will not injure our system, wait before eating again, until the first meal has been properly digested. Unfortunately, this is seldom done, especially as our daily habits are antagonistic to such apparent *fasting*. The true significance of fasting is thus practically unknown to us today. Man disregards altogether, as a rule, the fasts laid down by nature. On the contrary, we see him in winter, where, generally speaking, he has more time than in summer, eating oftener and more than in the latter season. We find almost everywhere the erroneous opinion prevailing that in winter one should eat well and consume plenty fat, in order to be able to withstand the cold. This, however, is in flat contradiction to all natural laws. How often, very often, have I had occasion to observe the injurious effect of eating and drinking too much during the winter. In nature, we find everywhere a certain period of fasting. We see how snakes fast often for weeks, after having taken a good meal. We see how deer and hares for weeks and months live most sparely, and yet overcome all the fatigues of a raw, cold winter. Were these animals in the situation to obtain the same amount of food as in summer, they would without doubt become ill and be unable to withstand the winter cold. Cold retards, as we know, every process of fermentation, and therefore digestion. Thus a quantity of food which in summer would be easily digested, in winter is much more difficult to digest. Hence the reason for the fact that our domestic animals, which for the most part are fed in the stall, almost always suffer from over-nutrition, are unable to stand the winter cold in the open; whilst animals in a state of nature, can endure even the fiercest storm, for they possess a power of bodily resistance unfortunately far too little regarded to-day.

These expositions now make it obvious to us, that disease only arises through a kind of over-nutrition. And we come thus naturally to the conviction that it is by no means a matter of indifference *what we consume, in which form we consume it, and where we consume it.*

To render the matter clearer, I will again introduce some examples.

If we drink boiled water, it tastes flat and disagreeable. How refreshing, on the other hand, is a draught of fresh water, how invigorating an apple! Just so with the air. Oppressive and relaxing, producing in many a headache—such is the effect of the stuffy, used up air of the average room, especially if the chamber be small, and a number of persons have been sitting in it. How one longs in such a case for the fresh, animating outside air.

And of like importance is where we consume our food. That which we eat in the open air, is always more easily digested than that consumed in the house; because in chewing, the food is mixed with air, and fresh air acts quite differently upon the digestibility of the food than the bad air of our rooms does.

As already stated, those foods which are most easily digestible, are exactly those which are best suited to nourish the body. Over-nutrition, also, is *least liable* to occur where the food is easily digested. It is, then, our first point to determine what the most readily digested foods are, that is, those which supply us with most vitality. The answer to this all-important and much debated question is as simple as it is natural.

THE INDIGESTIBILITY OF DENATURED FOOD

Those foods which taste good in their natural state, and tempt us to eat, are always whose which are most easy of digestion, and which supply us with the most vitality.

All food which we have to *change by cooking, smoking, spicing, salting, pickling, and putting in vinegar,* lose in digestibility, and as regards *vitality,* are far inferior to food in its natural condition, even though the above-named processes may enable the foods to keep longer.

Of *cooked* and *prepared foods, those are most easy of digestion,* which are *most simply prepared* or *cooked,* and *least salted* or *spiced.*

Food in fluid form, such as soups, and beverages, as beer, wine, cocoa, etc., are *much more difficult to digest* than those which in their *natural condition are solid,* and capable of being chewed. For this reason, continued use of fluid nutriment tends to dilatation of the stomach and disturbances of the digestion.

Those *foods* which in their *natural form* create *disgust* and *nausea,* are always *injurious to the health,* however good they may taste when in a prepared and cooked condition. And above all, flesh-meat comes under this class of food. No one would ever think of biting into a living ox, or eating raw sheep's flesh. Our instinct and natural feeling may be misled by seasoning and dressing; but foods repulsive to our true instincts, smell and taste, can never be rendered wholesome by such means.

For a clearer comprehension of the principles of a natural diet, the following points must be remarked.

All foods are easier of digestion, and more strengthening, when not fully ripe, *i.e.,* in a not yet fully developed state, than if already over-ripe. Unfortunately, the general public has got the erroneous idea that unripe food is unhealthy, because it causes diarrhea, flux and dysentery. This is quite a mistake. To be sure, a person who is accustomed chiefly to flesh-foods, and who then, by chance, eats an unripe apple, or other unripe fruit, gets diarrhea. But, on the other hand, we have exactly here an excellent proof of the easy digestibility of unripe fruit. Every easily digestible food is rapidly transformed by the fermentive process of digestion, in a manner such as is not the case with foods which are difficult of digestion. If now in the organs of digestion there are foods which are difficult to digest, or to transform by fermentation, they will be acted upon by the quicker fermentive process of the unripe fruit, in such a way that they also will be set in a state of decomposition and fermentation. In this manner arises the diarrhea which is so much, though wrongly, feared. Such a crisis of diarrhea often rids the body in a surprisingly short time of great deal of the foreign matter in it, and is accordingly to my experience, of the greatest benefit to the organism.

It will be well known to the reader, that dogs, which through the over attention of their owners become too fat, very frequently eat grass, a food which is not properly intended for a carnivorous animal. The reason for this conduct is, that the instinct of the dog teaches him that the grass, by reason of its ready digestibility, is the best aid for his digestion, overloaded with too rich food.

Thus to persons suffering from affections of the stomach, or troubles of the digestion, unripe fruit is to be recommended instead of ripe; and the use of such should be continued until the stomach is so far strengthened as to be again able to digest the fruit ripe.

As with fruits and other foods, so are grains (likewise of very different degrees of digestibility, according to their preparation, and the manner in which we eat them), always most easily digested in their most natural state, that is, as whole grains. Naturally the grinding of grain gives the teeth much work, but it is exactly the chewing and the thorough insalivation thus caused, that mainly promotes the digestion. Of course, only those people who are the fortunate possessors of a good set of teeth can consume grain in this form; those who have lost their dental organs to a greater or less extent, will not be able to perform the work. Such patients must chew the grains previously ground. Where the circumstances permit it, ground corn is a very important food for the seriously ill, and should always be used where wholemeal bread cannot yet be digested. In such a case, coarse ground meal with unripe fruit is of the greatest service, and wherever the patient is capable of recovery at all, improvement will very soon take place. In the form of wholemeal bread, the grains are not so easily digestible as when eaten raw, as above mentioned. Of all kinds of bread, however, whole wheatmeal bread is easiest to digest. For most breads, only the white, mealy interior of the grain is used, the outside parts being nearly always utilized for other purposes. In this way a fine meal is obtained, but the bread made from it gives the digestion far more work to do, than does wholemeal bread. It thus leads to constipation, the bran, the most important part of the grain, having been rejected.

Oats, as everyone knows, are an excellent food for horses. But how much depends upon the form in which the oats are given, in order that they may prove a valuable food, every horse-owner will confirm. If we fodder the horses on oats mixed with chaff, they will be able to digest them most easily and will be best nourished. If, on the contrary, we give the animals oats *without chaff*, we shall soon find that they can no longer digest the fodder so easily. If, finally, we give as fodder other grains such as wheat or rye, without the addition of chaff, we shall see still more clearly than before, from the digestion of the horses, that those foods alone are too heavy. Still more clearly is the difficulty of digestion seen, if we supply the horses only with oats from which the husk has been removed. The animals grow fat on them, but on the other hand become constipated and unfit for work.

The easy digestibility of grain is due chiefly to its shell or husk; the more shell or husk, the better for the digestion. The oat, is, of all grains, that which has the greatest amount of shell, and therefore much better adapted as horse-food than wheat or rye.

Although in the dung, oat-husks and chaff are found apparently unchanged, it is not therefore to be assumed that these have been worthless ballast as far as the horse's digestion is concerned. That would be a serious error. This ballast is as necessary to the horse for his normal digestion, as the interior part of the grain. *Food precisely in the form nature gives it to us,* is always the best for digestion.

For mankind, likewise it is of the utmost importance in *what form* we take our food. Often we hear people saying: "I cannot digest the pulses, they give me flatulence." But this depends greatly upon the manner in which they have been prepared. In the form of a puree or soup, as they are generally eaten, they certainly are difficult to digest, so that it is no wonder if they cause trouble. As soup, especially, they are objectionable, for soup reaches the stomach *unchewed*, and therefore in a state unprepared for digestion. If, on the contrary, we boil, for instance, the peas, in only a little water, so that when cooked they have absorbed nearly all the moisture, and appear in their natural round form, we shall scarcely consume one third of the quantity that we swallowed down as soup. Furthermore, we shall notice that this smaller quantity, although eaten with the shell, causes no unpleasantness, and is far more strengthening than soup.

I am reminded of a laborer who, from necessity, was obliged to live for some three months on nothing else than a handful of raw peas daily. With evident delight, this man used to relate to me the episodes of that dreadful time, when he often had for hours to let the peas soak in his mouth, in order to get them soft enough to chew. Yet in spite of this scanty food, he maintained that he felt the highest degree well, and was, in fact, never better in his life. This instance speaks to the high nutritive value of food in its natural condition. It teaches us further, that also when we are dealing with nutrition, the principle of nature which we recognize everywhere, is again to be found: to perform the most, with the simplest and smallest means.

My expositions may now have made it clear to my readers, how over-nutrition is to be prevented. Of course, I am not able to state exactly what and how much every person, or every patient should eat, in order to avoid over-nutrition again. There are scarcely two patients whose digestive powers are quite alike, so that the exact quantity, or kind, of food can never be decided offhand. Each must find out for himself what suits him best. It must, therefore, suffice to give the relative digestibility of the various foods.

As regards the digestive process itself, the orthodox school gives us no certain basis to go upon. Even the magnificent discoveries of chemistry, by the aid of retorts, balances, and all kinds of other apparatus, are of little significance for the New Science of Healing.

Digestion itself is a process of fermentation in the body. By it, foods are converted into quite different materials within the human system. The body appropriates for itself as much of them as are suitable, that is, assimilable. All foods, the fermentability of which we alter by artificial preparation, or suppress by means of salt, sugar or cooking are difficult of digestion; that is, the body can only assimilate them with difficulty. Their fermentability being thus influenced, they require a longer time than ordinarily, before they come in a state suitable for digestion. In other words, in order to reach the required condition, they remain much longer in the digestive canal than they should, whereby a higher condition of fermentation and consequently a higher temperature is caused. The greater development of internal heat caused by this condition, contribute finally to the firmer consistency and darker coloration of the faeces in the intestine.

Digestion begins as is well known, in the mouth. The foods then reach the stomach, where they mix with the gastric juice, and are thoroughly acted upon. They thus come into a state of decomposition or fermentation which essentially changes them. In the intestines, the process of fermentation increases in intensity, and the fermenting food is further mixed with the secretions of the pancreas, and other digestive juices.

That which is useless for the body is secreted again through the intestines, kidneys and skin. Sometimes we observe how animals completely digest, in a very short time, such apparently altogether indigestible things as tendons and bones. If now we examine the excrements of such animals, we will find absolutely no undigested pieces of bone. With men, on the contrary, we find that food often remains a whole week in the digestive canal. This gives rise to an abnormal condition of fermentation. The gases developed by this fermentation, which are not at all concerned in building up the body, are conducted to the skin, and are expelled as perspiration and effluvia, and on the other hand as wind. This wind should never be suppressed, since it is highly injurious to the body.

The digestion is normal when the excrements are *light brown, soft* and compact, and covered with a mucous coating, clearly showing the slimy nature of the various juices of the body. They should be of sausage form and leave the body absolutely unsoiled. We observe this in the case of all healthy animals; and so it should be in the case of healthy men. The end of the rectum is of such appropriate form, that when the digestion is normal, the excrements are exerted without the parts being in any way dirtied. Closet paper [toilet paper] is an acquisition for *diseased humanity,* as I have already remarked; the *healthy* country population does not use it. Furthermore, the excrements should never emit an *obnoxious, disgusting odor.*

If this is the case, we must conclude that the fermentive process of the digestion is here more or less abnormal. This leads to constipation or costiveness. The faeces stick firmly in the dried up intestines and can not be moved at all. The fermentation nevertheless still goes on within. It compels the hard faeces to change in form, and causes an active evolution of gas, which finally begins to penetrate throughout the body. The internal pressure, and tension caused by this condition of fermentation, tends towards the extremities and skin. If now, the latter no longer performs its functions, so that the gaseous foreign matter find no exit, more and more of it is deposited under the skin. The latter now becomes still more sluggish and its temperature decreases below the normal. Its fine blood-vessels become so saturated with foreign matter that healthy blood, which alone can warm the skin, is no longer able to circulate to the outside of the body. Hence, the external temperature of the latter falls, and the skin assumes a chlorotic color of one kind or another. Usually, there is a pale, corpse-like appearance (see the remarks on Chlorosis, Part II), but the exact color differs, according to the quality of the foreign matter and of the blood. Large quantities of urine in the blood causes the skin to appear red; in other cases the skin may be yellow, brown or greenish. The external colder temperature, in opposition to the internal heat, causes the gaseous foreign matter to become still harder; compressed together by the united action of the internal pressure and the low external temperature, it fills the surface of the body. In this way, a change is gradually brought about in the form of the body, which we call encumbrance with foreign matter. The extent of such encumbrance can be ascertained by my new system of diagnosis, the Science of Facial Expression. It is in this manner that all affections of the head, such as diseases of the eyes, ears and brain, mental debility, headaches, and the like arise. With the recognition of the unassailable fact, we solve at once one of the most puzzling riddles to be met with in the treatment of suffering humanity, and at the same time perceive the utter futility of the teachings of that medical school which will cure disease by a purely local treatment.

It is really remarkable what opinions the public has today concerning normal digestion. We often hear people saying, for instance: "My digestion is capital, I can eat so and so many beef-steaks and drink so and so many glasses of wine, without experiencing any indigestion. Everything agrees with me; I have a first-rate appetite." All this may be granted, yet, such habits are quite as injurious as smoking, say, ten cigars daily. Tobacco is, and ever will be, a poison to the body, and the body which has to occupy itself in the endeavor to expel nicotine, must, as a matter of course suffer in consequence. It is just the same with eating and drinking. A perfectly healthy stomach will refuse to retain even the smallest quantity of inappropriate food. By such complaints as eructation, heartburn and oppression, it indicates immediately that too much has been exacted. A debilitated stomach, on the other hand, tolerates apparently everything, that is to say, it has not the power to resist either suitable or superfluous food. In other words, the natural function, the natural instinct is lost. The food leaves the body insufficiently digested, without the latter having received any benefit from it.

The human body is able to extract from the simplest ailments, such as grains of corn, all those constituents which chemistry has pointed to as indispensable for its structure. Grain, such as we find in wholemeal bread, well chewed and insalivated, becomes sour immediately it enters the stomach. Through the process of digestion it is converted into important nutritive material for the body, alcohol, sugar, etc., being formed. *Such material is readily assimilated by the body, because it has been formed by it.* Those constituents of the grain which cannot be assimilated, are expelled again from the body in a certain definite form and of definite color.

Although the proofs, brought forward by me often do not find acknowledgement, the army of continually increasing diseases certainly does not exactly bear favorable witness to the progress of medical science. The public has here a gauge by which to measure the results of the practice of the orthodox medical school. How many have allowed themselves to be led astray by the false teachings of the medical profession; how many have broke Nature's laws in the food faith that they were acting well and wisely. But every transgression brings its own natural punishment in the form of disease or sickliness.

I cannot refrain here from publishing part of a letter received by me from a distant land, from an enthusiastic missionary in Honolulu. He wrote: "The natives here, before the whiteman was known, lived exclusively upon poi (the national dish of Honolulu, consisting of taro root beaten into a paste with water, forming an exceedingly nutritious food), with bananas and other fruits. Their only drink was pure water. They thus lived on a purely natural diet and their stature was gigantic, they were overflowing with health and strength. Then came the whiteman and taught the native that only flesh could give strength and only alcohol, particularly gin, produces energy. It did not continue long before the first cattle were imported and gin was spreading its blessing through the land. In the annals of Hawaii, the name is even recorded of the Hawaiian chief who first—on May 18th, 1819—openly changed his former manner of living. Pork has now become the national food and gin the national beverage; *but with what results!* The majority of the natives (Kanakas) suffer from eruption of the skin, and asthma; sexual disease are common and there is a great tendency to leprosy, which reaps a rich harvest amongst them." We see, then, how the natives on the new manner of living, brought to them by our much-lauded civilization, at once became diseased. The fact is another proof of the utter falsity of the theory of dietetics taught by the medical profession. In this case, naturally, the warm tropical climate was most favorable to the propagation of the disease which, in cold climate like ours, would have been much slower in making its appearance.

Let us now consider the theoretical principles upon which a natural system of diet is based.

THEORETICAL PRINCIPLES THAT DEMAND A RATIONAL, NATURAL SYSTEM OF DIET

We sustain our bodies through two organs: the lungs and the stomach. The reception of substances through inoculation with fluids is contrary to nature, and therefore always accompanied by injurious effects. The body has a sentinel for each: the nose for the former, and the tongue for the latter. Unhappily, as experience teaches us, neither is thoroughly incorruptible. There can hardly be a doubt that the fresh mountain air is the best food for our lungs; and in breathing such, our sense of smell is fully satisfied. He who has always lived in this pure air finds it quite impossible to remain for hours in smoky rooms, for his sense of smell warns him at each breath he draws. But if he often frequents such places, the warning voice gradually comes so accustomed to the bad air that this even appears pleasant. The sense has been corrupted and time is required before this morbid appetite can again be cured.

But, as we breathe from 16 to 20 times every minute, the ill effects of the direct absorption of foreign matter rapidly make themselves apparent, and thus it probably is that our understanding soon assumes the guidance, when our sense of smell has deserted us.

It is even worse with the tongue, which is unfortunately corrupted from our childhood, and which can, therefore hardly be regarded as reliable at all. It is well known, indeed, how the sense of taste can be made to conform to our habits. Nevertheless, it is of prime importance that the body should receive the right kind of nutriment; for all unnatural foods contain substances which are foreign to the body, and thus give rise to disease, as we have already seen.

Let us, then, consider the question: "What diet is the natural one?"

As we can no longer place full reliance on the tongue, we must seek to obtain an answer to this question by the aid of careful observations and conclusions in other directions.

Considered as a whole, the question is a purely scientific one. For its solution, therefore, we must adopt the only method admissible in science, the so-called inductive method, drawing general conclusions from particular cases. We may divide our task into three parts; we must

(1.) Collect observations;

(2.) Draw conclusions therefrom;

(3.) Make experiments.

The field of observation is an extremely wide one, and it is quite impossible for any one person to familiarize himself with every part. We must, therefore, content ourselves with a few excursions, just as one might make, if one desired to acquaint oneself with the flora of a country.

The ground to be traversed, in making a scientific enquiry into the question of diet, is so extensive that we must decide from the very commencement to keep our consideration within the closest bounds. For, to view the matter more comprehensively, we should have to inquire into the food of every organic being whatever. It will, however, suffice for us, if, in order to draw conclusions and to gain a foundation for systematic experiments, we consider only the higher forms of animals, that is, those nearer akin to ourselves. But to save digressions, I shall assume that you are familiar with all points on which general agreement prevails, and which are evident from observations, or have been proved beyond doubt.

A single glance at life in nature tells us that beings, in order to maintain the transformation of material going on, must, necessarily, obtain nourishment, in the choice of which, however, they are decidedly limited. A plant which grows luxuriously in the saliferous soil of the sea-coasts, dies when transplanted inland; one which flourishes in dry sandy ground, withers in the garden; and cultivated plants accustomed to rich humus, on the contrary, cannot grow in sand.

We observe quite the same thing in the animal kingdom, and in such a marked degree, that we can accurately classify animals according to their food. The classification of animals into those which feed on flesh and those which eat vegetable food only, is known to all; but this division is only a superficial one. On examining the matter closely, we find that we must separate the insect-eaters (insectivora) from the flesh-eaters proper (carnivora); and that the vegetable-eaters may be divided into those which live on herbs, grass and the like (herbivora) and those which live on fruit (frugivora). Besides these, we find some few which live on both kinds of food (omnivora). Our observations must also extend to the organs which aid in nutrition, in the case of each class. These afford us so good a clue to the diet, that we can determine, even from the skeleton, to what class the animal belongs. We will turn our attention chiefly to the *teeth*, the *digestive canal*, the *organs of sense* which guide the animal to its food, and the *manner in which it nourishes* its young. Thus, there are four excursions which we propose to make into the territory we have marked for observation.

As you are aware, teeth are divided into three classes: Incisors or cutting teeth, canines or dog-teeth, and molars or grinding teeth. The incisors of carnivorous animals are little developed, and hardly used at all, whereas the canines are of striking length. They project far beyond the rest and in the opposite row a special gap is necessary for their reception. They are pointed, smooth, and slightly curved. They are in no way suited for chewing, but especially adapted for *seizing* and *holding* the prey. In the case of predatory animals we call these teeth fangs, and can observe how they really are used as such. For dividing the flesh into small pieces, the back teeth are employed, the surface of which is covered with points. These points do not meet, but fit closely side by side, so that in the operation of chewing they only mechanically separate the muscular fibres of the flesh. A lateral motion of the jaw would hinder this process, nor is it possible in the carnivora. It is therefore clear that animals of this class cannot grind their food. We see, for instance, how hard it is for dogs to well masticate pieces of bread, so that they have finally to swallow the food nearly unchewed.

In the herbivorous animals, the incisors are developed for biting off grass and herbs. The canine teeth are usually stunted, the molars are broad, and well adapted for *crushing* and *grinding* herbaceous food.

MAN A FRUGIVOROUS ANIMAL

There are not many frugivorous animals; for us, the anthropoid (man-like) apes are the most important. It is in the frugivora that we find the teeth most evenly developed. They have nearly all the same height, only the canines projecting a little beyond the others, though not enough to enable them to serve the same purpose as in the carnivora. They are conical, but blunt at the top and not smooth, so that they could not serve for seizing prey. One can see that they are very powerful; indeed, we know that the anthropoid apes can perform astonishing feats with their teeth. The molars of these animals are furnished at the top with fold of enamel, and as the lower jaw admits of ample lateral motion, their action may be compared to that of millstones. The circumstance that not a single molar is pointed, is of special significance, for thus we see that they have not one tooth intended for chewing flesh. This is the more remarkable, because the omnivora, to which only the bears, properly speaking, belong, have both pointed and broad-topped molars. Of course, bears also have canines, like those of carnivora, without which they could not seize their prey; the incisors, on the contrary, resembling those of frugivora.

Now, which of these sets of teeth most resembles that of man? There is no room for doubt, for we can perceive without difficulty that the human teeth are formed almost precisely like those of the frugivorous animals. In man the canines do not grow quite so long as they do in the frugivora, and project very little, or not at all, beyond the others, but this difference is not material. It has often been concluded, from the mere presence of the canine teeth, that the human body is also organized for a flesh diet. This conclusion, however, would be justified only if the canines in man were able to fulfill the same function as the canines of the carnivora; and if, like the bears, we had at least a few corresponding back-teeth for dividing flesh.

The conclusions which we must draw from our observations are as follows:

1. Man's teeth do not resemble those of the carnivora, therefore he is not a carnivorous animal;

2. Man's teeth do not resemble those of the herbivora, therefore he is not an herbivorous animal;

3. Man's teeth do not resemble those of the omnivora, therefore he is not an omnivorous animal;

4. Man's teeth almost exactly resemble those of the anthropoid frugivora, therefore it is highly probable that he is a frugivorous animal.

The false deduction mentioned above, is frequently brought forward in another form as follows: "Judging by his teeth, man is neither a carnivorous, nor an herbivorous animal, but stand in the middle position between the two, therefore he is both." We need scarcely point out, that this conclusion is logically quite untenable. The notion of a middle position is much too general and indefinite to find application where scientific proof is required; only in mathematics does it admit of a definite conception.

Let us now enter upon our second excursion through the rich field of observation, and turn our attention to the digestive canal of the animals. Predatory animals have a small, almost round stomach, and the intestines are from 3 to 5 times as long as the body, measuring the latter from the mouth to the root of the tail. The herbivora, particularly the ruminants, have a large compound stomach, and the intestines are from 20 to 28 times the length of the body. In the frugivora, the stomach is somewhat broader than in the carnivora, and in the duodenum they possess a continuation of it, which may be described as a second stomach. The length of the intestines is about 10 to 12 times that of the body. In anatomical works it is often stated that the intestinal canal in man is from 3 to 5 times as long as the body and consequently more suited for a flesh diet. This is to accuse Nature of a flat contradiction: as regards the teeth she had formed man, in the popular opinion, as an omnivorous animal; as regards his intestines as a carnivorous one. But this contradiction is only apparent. In the above comparison, the length of the human body had been measured from crown to sole; whereas to conform with the other cases, only the distance from the mouth to the end of the spine ought to be measured. The conclusion drawn therefore, is a false one. The length of the human intestines is from 18-28 feet, depending upon the height of the individual, and the body from head to the end of spine 1 ½ to 2 ½ feet, a division yielding a quotient of about 10 or 11. Hence, we arrive at the conclusion that MAN IS A FRUGIVOROUS ANIMAL.

On beginning our third excursion, let us consult the sign posts to our diet—the senses. It is chiefly by the senses of smell and taste that animals are directed to their food and at the same time incited to eat. When a predatory animal finds the scent of game, his eyes begin to sparkle, he follows the trail with eagerness, springs upon his prey and greedily laps up the warm blood, all this evidently affording him the keenest pleasure. The herbivorous animal, on the contrary, passes quietly by his fellow creatures, and can at most be induced by other reasons to attack them, his sense of smell would never betray him into eating flesh; he will even leave his natural food untouched if it is sprinkled with blood. The sense of smell and sight lead him to grass and herbs, which also gratify his taste. We notice the same thing in the case of the frugivora, whose senses direct them to the fruits of the tree and field.

But how do human organs of sense act? Do the senses of sight and smell ever entice us into slaughtering an ox? Would a child, who had never heard anything of the slaughtering of animals, even if it had already eaten meat, ever think, on looking at a fatted ox: "That would be a tid-bit for me"? Only when we can associate in our mind the connection between the living animal and the roast as it comes upon the table, are we capable of such thoughts; they are not given to us by Nature.

The very idea of killing is abhorrent to our senses, and raw flesh is agreeable neither to the eyes nor the nose. Why are slaughter-houses always being removed further and further from our towns? Why are there, in many places, laws forbidding the transportation of flesh uncovered? Can this in point of fact be styled a natural food, when it is so offensive both to eye and nose? Before being eaten, it has, by means of condiments, to be rendered attractive to the senses of smell and taste, unless indeed these have already been abnormally deadened. How delightful, on the other hand, do we find the fragrance of fruit. It is surely no accident that reporters at fruit-shows almost invariably express their feelings in the set phrase: "The sight of the fruit make one's mouth water." I may remark that the various grains also possess an agreeable, if faint, odor, and have also pleasant taste, even in the raw state. There is nothing repulsive to us in harvesting and in cooking grain; and not without reason has the country-man been called a happy and contented rustic. Thus, for the second time, we must draw the conclusion: "By nature man is decidedly a frugivorous animal."

In examining, on our third excursion, the arrangements made by

Nature for the propagation of the species, the observations are more difficult. All animals, on their entrance into life, are provided with a food which favors their rapid development. For new-born babes, the mother's milk is undoubtedly the only natural food. And here we observe that a great many mother are quite incapable of performing their sacred duties, their organism not being in a condition to produce the nutrition for the child. This is especially deplorable, because such children are thus deprived at the very commencement of their life of the natural standard for sensuous impressions, no artificial food resembling the natural one in every respect. Observation shows us that the mother of so-called "better classes," whose chief nourishment is flesh-meat, suffer most in this respect, and are obliged to employ wet-nurses from the country, where very little flesh-meat is eaten. As a rule, such nurses on securing a situation, then live on the same food as the other inmates of the town house, and as a consequence not seldom lost the ability to suckle the child. On voyages, oat-meal gruel is given to nursing mother; for on the diet usually supplied on board ship, consisting as it does largely of flesh-diet, their breasts would soon dry up.

From these observations we draw the conclusion, that flesh-diet affords little or no aid in the production of mother's milk. (We do not mean to say, that on a vegetarian diet every mother could nurse her own child; for this, a certain degree of health is also requisite, which cannot be attained all at once.)

If our conclusion be correct, it necessarily follows that the greater part of mankind has wandered more or less from a natural diet. Creatures of Nature have turned aside from their natural food! That sounds monstrous, and needs still further proofs. Is it possible, then, that other creatures can likewise forsake their natural food; and what consequences would this have? This question must be answered before we can proceed.

We are well aware that dogs and cats can be accustomed to *vegetable* diet; but can we also adduce instances of vegetable feeding animals have become accustomed to flesh diet? I was once enabled to observe an extremely interesting case. A family reared a young deer, which soon made friends with the house-dog. She often saw the latter lapping meat-broth, and soon attempted to take her share at meal-times. At first, she always turned away with signs of disgust at the mere taste of the broth; but she repeated the attempts, and in a few weeks ate her share with relish. In a few weeks more she could even eat fleshmeat, which she at length preferred to her natural food. But the effects were soon observable; the animal become ill and died before it was a year old. I may add that this deer was not confined but ran about at will in the garden and woods.

We know, too, that the frugivorous apes can be easily habituated in confinement to a flesh diet, but then as a rule, die of consumption within a year or two. This is usually attributed to the climate, but as the other denizens of the tropics thrive quite well in our zone, we are justified in assuming that it is the unnatural food which is principally to blame. Recent investigations also confirm this view.

It is, therefore, certain that animals may turn from their natural food; and thus the assumption that a great part of mankind has done the same, becomes still more probable. But if this be the case, the consequences must also be perceptible to us—disease must surely appear, or have already appeared.

Should we ask in sober truth, how many persons have never required a physician, I believe we would find very few indeed. And how many are there who really die of old age? The cases are so rare that the newspapers usually record them. There are extremely few persons to be found who are not encumbered with foreign matter. In general, the more frugivorous country-folk, though not living strictly in accordance with Nature, are more fortunate in that respect; and though fresh air may play its part, food is here the prime factor. Although it is certain, that the unsatisfactory condition of our health is partly the result of other causes, we can ascertain by a comparison with the animal kingdom, the food is the most important cause. For instance, animals kept in the stable live in the most unfavorable hygienic conditions imaginable; they are forced to breathe continually the gases issuing from their excrements, and are almost wholly deprived of free exercise. They must naturally become diseased in consequence, and one can take it for granted, that such cattle are never quite healthy. But despite these unfavorably hygienic conditions, there are not so many disease prevalent amongst these animals as amongst men, who in all these respects can and do take much better care of themselves. The blame, therefore, must by laid chiefly on the food consumed.

Louis Kuhne (1835-1901) gave his first public course and instruction in 1888 on his *New Science of Healing* in Leipzig, Germany. The first edition of the book was published in 1891 in German in Leipzig. The first English edition was published in 1893 and Benedict Lust re-published Kuhne's book in 1917 with a modified title: *Neo-Naturopathy: the New Science of Healing. Ed.*

But as we know that foreign matter only forms as the result of wrong food, that is, can only arise in the body as the result of bad digestion, it must be our task to avoid such wrong foods and such bad digestion.

We find almost everywhere the erroneous opinion prevailing that in winter one should eat well and consume plenty fat, in order to be able to withstand the cold. This, however, is in flat contradiction to all natural laws.

All food which we have to change by cooking, smoking, spicing, salting, pickling, and putting in vinegar, lose in digestibility, and as regards vitality, are far inferior to food in its natural condition, even though the above-named processes may enable the foods to keep longer.

Thus to persons suffering from affections of the stomach, or troubles of the digestion, unripe fruit is to be recommended instead of ripe; and the use of such should be continued until the stomach is so far strengthened as to be again able to digest the fruit ripe.

Food precisely in the form nature gives it to us, is always the best for digestion.

The digestion is normal when the excrements are light brown, soft and compact, and covered with a mucous coating, clearly showing the slimy nature of the various juices of the body. They should be of sausage form and leave the body absolutely unsoiled.

Man's teeth almost exactly resemble those of the anthropoid frugivora, therefore it is highly probable that he is a frugivorous animal.

COCOA BREAD

Translated from the German by David Ammann

Herald of Health and Naturopath, XXIII(2), 175-177. (1918)

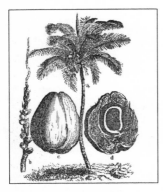

Cocoa bread referred to coconut bread.

Vegetarianism, in its endeavor to arrive at pure, unadulterated nourishment i.e., that the form of food, as we find it prepared by nature, takes more and more a partly conscious, partly involuntary tendency toward Raw Food. The greatest obstacle lies in the conservatism of our digestive organs. They are the weak flesh unable to keep up with the willing spirit, following by force, habits and traditions more than thousands of years old. This fact must naturally be taken into consideration. The transition to raw food can be but slow, but the obstacle can be overcome. It is the intention of this article to show a method of reconciliation with which even a very weak digestive organism may agree, and which means a step ahead on the road whose goal is **Uncooked Food**.

Another obstacle is a lack of proper comprehension of what is pure natural food. Most new disciples of the gospel of raw food think that they should become healthy and strong, if they eat plenty of fruit, because they regard fruit as the pure food of nature; they do not realize that almost all fruit that comes on the market, is not nature's but an artificial product, as for instance, apples, pears, grapes, prunes, oranges, apricots, peaches, nuts, etc. In their natural form, that is, in their primitive state, most fruits are sour, hard and almost unpalatable.

A wild apple does not at all agree with our taste, nor do wild prunes in the form of sloe-berries, nor wild peaches in the form of bitter almonds. Man's endeavor to improve on nature has, by means of horticulture, created artificial products which give more pleasure to the palate. Delicious, sweet fruits are these products. The peach, more than other fruits, shows how art has improved on nature's product. Here the green, unpalatable skin of the almond has been developed into a magnificent rich flesh. It gives great enjoyment, but the kernel, the most nourishing part, is thrown away.

Too much partiality to artificial fruits makes us lose the right direction. In their belief that fruits are pure nature food and therefore perfect in themselves, fruit-eaters partake of far too much sugar and too little albumen and fat. Therefore, with all due appreciation of fruit, it is timely to warn against the consumption of too great quantities of sweet fruit. Too much sugar in the blood prevents the assimilation of the albumen. The result of this is decay of the teeth, a frequent complaint with fruit-eaters. The proportion of sugar to albumen and fat should be the same as in the milk. This proportion must be considered as the normal one, scientific formulas to the contrary and exaggerations of super-nature men notwithstanding.

The nourishing value of fruit would be greater, if the kernels were, or could also be eaten. As long as this is not the case, fruit cannot be regarded as the principal food, but must remain a side-dish.

Nuts, however, contain all the nourishing elements which we require, in about the same proportion as milk, and must, therefore, be the principal food of those who desire to live on the raw products of nature. But the ordinary nut cannot be eaten with absolute impunity; black teeth and troubles of the digestive organs are the frequent result. Hazelnuts are excellent food, but, like most other nuts, are a rather expensive article. The cocoanut* is the finest, most agreeable, and—last but not least—cheapest of all nuts, and worthy to be designated the queen amongst them. It is a pure product of nature. It is at home not only in the gardens, but also in the virgin forests of tropical regions. In my household, the cocoanut has held since many years a place of honor. We have tried to make it our principal food. All possible experiments in cutting it up and mixing it with other foods gave very tasty dishes, but not the looked for form, in which it could serve as the staff of life. This result was reached only when I succeeded in making the cocoa-bread. Everybody enjoyed it, particularly the children whose taste, in my opinion, is a better criterion than that of adults who have spoiled theirs by too much "refinement."

COCOA-BREAD IS PREPARED IN THE FOLLOWING MANNER:

Cocoanuts are grated and thoroughly mixed with an equal quantity of raw rolled oats. Salt may be added or omitted according to taste. No liquid is added, neither the milk of nut, nor any other. This dry mixture, wrapped up in a cotton cloth, is put into a flat form, either round or square, smoothed out so as to be of the same thickness all over, sandwiched in between two boards and then left under a rather intense pressure for from 3 to 10 hours. A solid bread, the delight of everyone who partakes of it, is the result. No meat-eater ever tried it without giving it unstinted praise. The flavors of cocoanut and oats are blended in a perfect mixture to the satisfaction not only of the palate, but also of the stomach.

---

*Cocoanut refers to coconut. Ed.

This bread has the advantage that it must be thoroughly masticated, and it then tastes like pure milk. It has become our daily bread, our staff of life. It is a question only of very little time for one to become used to this simple raw bread. It gives a feeling of satisfaction and increased strength, and at the same time decreases always the desire for cooked food. As to quantity, it may be said that a pound a day for each person is a good average. In the experiments which led to the cocoa-bread, all possible combinations of different species of nuts with different sorts of flour have been tried, and even hashed dry fruit has been added to the mixture, but nothing gave the same satisfaction as cocoanut with oats.

Cocoa-bread has a very beneficent effect on the action of the bowels, the same as cocoamilk. In the latter, which is best partaken of in the morning, nature offers an absolutely harmless laxative.

As to cheapness, no other nut can be compared to the cocoanut. Until recently, in the port cities of this country where they are imported directly from the tropics, one hundred could be bought for $3 or $4, according to the size of the nuts. As the net weight of one nut—without shell or milk—is on an average 1 pound it may be said that the price was from 3 to 4 cents a pound.

Where fresh cocoanuts cannot be had, copra, or some of the other forms in which the fruit of the coca-palm reaches the market, can be used in the making of cocoa-bread.

It has been shown here how a cheap bread can be made which in taste and nourishing power is far above any other kind. Its preparation is so simple that every bachelor can make it for himself. Cocoa-bread is good only when fresh, and therefore, the supply for the day should be made either on the night before or early in the morning. If anything is left, the dog and the family cat will take it as eagerly as if it were meat. If it is impossible to get rolled oats, which should be about as thin as heavy paper, fresh ground oatmeal may be substituted. The fresher the oats, the better the bread. Anything can serve the purpose of a press, a copying press, a wine-press, or, in an emergency, a heavy board stone or other flat, heavy object. To give the bread a fine round or square form with sharp lines, a frame should be made of wood into which the two boards, between which the bread is pressed, must fit precisely. For the grating process, the ordinary utensil can be used; better still is a rotary grating mill, because it does better and quicker work.

> *The cocoanut is the finest, most agreeable, and—last but not least—cheapest of all nuts, and worthy to be designated the queen amongst them.*

Kitchen And Table, Menus For Purifiction

by Mrs. Louisa Lust

Herald of Health and Naturopath, XXIII(3), 278. (1918)

With the beginning of Lent, we approach the season of purification. Every season brings its own rules and regulation, and in order to keep healthy, we must observe and follow nature. During the winter—the season of feasting—when heavier dishes rich in oils, starches and proteins, are in order, the system naturally accumulates a certain amount of morbid waste matter. Unless the diet is changed with the early Spring, these waste products will be thrown to the surface of the body, producing skin eruptions, pimples, boils, carbuncles, etc.

Lent has more than a spiritual significance. It is an entirely practical institution—it is the season of body purification.

It comes a little too early this year for our climate and the first of March is ample time for the healthy to begin a purifying diet.

Eliminate salt from all dishes. Oils and nuts should be excluded from the diet as well as dairy products. Breadstuffs should be eaten sparingly. Hard baked breads or quickly made biscuits or matzos are the best kind of breadstuffs to indulge in.

Fruits and vegetables should be the principal articles of diet, and these should be prepared and eaten in their raw state.

Occasional fasts are in order at least one day each week with a three day fast at the end of the season. A regimen such as this followed for six weeks right now will assure you of health for the coming summer.

Menus For Purification

Breakfast

Fruit only; grape fruit, oranges, grated apple with orange juice, or dried fruits.

Lunch

Cereal or matzos and a fruit or vegetable salad.

Dinner

Fresh green vegetables, vegetable salad. Crackers, matzos or quick biscuits. Occasionally cottage cheese with chopped chives and onions.

Garlic and onions at this season can be used with good effect as intestinal purifiers.

THE SECRET IS OUT

A Treat for the Epicure   *A Triumph of Culinary Art*

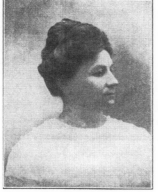

LOUISA LUST, N. D.

The Naturopathic Resort "Yung-born" at Butler, New Jersey, and the Florida Yungborn "Quisisana" at Tangerine have long been famous for the originality and excellence of their vegetarian diet. Visitors have described the meals as "masterpieces of the culinary art," and many have sought to discover the secret of the succulent and delicious viands which grace our table. All the vegetables, fruits and nuts of a bounteous Nature seem to have combined at the touch of a magician's wand into a profuse variety of new and savory dishes which tickle the palate and bring the smile of inward contentment to those assembled round the festive board. Selfishness has no place in Naturopathic ideals. Being willing, therefore, that our friends should have the secret of this dainty and nutritious cooking, Mrs. Lust has decided to place before the public the result of her labor and study of years in this particular branch, in the form of a complete Naturopathic - Vegetarian cook book, aptly entitled the

GOOD DINNER COOK BOOK

Vegetarian cooking takes on a new meaning after you have tried some of the recipes in this book and the gastronomic horizon of the vegetarian is broadened by new and unthought-of combinations, even the reading of which makes your mouth water with joyful anticipation. You are real mean to yourself if you don't get this book. Send for it to-day and give your friends a treat.

PARTIAL CONTENTS

Section 1—Cooked and Uncooked Foods. Section 2—Substitutes for Animal Foods. Section 3—Egg Plants, Potato Croquettes, etc. Section 4—Rice or Farina Fritters, Rice with Tomatoes, etc. Section 5—Mushroom Pie, Cabbage Pie, Spinach and Eggs, Stuffed Peppers, etc. Section 6—Soups and Gruels. Section 7—Vegetables and what may be done with them. Section 8—Sauces and their importance to a good dinner, etc., etc. Sixteen Sections with table of Food Values from reliable authorities.

Price, 75 cents; Cloth, $1.00. Postpaid with a year's subscription to THE NATUROPATH $2.25. Send all orders to

NATURE CURE PUBLISHING COMPANY, BUTLER, N. J.

Ad for Louisa Lust's *Good Dinner Cook Book*.

Horse-radish as well as grated raw turnips will help the liver action, accomplishing the removal of uric acid and other irritating protein wastes from the blood.

Rhubarb, skinned and chopped in small pieces on salads, is a splendid stomach and liver tonic. Use all the greens as they come into the market, including spinach, mustard, dandelion and sorrel as salads.

Aromatic seeds, such as fennel, anise, caraway, dill and celery, should be sprinkled over salads, not only for flavoring, but to rid the alimentary tract of bacteria, parasites and to allay putrefaction.

If constipated, resort to colon irrigation.

A Nut And Fruit Dietary For Brain Workers

by Sophie Leppel (England)

Herald of Health and Naturopath, XXIII(6), 575-576. (1918)

[Note that a particular fruit or nut contains "no" heat; brain food, etc. is only said relatively. It is meant that it contains none practically, or in comparison with the other elements it possesses.]

Properties Of Some Fruits And Nuts

Blanched Almonds give the higher nerve or brain and muscle food (no heat nor waste).

Walnuts give nerve or brain and muscle food, also heat and waste.

Pine Kernels give heat and food. They serve as a substitute for bread.

Green Water Grapes are blood-purifying, but of little food value. (Reject pips and skins).

Blue Grapes are feeding and blood-purifying. For those who suffer from the liver they are too rich.

Tomatoes (English) are a higher nerve or brain food, also waste. No heat. They are thinning, also stimulating. (Do not swallow skins).

Juicy Fruits give more or less the higher nerve or brain food, and some few, muscle food and waste. No heat.

Apples
(English eating) supply the higher nerve and muscle food, but do not give stay.

Prunes afford the higher nerve or brain food. They supply heat and waste, but are not muscle-feeding. They should be avoided by those who suffer from the liver.

Oranges are refreshing and feeding, but are not recommended if the liver is out of order.

Green Figs are excellent food.

Dried Figs contain nerve and muscle food, heat, and waste, but they are bad for the liver.

The great majority of small fresh seed fruits are laxative.

All stone fruits are injurious for those who suffer from the liver.

Lemons and tomatoes should be used cautiously in cold weather. They have a thinning and cooling effect.

Raisins are stimulating in proportion to their quality.

A Nut And Fruit Meal For Brain Workers

1 oz. table raisins (muscatels).

3 French prunes (supplied in glass jars).

1 Fig (if not found too laxative).

Nut cream (see "Recipes").

Apples (raw, peeled, or baked), as many as relished.

1 orange, and as many grapes, soft pears, tomatoes, or any other small seed fruits as relished, bearing in mind that the kidneys should not be over-taxed by too much juicy fruit. This meal can be taken three times a day.

Brainworkers who have hard physical work to do as well should, to the nut cream, add more pine kernels, and they should also take some Brazil nuts.

General Rules

If a sense of faintness (indicating inadequate nutrition) is felt between meals, raw apples or any small seed fruit, grapes, or pears can be taken, also pine kernel and lemon, orange, fig, or apple cream or "ambrosia" (see "Recipes"), till the exact quantity of fruit and nut cream is determined which the system requires at each meal.

Great caution should be used not to take too much nut cream. Roasted or boiled nuts will be found more digestible than those in their natural state.

Green Grapes are the best food for night worn. If, however, they are out of season, sweet baked apples, oranges, and, if relished, a few table raisins, form a good substitute.

All the fruits may be taken uncooked if the system can assimilate them.

When no great hunger is felt at a meal, nut cream should never be eaten, but only a little juicy fruit, baked or raw apples, green grapes or tomatoes being always the safest.

If sores appear with watery exudation, too much acid is being taken.

If irritation is felt, or skin eruption appears, too much nut cream is being taken.

Should constipation set in, less nut cream and more juicy fruits should be eaten. If the bowels are too much relaxed, less fruit and more nuts, such as pine kernels, are needed. At each meal, some acid or sub-acid fruit should be taken.

At each meal, some waste must be taken. This is found in the skins of nuts and fruits. Too much waste should be avoided.

Sweet, soft, good English eating apples may be considered the safest fruit foods for healthy people.

The better the quality of the fruits and nuts taken, the better the health, work, thoughts, clearness of mind, and keenness of perception.

RECIPES

NUT CREAM FOR BRAIN WORKERS

(Quantity for One Meal)

3 blanched almonds

2 walnuts

2 eggcupsful of pine kernels (if pine kernels are not obtainable, roasted or boiled chestnuts may be used; but pine kernels are the best).

Pound all very fine, and then soak all night, in lemon or orange juice, or in half lemon and half orange juice.

The nuts will swell; hence sufficient juice should be allowed so as to form a thick cream when taken.

To save time and trouble, and, above all, to ensure thorough soaking, a sufficient quantity may be prepared in the evening for the three meals of the following day.

The lemon juice is a powerful digester (solvent) of the nuts.

PINE KERNEL AND LEMON CREAM

Pound pine kernels fine, and mix with lemon juice, so as to form a thick cream.

Eat when fruits are not satisfying. It will give stay. Lemon cream is good for those who suffer from the liver, but if the acid should not be relished, use half lemon and half orange juice.

PINE KERNEL AND ORANGE CREAM

Pound pine kernels and mix with orange juice.

This will give stay and also warmth.

PINE KERNEL AND FIG CREAM

Pound pine kernels and mix with steamed figs in equal proportions. (The figs should be quite soft.)

Fig cream gives great stay. It is very warming, and is nerve and muscle feeding; but it is laxative; while it is also bad for the liver.

PINE KERNEL AND APPLE CREAM

Pound pine kernels and mix with baked apples (three times the proportions of the apples to one of pine kernels). The baked apples may either be put through a colander (so that the pips, skins, and cores may be removed), or they may be mixed entirely with the pine kernels. The pips should not be crushed in the mouth, but ejected, with the cores and the skins.

This cream is warming, while it feeds the body and increases mental activity. (The cream keeps one well-balanced in body and mind.)

AMBROSIA

Mix baked apples passed through a colander with stewed pudding raisins (not sultanas). (Two parts of apples to one part of raisins.) The raisins should be stewed in as little water as possible till the skins are quite soft. Skins and pips must not be swallowed.

One small breakfast cupful of warm "ambrosia", one or two hours before breakfast, will act as a gentle aperient. It is good for those who suffer from the liver. When taken during the day at meals, or between meals, it will be found feeding, a little warming, and stimulating.

Healthful Eating

by E. Howard Tunison

Herald of Health and Naturopath. XXIII(7), 652. (1918)

Show me that young man or that young woman who eats habitually in an indiscreet and indiscriminate manner, and I will show you the person who is doomed at forty years of age, or shortly thereafter, to die of apoplexy, heart disease, kidney trouble, or cancer. A man should be his own physician, rather than be a fool, **before** forty.

Brillat Savarin, the popular French epicure of fifty years ago, once said, "Tell me what kind of food you eat, and I will tell you what kind of a man you are." This significant remark can be improved somewhat by a few interpolations. It should be, "Tell me what kind of food you eat, **when you eat, how you eat, how much you eat at a meal, and how you mix together your foods,**—and I will tell you what kind of man you are."

Everything in nature, man excepted, follows natural law. Nature, at creation, was lenient with mankind; she endowed him with the very often abused privilege of free will. Lower animals have been blessed with the power of instinct; they seldom err in their habits unless under man's direct, unskilled supervision. Man is free to follow or not, as he deems fit, Nature's dictates. When he obeys them, he prospers; when he disregards them, he suffers. Nature is just as strict in rules of dietetic concern as she is in anything else. It behooves us, then, if we desire physical welfare, to trust and to obey her in this respect.

Rules pertaining to diet have been gradually learned by painstaking observers during years of careful study. These rules have been discovered often by observing the eating habits of animals. Adherence to such rules has been found to result in the attainment of perfect digestion and pure blood—prime health requisites.

Concise, recognized rules for correct eating now follow.

1. *Eat only when you are hungry.*

    A vast difference between hunger and appetite exists. Hunger is a normal desire; appetite is an abnormal craving. Hunger relishes coarse, substantial food, while morbid appetite prefers only dainties.

2. *Eat preferably natural foods.*

    Natural foods are: Cereals (whole-meal wheat and rye products; natural brown rice; stoneground cornmeal and oatmeal, rolled or cut), Vegetables (green or salad vegetables, roots and legumes); Fruits,

Nuts, Melons, Berries, and Dairy Products (eggs, milk, cheese, and butter).

3. *Chew your food thoroughly; never bolt it.*

   Chew the taste out of your food; it should be so well liquefied that it will swallow by itself.

4. *Do not wash down your food, or soak it in any drink before you eat it.*

   If you desire water at meal time, drink it, but do so only when your mouth is free from food.

   Never gulp water down in a hurry; drink it slowly, warming each mouthful before you swallow it. Never drink ice water.

5. *Never eat when overtired, or when in the grip of depressing emotions.*

   Fatigue, worry, fear, anger, and intense sorrow greatly retard, or suspend altogether the secretion of digestive juices and motions of the digestive organs.

6. *Never eat while feeling ill.*

   Feeding during sickness handicaps nature; she indicates her will by removing the desire for food at such times.

7. *Stop eating when your appetite (true hunger) begins to wane.*

   Quit eating when you feel comfortably filled; do not continue to tickle your palate with delicacies. Overeating is a grave dietetic sin; avoid it.

8. *Do not eat too great a variety of things at a meal.*

   Too varied a number of foods, by overstimulating the sense of taste with so many flavors, tempts one without knowing it to overeat.

9. *Do not eat between meals.*

   Eating between meals is another form of overeating.

10. *Two substantial meals a day, with an interval of five or six hours, are better than three.*

    Those people who observe this rule, notably the Italians, possess most rugged health.

11. *Avoid late suppers; never eat just before going to bed.*

    The blood, more than any other time, renews during sleep the tired body cells. If the stomach requires the blood to assist it to digest food throughout one's period of sleep, he cannot help but awake unrefreshed.

12. *Avoid mental application or too active exercise immediately after eating.*

   Such activities, by withdrawing blood from the stomach at a critical time, interfere with digestion.

13. *Avoid spices and spiced foods, tea, coffee, and alcoholic drinks.*

   Spiced foods, by continuously overstimulating digestive glands, eventually produce a weakened and congested condition of the alimentary tract, thereby interfering with the digestion and absorption of food.

   Cocoa, cereal coffee and milk are the only permissible food-drinks. Cocoa and cereal coffee are almost dietetic outcasts, because they require the addition to them of sugar and milk to make them palatable. Thus, in the light of our rules relative to the proper combining of foods, these drinks will not harmonize well when taken with foods of a starchy nature. If you desire either cocoa or cereal coffee, it would be a good plan to indulge in an exclusive "cocoa meal" or "cereal coffee meal" by sipping slowly a generous cupful or two, according to your desire.

14. *Avoid bathing too close to meal time.*

   Bath one hour before meals, or three hours afterwards. Bathing too close to mealtime interferes with the blood-supply to the digestive organs.

15. *While eating, converse on pleasant topics, or think pleasant thoughts.*

   Cheerful states of mind aid digestion by stimulating the digestive glands to healthful activity.

16. *Do not mix starchy foods,* as bread, oatmeal, rice, cornmeal, macaroni, spaghetti, tapioca, sago, potatoes, parsnips, peas, lentils, beans, apples (mealy) pears and bananas—

   1. With sour-tasting (acid) foods, as apricots, blackberries, cherries, cranberries, gooseberries, grapes, huckleberries, lemons, limes, oranges, grapefruit, peaches, plums, prunes, raspberries, rhubarb, strawberries and tomatoes; buttermilk.

   2. Intimately with fatty or oily foods, as suet, lard, tallow, butter, cream, olive oil, peanut oil, cottonseed oil, or corn oil.

   3. With highly-sweet foods, as cane (granulated) sugar, maple sugar, molasses, candy, or honey.

Examples of inharmonious mixtures of starchy foods with:

Sour-tasting foods:

lemonade and cake, strawberry shortcake, peach cobbler, bread and jam, etc.

Fatty and oily foods:

fritters, gravy, dressing, doughnuts, pork and beans, etc.

Highly sweet foods:

syrup, coffee with buns or rolls, cake with icing, buckwheat cakes and syrup, gingerbread, etc.

Indiscriminate food mixtures dispose to fermentation. Fermentation is a souring process caused by bacteria in the presence of starchy or sugary food, moisture, and heat. Fermentation, according to the type of bacterium present, results in the formation of alcohol (vinous), acetic (vinegar), lactic acid (acid of buttermilk), butyric acid (acid in rancid butter), and carbonic acid gas. Fermentation products irritate the digestive tract, producing countless digestive disturbances; their absorption into the bloodstream acidifies it, producing blood "humors."

Lower animals have been blessed with the power of instinct; they seldom err in their habits unless under man's direct, unskilled supervision. Man is free to follow or not, as he deems fit, Nature's dictates. When he obeys them, he prospers; when he disregards them, he suffers.

Eat only when you are hungry.

Never eat when overtired, or when in the grip of depressing emotions.

Stop eating when your appetite (true hunger) begins to wane.

Indiscriminate food mixtures dispose to fermentation.

THE DIETETIC CURE FOR CANCER
AUGUSTIN L. EVANZIN, A.B. PH.D.

THE CAUSE OF DISEASE
IRVING JAMES EALES, M.D., D.O.

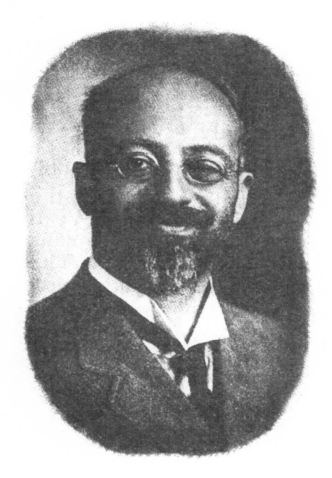

Prof. Augustin L. Evanzin, A.B., Ph.D.

THE DIETETIC CURE OF CANCER

by Prof. Augustin L. Evanzin, A.B., Ph.D.

Formerly Lecturer on Dietology at the College of Physicians and Surgeons of Boston, Mass. (copyrighted by the Author)

Herald of Health and Naturopath, XXIV(3), 125-128. (1919)

Cancer is still the autocratic king among diseases. Dr. J.H. Kellogg, of Battle Creek, calls it appropriately "The Monster Malady, the Coming Plague of the Race," and Dr. Robert Bell of London, England, calls it a "scourge." And it surely is, because it attacks not only mankind but also animals and plants, and in persons past thirty-five years of age one out of every eight women and one out of every eleven men dies of cancer. Its harvest of mortality is growing by leaps and bounds, and it exists in nearly every corner of the world. More than seventy-five thousand people die from cancer in the United States each year.

Cancer is the arch-enemy of mankind; and it behooves us to study its causes and the best means to prevent it and cure it; because otherwise, at its rate of increase, the extermination of the whole human race is not very far off. Half a million die annually from it in the civilized world, and the mortality is increasing at the rate of two and one-half per cent every year, according to Fred. L. Hoffman, statistician of the Prudential Insurance Company of New York.

This increase is undoubtedly due to the greater use of meat and other protein-rich foods in modern times and especially to the common use of foods deficient or lacking in vitamines, without which life, growth and reproduction are impossible.

After many years of study and experience there is no doubt left in my mind that the chief cause of cancer is the wrong way of eating of the majority of the people; and, therefore, its real cure cannot be effected by means of the knife, plasters, chemicals, drugs or by any other artificial contrivance, but simply by natural means; by the right diet, by the help of fresh air, of a moderate amount of sunshine and exercise, and by an optimistic mental attitude and a congenial environment.

That the chief cause of cancer is the wrong way of eating is not my exclusive opinion; several other eminent physicians are the same view. Dr. Elmer Lee, the well-informed editor of the *Health Culture Magazine*, in the September number of 1910, wrote: "Cancer appears to originate in improper feeding; it is then a **food-caused disease**. If bad foods ruin the digestion and produce the soil favorable to cancerous degeneration, it naturally follows that the only treatment worthy of serious consideration lies within the domain of good foods, diet and improved nutrition."

In London England, exists a "Society for the Prevention and Relief of Cancer," with a large membership of very intelligent and progressive physicians and laymen. The Duchess of Hamilton is the patroness and the famous cancer expert, Dr. Robert Bell, is the president. In the first Annual Report of this Society I read the following two important clauses:

1. "That the cause or causes of cancer may be more successfully sought by a careful investigation of the dietetic and other habits of the community than in the vivisection laboratory."

2. "That the treatment and cure of this disease may be more confidently looked for in the intelligent application of dietetic principles and the skill of the physician than in the surgeon's knife and operating-theatre." They insist especially on purity of foods and they have a hospital where cancer is being cured by dietetic means only, with wonderful results.

Dr. C.S. Carr, in *The Columbus Medical Journal*, wrote: "Gradually the fact that cancer, like consumption, is a disease of nutrition; and that it is, like consumption, preventable and curable if taken in time, is being established by many investigators. ... It is not this or that particular food that causes cancer, but defective nutrition, the chief physical factor in which is the unnatural mixing of so many different kinds of incompatible foods."

Dr. Horace Packard, M.D., in *The Boston Medical and Surgical Journal*, writes: "Some have attributed cancer to the eating of meat, but is it not possible that it is the combination of meat and white bread—the demineralization of the food? There is a close resemblance between certain tumor-growths on trees to human cancer; and these growths are especially common on trees growing on land deficient in the mineral elements of food."

Luther Burbank, the Wizard of Santa Rosa, in his *The Human Plant*, also writes that: "Plants that are fed on an unbalanced ration are quickly attacked by fungous diseases"; and the eminent Dr. W. Roger Williams, of England, attributes the cause of plant-cancers to soil rich in sewage, especially when the percentage of nitrogen is very high.

Eli G. Jones, M.D., of Dartmouth Medical College, in *The Scientific American*: of March 31, 1904, wrote: "I have made a special study of the cause and treatment of cancer for twenty-five years. The theory that inoculation by erysipelas would prevent or cure cancer has been exploded long ago. The treatment of cancer by the knife is purely mechanical, and has been described by our best authorities on surgery as only palliative and never a cure for the disease. I can say that in my own experience I have never known a single case of cancer cured by a surgical operation. About one-sixth of the cases that come under my treatment are hereditary.

We may lay it down as a general law in regard to the cause of cancer that anything that has a tendency to weaken the vitality of a person may predispose to the development of the cancer germs in the system. We then need only a local irritant to cause its appearance upon the surface. The successful treatment must then, of necessity, be constitutional and local. Nothing but a complete renovation of the blood and the annihilation of every cancer germ within its current can be counted as a cure. It has been claimed that certain kinds of food will cause cancer, namely, tomatoes, pork, etc. The first is in itself a very good blood purifier; the latter I do not think ever caused cancer, but there is a very common cause of cancer and that is the adulteration of food and drink that is used by the masses at the present day. I claim that this is one of the chief causes that account for the rapid increase of cancer. ... Worry weakens the nervous system and predisposes to the development of cancer or consumption. In England we find that cancer, in 1838, caused one death in 140 of the total mortality; in 1890 one in 28 of the total mortality. In the United states 36 out of one thousand deaths are due to cancer."

I do not agree with Dr. Jones, neither with Dr. Tenison Deane of San Francisco, that cancer is caused by specific germs, and I shall give fully my reasons later; but Dr. Jones is right when he says that adulteration has a great deal to do with the causation of cancer, because it destroys the valuable vitamines and organic salts as absolutely necessary for health, and introduces into the organism noxious poisons and unwholesome irritants.

Mr. Rollo Russell, an eminent English investigator, considers the habit of drinking hot liquids and of eating hot foods not only as unnatural and unhygienic, but also as one of the causes of cancer. He says that by relaxing the stomach, under the influence of heat, the food is kept longer, causing fermentation and dyspepsia, and as a consequence gastric ulcers and cancer. The British Medical Association investigated, some years ago, a case of extreme longevity in Bolivia, and found that the man had, besides eating once a day and eating no meat, always taken everything cold.

Mrs. Annie Besant, the Theosophical leader, who although not a physician is one of the most intelligent women of our age, attributes also to the use of meat many diseases, including cancer; and I cannot understand how genuine Theosophists can continue to eat meat, encouraging in this manner the unnecessary slaughter of animals. The following noble words ought to touch their hearts and enlighten their minds to drop such detrimental habit to their health and to their spiritual unfoldment. She writes: "Health is not gotten by poisonings, however carefully graduated. Health is brought about by pure living, pure food, moral self-control, and by becoming the master and not the slave of your appetites and passions. It is a road that leads to Death and not to Life, when you want to live evilly and be cured of the results of evil-living by things which are wrung from the tortured bodies of the animal kingdom."

Robert Bell, M.D., the eminent cancer specialist of London, England, writes in his book, *The Cancer Scourge*: "Cancer occurs in a group of devitalized, degenerate cells. The mutilation by the knife, though perhaps giving temporary relief, tends to leave the parts still less resistant to renewed attacks of the malady. As one who has devoted many years to the study of disease, and has had, therefore, rather unusual opportunity for close observation in many sufferers, I am loud in my pronouncement that it is a preventable, and usually a curable, malady where especially prescribed vegetarian diet is used and accepted. And I hold that a speedier cure will reward the use of the uncooked fruits of the earth, inasmuch as the vital elements have not been lessened or impaired by processes of cooking."

So far as I know Dr. John Bell was the first one not only to understand the true cause of cancer, viz., that it was due to wrong diet, but he was also the first one to advocate a vegetarian diet as a cure and to cure many cancer patients by dietetic treatments. These cases were reported nearly seventy years ago, and were recorded in a work entitled. *Regimen and Longevity*.

Dr. Kellogg of Battle Creek, in his *The Monster Malady*, speaking of Dr. Bell's remarkable work writes: "Among the first cases of spontaneous cure of cancer reported were a series of cases reported by John Bell, surgeon to one of the leading hospitals of London. ... Dr. Bell believed that close adherence to a vegetarian dietary would prevent cancer, and that the adoption of a non-flesh dietary would in many cases effect a cure. When I first read Dr. Bell's book, some forty years ago, I concluded that Dr. Bell, though an able and honorable physician, must be mistaken in his diagnosis. About ten years ago, however, I myself encountered a case which convinced me that under similar circumstances at least the body is able to successfully combat this awful disease. I was one day consulted by a gentleman, a bookkeeper by profession, who desired me to examine a growth on the back of his neck. He stated that he had been recently examined by one of my associates, who had suggested that the growth was of a cancerous nature and had slipped off small pieces of the growth to be submitted to our pathologist for examination. On inquiry I found that the growth had been present upon the neck for some four years. It had varied in size, sometimes nearly disappearing, then slightly increasing size. At the time I saw the growth it was about the size of a small pea and seemed to indicate that it was probably of a non-malignant nature. I so informed the gentleman, and suggested that if it were really cancerous it would probably have attained much greater proportions in four years and would not probably have shown any tendency toward recovery, as it had done several times.

I considered the matter, however, of sufficient importance to order a careful examination made. By accident, the report did not reach me until some four weeks later. The pathologist then reported that the growth was undoubtedly cancerous. I sent at once for the gentleman to come to my office and broke the news to him by saying: 'Good morning, Mr.— how is your cancer today?' He replied, 'It is gone.' On examination I found, greatly to my surprise, and no small satisfaction, that the growth had really disappeared, leaving behind only a small red surface about one-eighth of an inch in diameter. A few weeks later this had also disappeared, leaving only a small white scar which marked the point from which the portion of the growth had been removed. The case was under my personal observation for a number of years, as the gentleman later entered the employ of the institution as a bookkeeper, and while I have not seen the patient for a number of years I have reason to believe that he is still in good health. On inquiry of this patient I learned that when the presence of the growth upon his neck was discovered he made a radical change in his habits of life. Finding that the growth was very obstinate in character, not yielding to any of the various remedies which were applied, he became alarmed, thinking that it might be cancer, **renounced entirely the use of flesh foods,** began the practice of sleeping with the windows of his chamber widely opened, and also began taking vigorous active exercise out of doors every day. The result was a very great improvement in his general health, the growth ceased to develop, and, as has already been stated, alternately diminished and increased in size, and finally disappeared. To make certain that there could be no mistake in the diagnosis in this case, a portion of the tissue removed was sent to New York and submitted to the judgment of one of the best pathologists of the country, the professor of pathology of Cornell University. His report was to the effect **that the growth was unmistakeably cancerous in character."**

This is one of the many remarkable cures of cancer effected without knife and drugs, by simply adopting a vegetarian diet. As I said before, Dr. John Bell was the first one to cure patients by this natural method. If still alive, he ought to be generously remunerated for such a great discovery—the greatest and the most beneficial of modern times. He ought to be awarded the Nobel Prize. George Croker, the Californian magnate, who, with his wife, died of cancer after operation by the noted cancer specialist, Dr. Bull of New York (who himself has died of cancer), gave, in 1910, two million dollars to Columbia College to be used for investigation into the cause, prevention and cure of cancer. If Dr. Bell is still living he ought to have some of this money, because what the well-equipped laboratories of our big universities and medical colleges with their numerous staffs of expert and well-paid investigators have not done, was absolutely discovered and proved to the hilt by this humble English practitioner. His great discovery, as I am trying to prove by so many quotations, has been confirmed, directly or indirectly, by many eminent investigators, and I repeat that in my mind there is not left the least shadow of doubt that cancer is due to wrong ways of eating, especially to the excessive use of protein-rich foods, and of those foods that are lacking or deficient in vitamines and organic salts. If cancer, then, is caused by errors in diet, the most logical way to prevent it and cure it is to correct these errors.

Cancer is the arch-enemy of mankind; and it behooves us to study its causes and the best means to prevent it and cure it; because otherwise, at its rate of increase, the extermination of the whole human race is not very far off.

After many years of study and experience there is no doubt left in my mind that the chief cause of cancer is the wrong way of eating of the majority of the people; and, therefore, its real cure cannot be effected by means of the knife, plasters, chemicals, drugs or by any other artificial contrivance, but simply by natural means; by the right diet, by the help of fresh air, of a moderate amount of sunshine and exercise, and by an optimistic mental attitude and a congenial environment.

So far as I know Dr. John Bell was the first one not only to understand the true cause of cancer, viz., that it was due to wrong diet, but he was also the first one to advocate a vegetarian diet as a cure and to cure many cancer patients by dietetic treatments.

There is a very common cause of cancer that that is the adulteration of food and drink that is used by the masses at the present day. I claim that this is one of the chief causes that account for the rapid increase of cancer.

THE CAUSE OF DISEASE

by Irving James Eales, M.D., D.O.

Herald of Health and Naturopath, XXIV(6), 276. (1919)

To those who have given little if any thought to the matter of the abuse of the stomach and other digestive organs by over-eating and drinking, let me call your attention to a little statement prepared by Professor Soyer giving the quantity of food usually consumed by an ordinary man during sixty years of life, after early childhood. He placed the total at 33 ¾ tons of meat, vegetable, and farinaceous food (water-free food) during that period, which if computed in terms of animals would mean that a man at seventy had eaten 30 oxen, 200 sheep, 100 calves, 200 lambs, 50 hogs, 1,200 fowl, 300 turkeys, 24,000 eggs, 4 ½ tons of bread (9,000 loaves of one pound each) and 3,000 gallons of tea and coffee. A vegetarian would of course consume other than flesh food, but of the same weight. Another writer estimates that an adult male will consume of food and water 3,000 pounds every year—nearly eight pounds a day.

These computations are made according to ordinary standard dietary tables, allowing 118 grams (about 4 oz.) of proteins, 56 grams (nearly 2 oz.) of fats, and 500 grams (about 17oz.) of carbohydrates every twenty-four hours. This is according to professor Carl Voigt of Munich, whose tables have been quoted for fifty years as being about the average diet necessary. They vary but very little from any of the fifteen dietary tables by that many writers in different countries. According to investigations and facts determined within the last few years by Professor Chittenden, director of the Sheffield Scientific School of Yale University and professor of physiological chemistry, it has been very clearly and definitely proved that the nitrogen allowance (derived from the protein foods—meat, peas, beans, lentils, etc.)—is altogether too high in the Voigt and other standard dietary tables; that health, strength, nerve force, blood, and every bodily function is improved greatly under a low protein diet: 60 grams of protein (2 oz.), 50 grams if fats (1.66 oz.), and 480 grams of carbohydrates (16 oz.) is the Chittenden standard, and is amply sufficient for a good hard day's work. It will be noticed that the principal difference between Chittenden and the Voigt standard is that of the nitrogen—Voigt, 118 grams; Chittenden 60 grams, almost half. The Voigt diet gives 3,055 calories, and the Chittenden 2,679 calories in twenty-four hours.

But standards are of little value, as most people pay little attention to them or to the proteins, fats, and carbohydrates in their diet. They eat three square meals a day; weigh from twenty-five per cent to forty per cent in excess of what they should weigh according to standard life-insurance tables, and then wonder what is the matter with them when their stomach and other organs, after months and years of patient endurance of this abuse, break down. And this—in a few words—is the cause of disease. With the expenditure of the vital energy necessary to digest and assimilate such vast and unnecessary quantities of food, is it any wonder that degeneration of the vital organs should take place and disease manifest itself? We must also consider in connection with overeating, the demineralization of food by milling, manufacturing, canning, and cooking; food preservatives; the action of acid on tin in canned goods; an excess of protein food, and wrong combination of food as other potent causes of disease.

To those who have given little if any thought to the matter of the abuse of the stomach and other digestive organs by overeating and drinking, let me call your attention to a little statement prepared by Professor Soyer giving the quantity of food usually consumed by an ordinary man during sixty years of life, after early childhood. He placed the total at 33 ¾ tons of meat, vegetable, and farinaceous food (water-free food) during that period, which if computed in terms of animals would mean that a man at seventy had eaten 30 oxen, 200 sheep, 100 calves, 200 lambs, 50 hogs, 1,200 fowl, 300 turkeys, 24,000 eggs, 4 ½ tons of bread (9,000 loaves of one pound each) and 3,000 gallons of tea and coffee.

We must also consider in connection with overeating, the demineralization of food by milling, manufacturing, canning, and cooking; food preservatives; the action of acid on tin in canned goods; an excess of protein food, and wrong combination of food as other potent causes of disease.

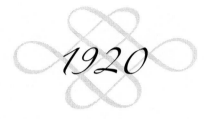

Fasting
William F. Havard, N.D.

Canning Without Sugar
Martha B. Opland, N.D.

The Curative Diet
William F. Havard, N.D.

POST GRADUATE INSTRUCTION

Physicians desiring to take instruction in any method of

Diagnosis or Rational Healing

are offered exceptional opportunities by the Academy of Healing Arts, located in Chicago. Students are accepted either ngly or in groups. Classes forming all the time. Rates and tuition fees will be quoted upon request. For details, communicate with

WM. F. HAVARD, N. D.
32 North State Street, Chicago, Ill.

Ad for post graduate instruction in Diagnosis of Rational Healing.

FASTING

by William F. Havard, N.D.

Herald of Health and Naturopath, XXV(6), 277-282. (1920)

The sick animal refuses food by instinct. Even domesticated animals, when sick, seek a quiet secluded retreat and rest, at the same time refusing to partake of food. Only man, the intellectual animal, persists in clinging to his daily habit after Nature has issued her warning that disorder exists in the body. Only man fails to properly interpret Nature's language. And yet, down through the ages, from the earliest dawn of recorded history, man has been constantly reminded that Nature is the safest guide to his welfare. Every ancient religion offered fasting not only as the means of attaining spiritual development but for the purpose of purifying the body as well.

Within the last two or three decades numerous demonstrations have been made proving the efficacy of fasting in the cure of chronic disease. Almost every variation of disease has been permanently cured by rational fasting and diet, all through the ability of these measures to assist the body to eliminate accumulated wastes and disease products, to rest depleted organs and to correct defective nutrition.

Many scientific treatises have been written of late years on the subject of Fasting, the most worthy of which are *The Philosophy of Fasting* by Purinton, *Vitality, Fasting and Nutrition* by Carrington, *How to Fast* by Hanish, and *Rational Fasting and Regeneration Diet* by Ehret. These books are well worth the most careful study.

Fasting means total abstinence from food for a period of days.

The philosophy involved is very simple. The digestive organs and anabolic function of the liver are given a complete rest, leaving the liver to the more thorough performance of its katabolic function while the eliminating organs—kidneys and sweat glands—are allowed full play to carry off the effete matter which has acted as an encumbrance to normal physiologic action.

A large volume could be written on fasting, explaining all the details of the procedure, but here we will cover only the main points. Fasting means complete, total abstinence from food.

Fasting is not advised unless the patient thoroughly understands his condition, or unless he is under the care of a competent physician. The average allopath is violently opposed to this method of cure, because he has the false impression that it impairs the patient's vitality. He makes no discrimination between the food requirements of the healthy person and the invalid, unless it be that he thinks the person when sick requires even more food. To the mind of the allopath, loss of strength and vitality always indicates a lack of food or improper digestion and for this reason there are no real dietitians in the allopathic profession and but few among our newer schools of healing. Their knowledge of food stops with alimentation. If you feel that fasting will benefit you, be sure to consult a physician who knows enough to conduct you safely through it.

THE CURATIVE FAST

To commence a fast, the patient should have the proper preparation, the most essential part of which is cleanliness of the alimentary tract. The patient should go on a raw vegetable diet for one or more days preceding the fast, during which time high enemas should be employed nightly. If it is to be a long fast, the patient should use fruit juices freely the first few days. The idea involved in this is to keep up the action of the alimentary tract to insure the complete evacuation of all waste food. The patient should have a movement of the bowels at least once in twenty-four hours, for the first seven days. Mucous is continually being secreted from the membranes of the stomach and intestines and the liver will continue to throw off bile. If this material is not promptly removed, it will decompose and give rise to systemic poisoning through it reabsorption, headache being a prominent symptom.

WATER DRINKING DURING A FAST

It is an erroneous idea to believe that the faster should drink large quantities of water. The patient should take only enough to satisfy his thirst. The water should be neither too hot nor too cold—50 degrees Fahrenheit is cool enough.

EXERCISE DURING FAST

Daily exercise should be taken in proportion to the patient's strength. Long walks and deep breathing exercises are preferable to any strenuous indoor exercises.

BATHS DURING FAST

A quick, cool friction bath is recommended in the morning followed by a vigorous towel rub. Very cold or very hot baths, particularly when prolonged, are generally to be avoided while fasting, as they tend to deplete the patient's strength. If skin action is very poor, salt rubs or Epsom salt baths or sponges may be resorted to. These measures should be left to the recommendation of the physician.

DURATION OF FAST

A fast may last anywhere from one to forty days, depending on the results desired. If a fast is decreed for the purpose of curing digestive disorders, usually from three to ten days will be sufficient. In obese individuals who have been heavy feeders all their lives, from fourteen to thirty days is required to effect any marked change in their conditions. In constitutional disorders such as rheumatism, arthritis, syphilis, diabetes, Bright's disease, etc., the fast may have to be continued up to forty days. The length of the fast should be determined by the physician.

For the individual who desires to fast, but who is obliged to continue to work, short intermittent fasts are best. A good plan is to adopt a strict elimination diet (fruits or vegetables) for seven days and follow it by a three days' fast, this procedure to be continued over a period of from six weeks to three months.

Breaking The Fast

This is the most important period of fasting, because on it depends whether or not the benefits secured will be lasting. The short fast of three or four days which is largely for the correction of digestive disorders should be broken on freshly popped corn (pop corn) without butter or salt, about a double handful three times the first day and ripe fruit. The second day the patient should eat fruit and well cooked cereals, thinned with milk or cream, returning to the prescribed diet on the third day.

After a longer fast, from three days to a week is required to properly break it. If the patient has fasted for ten days or more, great care must be exercised for at least three days. No bulky food should be allowed and nourishment should be taken in very small quantities at a time. Three cases selected out of my own experience should suffice as a warning.

Case No. 1.

A young man twenty-four years of age who had suffered from chronic constipation and indigestion, fasted twenty-seven days after reading an article in a popular health publication. On the 28th day he ate a meal of beef steak, potatoes, bread and butter and coffee. He was seized with violent vomiting spells and could not tolerate even a tablespoonful of water on the stomach. When called on the case I discovered an intense soreness of the entire abdomen and every indication as acute gastritis.

By the aid of high enemas and spinal inhibition, I succeeded during the night in relieving the distress. I then gave gum arabic water by the teaspoonful every half hour. The next day I fed him the water from boiled rice, beginning with a teaspoonful and gradually increasing the dose until by evening the patient could comfortably take one-half cupful. On the day following, I fed the beaten white of egg in teaspoonful doses every hour, with two tablespoonfuls of dilute orange juice (half and half) in between. The next day I began with milk, one quarter glass at a time, sipped very slowly and had the patient take one pint during the day with dilute fruit juice in between the milk feeding. The patient was kept on a diet of thin gruels, milk and fruit for ten days longer, as any coarse or bulky food would immediately cause distress.

Case No. 2.

A lady of thirty-five years was induced to fast because she had an obstruction of the intestines. On the 30th day of the fast an attempt was made to break it with the result that everything taken was shortly afterward vomited. On the 31st day, I was called in consultation and found the woman suffering from extreme toxemia. Due to the obstruction of the intestine, none of the waste material had passed off from the alimentary tract during the fast. The material which was there had undergone putrefaction and the absorption of this material had produced an extreme toxemia of the system. The patient died the following day, despite every effort which was made to clean out the alimentary tract and introduce nourishment.

Case No. 3.

A young man about thirty had fasted on his own initiative for forty-two days. Attempted to break the fast on coarse bread with the result that vomiting occurred and the stomach became so irritable that nothing could be retained. There was marked emaciation and extreme weakness and every indication for immediate nourishment. The stomach was given another day's rest, then a small amount (half teaspoonful) of white of egg well beaten, was given every hour. Dilute fruit juice was also given in small quantities. This was continued for two days, when very thin gruels were substituted. Grain was boiled for two or three hours and strained through a sieve. This was reduced with milk and water. The patient was kept on a semi-liquid diet consisting of thin gruels and soft fruits for ten days, after which coarser foods were gradually added. He rapidly gained in weight and the last seen of him he was stronger and healthier than he had ever been in his life.

These cases are cited to show the necessity for exercising the greatest of care, first in ordaining a fast and secondly in breaking it.

RULES FOR FASTING

1. Put aside all fear of starvation. Man can live many days without food. There are cases on record where individuals fasted for 60 or more days. Forty-day fasts are common.

2. Be properly prepared for the fasting ordeal by thoroughly cleansing the alimentary tract with a raw vegetable diet and nightly enemas for three days preceding the fast.

3. See to it that there is a bowel movement every day for the first seven days during the fast. Some patients develop diarrhea as late as the thirteenth day of fasting. Do not break the fast on this account and do not take anything to check it as it means good elimination.

4. Drink a moderate quantity of water when thirsty. If the kidney or bowel action is not good, use a moderate quantity of prune or fig juice.

5. Take daily exercise. Keep in the open air and sunshine as much as possible. Practice deep breathing.

6. Rest in bed ten to twelve or more hours out of each twenty-four.

7. Keep away from the kitchen and avoid the places where food is displayed.

8. If a headache develops take an enema.

9. Exercise care in breaking a fast, remembering that in many cases more harm than good will result from introducing too much food, or the wrong kind of food, after a fast.

10. In ordinary cases, fasting should be carried from day to day and no particular time limit should be set. If overtaken with extreme weakness that does not subside after rest in bed or if the pulse becomes feeble and the rate alarmingly high, the fast should be broken immediately.

DIET

A curative diet to be such must give rest to the digestive organs in the first or rest stage of the process of cure. It must assist fatigued and encumbered tissues to rid themselves of waste and foreign material. It must promote greater elimination.

A study of foods from this standpoint leads us to the conclusion that an eliminating diet must be free from any substances that generate too many irritating poisons in the body. The first of these materials that falls under the ban is meat, meaning by that term the flesh of living creatures. Every argument in favor of meat as food for man has been defeated by the practical demonstrations of those who have eliminated it from their diets. In the first place meat undergoes decomposition and putrefaction in the alimentary tract. It is broken down by bacterial action rather than by the normal digestive process, thus generating a great quantity of poisons. These poisons greatly overbalance the small amount of actual food substance that the meat affords. Meat adds more encumbrance to the body than it does food, consequently it cannot be considered of value either in a nutritive diet or an eliminating diet.

Eggs, cheese, very starchy substances including white flour products, polished rice and starchy vegetables such as potatoes; refined sugar; stimulants—tea, coffee, tobacco, alcoholic beverages; seasoning such as pepper, spices, vinegar and condiments, must all be scratched from the lists of permissible foods.

The substances that aid elimination are all found in fresh fruits and vegetables, consequently an eliminating diet must consist largely of fruits or vegetables in their natural, raw state. A small amount of grain or cereal food and milk may be included.

Acid Fruits As Eliminators

Grape-fruit, grapes, oranges, lemons, limes and pomegranates are ideal blood purifiers during the Fall, Winter and Spring. For liver troubles, pustular skin eruptions, obesity, rheumatism, septic poisoning, intestinal toxemia and chronic catarrh in obese people acid fruits should be given in abundance. An exclusive diet of seasonable acid fruits for ten to twenty-one days will often succeed in eliminating the most irritating poisons from the blood.

Sweet Fruits As Eliminators

The sweet fruits are less potent as eliminators than the acid fruits. They can be used to advantage in regulating bowel action but little would be gained in the way of greater elimination by using them as an exclusive diet. They serve a greater usefulness in the building or constructive diet but should be used mainly by those who are habitually under weight.

Leafy Vegetables As Eliminators

The vegetables which grow above the ground are superior to underground vegetables (roots and tubers) as eliminators. They are rich in the organic salts which are needed to preserve the alkaline reserve in the blood. It is these salts which serve to neutralize the acid wastes of protein metabolism. Lettuce, spinach, celery, kale, beet tops, asparagus, mustard leaves, dandelion, sorrel, cabbage, etc., should be used in large quantities to promote good elimination. Non-poisonous herbs fall in this class.

Underground Vegetables As Eliminators

Tubers in their raw state when grated and served as a salad on lettuce or cabbage leaves are good intestinal cleansers and in some instances serve as blood purifiers as well. Turnips, black radish and horse-radish help to eliminate uric acid from the blood.

A special word must be said for garlic and onions. The objectionable odor which these two vegetables impart to the breath has instilled in us a marked prejudice. However where health is at stake, such objection can readily be laid aside. These two vegetables are the best intestinal disinfectants known and serve as an antidote for the poisons generated through protein putrefaction in those who persist in eating meat. Garlic is a remedy for worms in children and is the best nerve tonic obtainable. The plentiful use of garlic and onions will redeem us from many dietetic errors.

To secure the best possible success with an eliminative diet, the following rules should be strictly observed:

Select only fresh fruits or vegetables; do not use even slightly spoiled fruits, wilted vegetables, canned or preserved stuff.

Do not use sugar or sweetening with fruits.

Do not boil vegetables. Boiling robs them of their soluble salts.

Do not salt or season vegetables; learn to appreciate their natural flavor.

Do not eat more than two kinds of fruits at a meal nor more than three kinds of vegetables.

Fasting is not advised unless the patient thoroughly understands his condition, or unless he is under the care of a competent physician.

The patient should go on a raw vegetable diet for one or more days preceding the fast, during which time high enemas should be employed nightly.

If the patient has fasted for ten days or more, great care must be exercised for at least three days. No bulky food should be allowed and nourishment should be taken in very small quantities at a time.

See to it that there is a bowel movement every day for the first seven days during the fast.

Eggs, cheese, very starchy substances including white flour products, polished rice and starchy vegetables such as potatoes; refined sugar; stimulants—tea, coffee, tobacco, alcoholic beverages; seasoning such as pepper, spices, vinegar and condiments, must all be scratched from the lists of permissible foods.

Turnips, black radish and horse-radish help to eliminate uric acid from the blood.

CANNING WITHOUT SUGAR

by Martha B. Opland, N.D
Herald of Health and Naturopath. XXV(9) 449. (1920)

Much fruit that ought to be canned or dried is going to waste. I have heard many women remark that they could not afford to put up fruit because sugar is so high.

Now if these women knew that fruit will keep perfectly without sugar, they would put it up. What about the pie-fruits put up by canneries all without sugar. Fruit is better **without** sugar, especially the white, bleached, granulated. Perfect sterilization is the principal factor in canning.

Vegetables are put up without sugar and being alkaline foods are much easier to ferment than fruits, most of which are of an acid nature. I do not believe in blanching (or scalding) fruits and vegetables, for in this process most of the flavor and mineral elements are thrown away. Mason jars with zinc covers ought never to be placed upside down as some of the food will come in contact with the zinc and also get under the porcelain cover. A six inch square of the emery cloth placed in the palm of the hand, helps you to tighten mason covers. Glass covers are the best.

Put up fruits and vegetables while reasonable, for after they have been in storage you will have to pay considerably more and they are not as good. Drying fruit is very little work if you have a cook stove fruit drier. Children as a rule will eat fruit in preference to vegetables, but they should also learn to eat vegetables, as they get old enough to masticate. Most of the dried fruits can be eaten raw, that is why they are better than canned fruits.

Wash dried fruit in several waters, then place in jar or porcelain dish, cover with cold water and let soak six or twelve hours. Be sure to cover the dish with a plate, granite or aluminum cover. Also keep your fruit covered while cooking for canning, this helps to retain the flavor, and there is less evaporation.

If you prefer sweetening either dried or canned fruit, strain off the juice in which you may dissolve some strained honey, maple sap, pure sugar cane sap or sorghum or some dark brown sugar. Try a tablespoon or two of sweet or sour cream on each side of fruit sauce instead of sweetening, do not mix it except as you eat it or the cream will curdle and spoil the appearance. Milk or cream can be taken with fruits, even though they curdle it, because the gastric juice of the stomach is acid and milk and cream curdles as soon as it reaches that. The only precaution is to drink milk slowly, a teaspoonful at a time.

Another way to sweeten fruit sauce, that is not sweet enough by itself. Take one fourth pound of seedless raisin, (or more) wash well, then run

**For *real nutriment* and the
pleasures of eating, try**

BANANA FIGS

our luscious cured bananas, rich in
natural fruit sugars and body-building
materials.

Banana Figs are good because they
taste good—because they are pure, free
from all foreign compounds and preservatives.

If it is *real nutriment* you want, combined with an appetizing, *toothsome*
food, eat Banana Figs, enjoy your meals
and be well nourished.

A large trial package will be mailed
for 20 cents and the name of your
grocer.

TROPICAL FOOD COMPANY
Mayaguez, Porto Rico
(Note our new address.)

Ad for banana figs rich in natural sugars.

through food chopper, add the juice from a quart of dried or canned fruit, mix well, then pour over fruit, mix in carefully with a fork and let stand a few hours or over night. Apples, pears, peaches, plums, berries, etc., can be sweetened this way. The raisins should be chopped or ground up as they sweeten so much better than when left whole and there is no danger of children swallowing without chewing, which if they do will tend towards gas formation.

All fruits and vegetables should be well washed before using as they have been handled many times before they get to your kitchen.

Fruit And Nut Candy

One half pound of unbleached, seedless raisin. One quarter pound of black figs. One quarter pound of dates or prunes or both. Two ounces finely chopped or coarsely broken nuts or two ounces of fresh grated cocoanut or bakers' dried cocoanut.*

Wash fruit well, then put through food chopper, add nuts, then form into large or individual cakes, rolling in cocoanut or finely chopped nuts if desired.

Wash dried fruit in several waters, then place in jar or porcelain dish, cover with cold water and let soak six or twelve hours.

---

*Cocoanut refers to coconut. *Ed.*

THE CURATIVE DIET

by William F. Havard, N.D.

Herald of Health and Naturopath. XXV(10), 504-508. (1920)

A little treatise on health-producing foods, written as a guide for those who are going through the process of regaining health.

A FEW DEFINITIONS

METABOLISM:

The act or process by which, on the one hand, food is built up into complex and unstable living material, and by which on the other hand, the living matter in protoplasm is broken down into less complex and more stable substances, within a cell organism. ANABOLISM: The process by which food is converted into protoplasm. KATABOLSIM: The process by which protoplasm breaks down into waste or excretory products

PROTEIN:

The entire amount of nitrogenous material in organic substances or components, whether of nutritive value or not, consisting of nitrogen, carbon, hydrogen, oxygen, sulphur and phosphorus.

STARCH:

A compound of carbon, hydrogen and oxygen (CHO) found in seeds, pith or tubers of all plants except fungi. Rice contains 76%, corn 56, wheat 54.75, barley 46.3, rye 45, beans 37.7, oats 36.5, potatoes 18.5. Changed to sugars (maltose and dextrin) by the action of digestives juices.

SUGAR:

Compounds of carbon, hydrogen and oxygen, containing double the amount of hydrogen as of oxygen. Crystalline, containing double the amount of hydrogen as of oxygen, soluble in water and subject to fermentation. Found in vegetable kingdom and is an animal food furnishing heat through combustion in animal tissue.

FAT:

Oily, greasy substances containing carbon, hydrogen, oxygen used in the body to impregnate certain tissues to afford protection to delicate parts and as fuel to provide heat.

SALTS:

Any compound produced when all or part of the acid hydrogen of an acid is replaced by an electro-positive radical or a metal.

WASTE:

Produced in excess of consumption; surplus or useless stuff; debris, refuse, remains. Body wastes; materials of no further economic value in the body.

DIGESTION:

The process by which food is chemicalized and dissolved in the alimentary canal to prepare it for assimilation by the blood.

WHAT ARE VEGETABLES?

The proper definition of a vegetable is that natural product of the soil which grows from the seed and bears in one year or less.

WHAT IS A FRUIT?

A fruit is that natural product of the soil which is produced from the same plant, year after year.

There are some few fruits possessing vegetable properties and some vegetables possessing fruit characteristics. Is a tomato fruit or vegetable? Tomato is a vegetable with some fruit properties.

How about a Pineapple? A pineapple is a vegetable with fruit properties. Both may be used as fruits in certain combinations.

A Banana is a fruit with vegetable properties.

PROPER FOOD

It is extremely difficult to impress even the student of food chemistry and dietetics that there is a difference between proper food for the well person and proper food for the sick. The popular conception of food is that it is anything that can be chewed and swallowed and the only reason the average person sees for special dieting is to relieve digestive trouble.

The function of food is to afford nourishment to the cells of the body and by popular standards its value is measured in the number of heat units which it gives off during combustion.

That is even less than half the Story

In the first place, when cell-building material (protein) is put to proper use, it produces little heat and its real value cannot be measured in calories (heat units). The only materials we can measure in calories are sugars and fats—the sources of body heat. That surplus protein in the body does undergo combustion and liberates heat, goes without saying, but this only occurs when it is in excess of the body's requirement and must be utilized in some manner.

Secondly, the other side of the story of nutrition deals with the elimination of waste materials from the blood and tissues. This is accomplished by the aid of materials which generate no heat and never in reality become a part of the cellular structure of the body except in the making of bones and teeth. These substances should ever be present in the blood as a reserve and in the form of salts so that they are on hand when the liver requires them, in order to effect their combination with the wastes from protein metabolism. Through this chemical process the acid protein wastes are changed into soluble salts which are readily eliminated through the kidneys and sweat glands.

Because of the lack of knowledge regarding physiological chemistry there are few dieticians in the world. Most of our food scientists are merely alimenticians. They content themselves with studying out food combinations that are agreeable to the stomach and intestines. Many of them, even in this field, start with false premises and false notions regarding what is and what is not fit food, for humanity. Some make little or no distinction between sick and well people, but try to bend everyone to their ideas of a "balanced diet".

There is abundant evidence surrounding us to support the statement that "man eats his way to disease". On the other hand, it is quite possible for the sufferer to eat his way to health.

The consideration of diet may be divided into three parts:

   i. The building diet or the diet of physical growth, which is also the diet of convalescence, reconstruction and recuperation.

   ii. The diet of maturity or the diet of maintenance; the diet of adolescence.

   iii. The curative diet.

I. Diet Of Growth

During the growing, developing years of a child's life, the character of food required is such as to supply the materials of growth. The cells of the body are undergoing expansion; tissues are growing and much building material is required. It is during this period of life, when nutrition is at its highest (except during the period of pregnancy in women) that food is required in larger quantities and in more concentrated form than at any other period of life, unless it be that period following a long illness or immediately after an acute disease (healing crisis).

II. Diet Of Maturity

Following our period of physical growth, we enter upon the age of adolescence. The food requirements of the adult body are vastly different from the requirements of youth. It takes much less material to maintain a body than it does to build one, just as it requires little material to maintain a building in comparison with that which was needed to construct it. The main requirements of any structure, animate or inanimate, are prompt attention to repair of damage and wear and tear, cleanliness and careful preservation. An automobile given proper attention, will last much longer than one which is abused and neglected.

The adult boy needs building material in the form of protein, only in sufficient quantities to repair waste, which is extremely small where the body is given the right attention. Its greatest need is cleansing internally to prevent obstruction to a cellular action, circulation and nerve flow. By internal cleanliness is meant the prompt removal of waste products from around the cells and their elimination from the circulation by way of lungs, skin and kidneys.

The adult diet must be regulated according to normal body weight and to the character of work performed, the physical worker requiring more protein, sugar and fat than the person of sedentary habits. The eliminators in both cases must overbalance the protein, starch, sugar and fat in the diet.

Health then, can be maintained in an adult body on much less food of the building variety, than is required by the growing body.

III. The Diet Of Cure

This is the phase of dietetics in which we are especially interested and on which we shall dwell to the greatest extent. But before proceeding to its consideration, let us try to see the difference between a body in health and a diseased body.

There is fundamental physiological law which says, "If every cell in a body receives the proper quantity and quality of food material and oxygen and has its waste products promptly removed, that body will maintain a state of health." This law, of course, leaves out of consideration exposures to extremes of temperature and injury by violence.

We may state our law in the following manner. "Every organism will perform the function for which it was designed, provided it is supplied with the necessary materials and is free from interference."

Health then, is that state in which an organism is free to perform its function unimpeded.

Disease is the result of obstruction to normal function.

However, what we commonly mistake for and miscall disease, is nature's reaction to obstruction and irritation. These reactions are called acute diseases, but are properly healing efforts of nature.

The food requirements of a body in health are quite different from the requirements during a process of cure.

In health the body needs protein, sugar, fat, organic salts and water in right proportions to maintain cellular action and to take care of necessary repairs.

In disease the body requires principally organic salts to effect the elimination of accumulated wastes before proper metabolism can be re-established.

Protein contains the elements necessary to build tissue, or in other words to make animal protoplasm. Sugar and fat provide heat by being oxidized in the tissues. Salts provide substance for bone making and are the products necessary to promote the process of metabolism. They with water are the most transient materials with which the body has to deal.

The waste from protein metabolism consists of acids of a more or less irritating character. They are in such form however, as to make their elimination most difficult if not impossible unless further chemicalized.

The liver prepares them for elimination by reducing them and recombining them with soluble salts. These salts also play the role of maintaining the proper specific gravity to the blood. This is a most important function as the whole process of cellular metabolism is governed largely by the destiny of the fluids of the body.

For the purpose then of assuring perfect metabolism, the blood must maintain a certain alkaline reserve which is only possible by eating daily a sufficient quantity of foods rich in organic salts.

THE NECESSITY FOR CURATIVE FOOD

A body undergoing a disease process is heavily encumbered with waste products and accumulations of morbid matter, which require to be eliminated before the body can build itself back into a state of health. The initial steps then, in a process of cure must be those leading to the complete eradication of all such accumulations.

Waste products form and accumulate not so much as the result of faulty elimination as of incomplete metabolism. In other words, the organs of elimination (lungs, kidneys and skin) may not be primarily at fault. They are confined in their work of elimination to those products which have been previously prepared by the liver and other glands. We find these waste products in an incomplete state of preparation for elimination; consequently their escape from the body is impeded. Nor is the liver always at fault, for it may be that the cellular action on these foods has been incomplete, owing to their superabundance, or that they are of an abnormal quality in the first place. In this treatise we will not attempt to deal with the first causes of disease, as that would require too long a dissertation on pathology. Let it suffice to say that practically all disease is the result of, or is accompanied by, disturbances of metabolism and if such a condition needs anything it needs dietetic correction.

ELIMINATION

There are two phases to dietetics as a study. One which takes in the body's cellular requirements and the other which takes into account the manner in which the wastes are removed from the body.

In disease all effort must be concentrated upon the removal of waste accumulations, on the removal of encumbrance and the purification of the blood.

There are three steps preliminary to the process of eliminating waste material from the fluids of the body:

1. Oxidation
2. Neutralization
3. Chemicalization

Oxidation takes place in the tissues and in the liver; neutralization largely in the lymphatics and chemicalization chiefly in the liver.

If these steps are complete, elimination by way of the kidneys and sweat glands is made easy.

Oxidation of waste products is effected by virtue of lung action and the haemoglobin of the red blood corpuscles. The more waste material a person creates, the more oxygen he requires. Neutralization and chemicalization are effected by the proper functioning of the lymphatic structures and the liver. These organs require certain materials in order to properly function and such products are all found in vegetables and fruits.

A curative diet to be such must be one which aids elimination, consequently, largely a fruit or vegetable diet.

Food Requirements During the Process of Cure

Our researches and experiments in physiological chemistry have proved to us that with few exceptions a curative diet must first of all be an eliminative diet. It must aim to remove all irritants and encumbrances from the blood. It must be free as possible from acid forming products, consequently proteins and starches must be either reduced to a minimum or eliminated from the diet entirely.

Fruits and vegetables by virtue of the fact that they contain large quantities of soluble organic salts, should constitute the principal foods for the invalid.

Waste Always Causes Trouble

Waste products in the animal body are of two kinds:

1. Normal waste from the proper, complete metabolism of foods and from the breaking down of cell protoplasm during normal activity; they are readily eliminated;
2. Abnormal wastes resulting from an abnormal quality of food or the digestion of quantities in excess of the body's need or from the

excessive breaking down of the body's own tissue, as occurs in some disease manifestations. These are the most difficult to eliminate and where they occur, require special action on the part of lymphatics and the liver.

In disease, these waste products have a tendency to accumulate in the tissues, clogging capillaries, lymphatics, intercellular spaces and in advanced chronic disease, they become incorporated into the protoplasm of the cells, causing degeneration and disintegration.

Blood is the common carrier both of food and waste. It carries the food material and oxygen to the cells and gathers the waste products from the cells by the way of the veins and lymph vessels.

The liver's principal functions are to prepare food products, which have been digested, for cellular consumption and to prepare waste products of cellular activity for elimination by way of the kidneys and sweat glands. The liver is the body's chemical laboratory, but needs special materials in order to carry on the necessary chemical reactions. The more waste accumulations there are in the body, the more of these special substances the liver requires in order to oxidize, neutralize and dissolve them. These special products are salts of sodium, iron, calcium (lime) potassium, manganese and silicon, as found in their organic state in fruits and vegetables.

It sometimes happens that the body is so heavily encumbered and the digestive organs so depleted that even though the diet is most carefully regulated for elimination such will not take place until the organs of both digestion and elimination have had a sufficient period of rest in which to recuperate their energies. A period of fasting (total abstinence from food) must then be decreed.

Fasting

Cure or healing is a process which begins with the elimination of old accumulations of waste products and disease refuse, and one of the most valuable procedures to effect complete elimination is rational fasting. The philosophy involved is very simple. The digestive organs and anabolic function of the liver are given a complete rest, leaving the liver to the more thorough performance of its katabolic function while the eliminating organs—kidneys and sweat glands—are allowed full play to carry off the effete matter which has acted as an encumbrance to normal physiologic action.

A large volume could be written on fasting, explaining all the details of the procedure, but here we will cover only the main points. Fasting means complete, total abstinence from food.

Fasting is not advised unless the patient thoroughly understands his condition, or unless he is under the care of a competent physician.

The average allopath is violently opposed to this method of cure, because he has the false impression that it impairs the patient's vitality. He makes no discrimination between the food requirements of the healthy person and the invalid, unless it be that he thinks the person when sick require even more food. To the mind of the allopath, loss of strength and vitality always indicates a lack of food or improper digestion and for this reason there are no real dietitians in the allopathic profession and but few among our newer schools of healing. Their knowledge of food stops with alimentation. If you feel that fasting will benefit you, be sure to consult a naturopathic physician who knows enough to conduct you safely through it.

The Curative Fast

To commence a fast, the patient should have the proper preparation, the most essential part of which is cleanliness of the alimentary tract. The patient should go on a raw vegetable diet for one or more days preceding the fast, during which time high enemas should be employed nightly. If it is to be a long fast, the patient should use fruit juices freely the first few days. The idea involved in this is to keep up the action of the alimentary tract to insure the complete evacuation of all waste food. The patient should have a movement of the bowels at least once in twenty-four hours, for the first seven days. Mucous is continually being secreted from the membranes of the stomach and intestines and the liver will continue to throw off bile. If this material is not promptly removed, it will decompose and give rise to systemic poisoning through its reabsorption, headache being a prominent symptom.

Let it suffice to say that practically all disease is the result of, or is accompanied by, disturbances of metabolism and if such a condition needs anything it needs dietetic correction.

Waste products form and accumulate not so much as the result of faulty elimination as of incomplete metabolism. In other words, the organs of elimination (lungs, kidneys and skin) may not be primarily at fault. They are confined in their work of elimination to those products which have been previously prepared by the liver and other glands. We find these waste products in an incomplete state of preparation for elimination; consequently their escape from the body is impeded.

GRITS VERSUS BREAD
BENEDICT LUST

THE CURATIVE DIET
(CONTINUATION)
WILLIAM F. HAVARD, N.D.

SOME THOUGHTS ON THE VALUE OF VEGETARIANISM
AND RAW FOODS IN HEALTH AND DISEASE
LOUISE LUST, N.D.

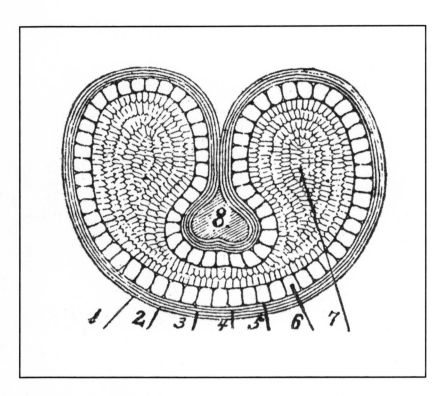

"The outer line 1 is the bran coat which furnishes but little nourishment, but is necessary in the digestive process as bulk; layers 2 and 3 contain nitrogenous matter and the indispensable salts of phosphorus and potassium which build bones and teeth; in 4 and 5 we find a cerealine substance which gives color and flavor to the kernel; layer 6 consists mostly of gluten, while 7 contains principally starch; 8 is the germ, containing the easily soluble organic salts which supply vitality and the first nourishment to embryo-plant. In white flour, parts 1 to 6 and 8 are removed, leaving a product which is entirely insufficient as a food. (Miller, 1907, 168)

GRITS VERSUS BREAD

by Henry E. Lahn, M.D.

Herald of Health and Naturopath, XXVI(2), 67-72. (1921)

The statement has been made that there is nothing harder to solve than an easy problem in an easy way. As a rule, the more who try to assist, the more complicated the problem becomes, particularly in high-sounding formulas and so-called scientific deductions are the bases of reasoning. Hyrtl, the noted Austrian anatomist and anti-vivisectionist, has said that the exclusive use of the microscope prevents real progress in science. A harsh statement, but true! When we "cannot see the woods for the trees", the sum total of our investigations is likely to yield us nothing but a mass of conflicting, hair-splitting opinions with no tangible results.

It is mainly along these lines that present-day investigators labor, and the late inquiries into the food question have proved no exception. The requirements of the different packers, millers, food manufacturers, etc., are ever uppermost in the minds of the so-called "food experts" and "chemists", in the pay, as they are, of these "food interests". Is it any wonder that the average open minded person, after reading these "findings", is not more enlightened than before? We read, for instance, that the United States Bureau of Chemistry has succeeded in creating forty different kinds of "tasteful" bread, yet any experienced housewife or practical baker is better able to give first hand information on this important subject. For the requirements of life, life itself, is our best teacher.

Except in the farthest north, bread has been regarded as the staff of life—the one staple article of food for civilized man. This, however, is not true; for that place must be reserved for the old-fashioned **whole grain grits**. The important place held by bread on the menu of to-day, is largely due to the increased facilities for travel during the past forty or fifty years. The handy form of bread and its good keeping qualities render it particularly suitable for that purpose.

This increased demand hastened the development of the roller mill system (1878), and made possible the production of the refined white flour consumed in such enormous quantities by a misguided public to-day. The fact that the fine white flour has much greater keeping qualities than the darker whole grain flour, thus allowing greater amounts to be milled and stored, had an important bearing on this increased production. The farmer, even, is eating white bread, baked in the city—a state of affairs that would have been unbelievable, a generation ago. The slogan at that time was, "home grown and home ground", the farmer taking his grain to the nearest mill, one of which could be found in almost every settlement. A relatively small amount, a bushel or so, was ground at one time, the miller reserving a portion for his toil. This flour of a generation ago was in every way superior to the superfine white flour of to-day, for it was the color of amber and had a pleasant odor and rich, nutty flavor. Bread, baked from such flour, well deserved the term, "Staff of Life".

Another and most excellent method of using the whole grain is in the form of a pancake. The Bible, when it speaks of the crumbs which fell from the Master's table, refers to the pancake which served the double purpose of being used as an article of food and as a napkin. As was the custom in those days, the residue was discarded under the table. At the present time, the pancake is to be found in the southern parts of Europe, in Asia Minor and in Africa. In Central and South America, the Indians fashion it in exactly the same manner—their sole method of preparing grains to be used as food. The Mexicans have a bread substitute, called Tortilla, which is made as follows: After the dried corn has been more or less softened by soaking or boiling in lime water, the woman, whose duty it is to prepare the daily bread, reduces it to a stiff paste under a special kind of grinding stone, adding water from time to time to control the consistency. This grinding implement, inherited from the ancient Aztecs, consists of two parts, the lower grinding stone or flat mortar, and the upper grinding stone. The dough or paste is then patted into thin cakes and baked without grease in an earthenware dish or on a sheet of iron over an open fire. These cakes are also combined with other food, as beans, etc.

As already stated, neither the loaf nor the pancake takes precedence over the whole grain grits. These consist of the whole grain kernel, which has been ground or cracked to a degree of fineness resembling sea sand. As shown so frequently in history, this was the true food of the ancients, both civilized and uncivilized nations. It was the food of the fair-haired Teutons, unsurpassed in strength and vitality, whom the navigator Pytheas in the time of Alexander the Great, found inhabiting the northern shores of Germany, and whom he described as the wonderful blue-eyed giants, stronger and taller than any other people he had seen. The Cimbrics (Celts) and Teutons, who caused over-civilized Rome to tremble two hundred years later, subsisted on this diet, as well as did the Germanic tribes that, in a few hundred years more, destroyed the world power of Rome. The "dark soup" of the Spartans was whole grain grits darkened by the addition of whole rye flour.

Even to-day, whole grain grits are a staple food for a large part of humanity. Their consumers are among our best workers—with marrow in their bones, and able to withstand the scorching heat of the sun and the freezing cold of winter. The Germans inhabiting the Alps use bread only occasionally, as they mainly live on grits, for which they use the term, "Staerz". In other parts of Germany and Austria they are called "Gruitze", or "Graupe": the Scandinavians know them as "Grit"; the Irish,

"Stirabout", or "Gruel"; the Scotch, "Porridge"; the English, "Mush".
In Italy, as "Polenta", they form a main dish; in Russia they are popular
under the name "Przenow graupa". The high estimation in which they
have been held is affirmed by the fact that the poets of all nations have
sung their praise, and that their consumption has been recommended by
the best physicians as well as by teachers of economics.

"Avoid food waste" is one of the slogans of to-day, as the late war
has brought an unparalleled world shortage of food, and as a great part
of war-swept Europe will have to depend upon or at least supplement
their own slender food resources from the two Americas for some time
to come. The doctrine of the clean plate has helped to a certain extent;
but while it is almost impossible to avoid some food waste in restaurants
and other public eating places, in the home, at least, our eyes should not
be larger than our stomachs. When we overcome the habit of leaving a
portion on the plate, a great deal more will have been accomplished in
this direction. Many suggestions have been made, but, as hinted at in the
beginning, no uniformity of opinion has been reached.

One group of food reformers advocates the use of more rice, especially unpolished rice, the only kind that can be taken into consideration.
While the employment of this cereal in its natural state is surely to be recommended, particularly from the physician's viewpoint, its most ardent
defenders have to admit certain obstacle to its more universal acceptance
to-day. First, although there are comparatively large areas in the United
States suitable to rice culture, it has too often been looked upon as a
foreign food, to be regarded as a staple article of diet. The greater bulk
of it being imported, it is necessarily high priced and has not become
widely distributed. Added to this, the American housewife seems to lack
ingenuity in preparing it, the little we do eat usually being treated as a dessert, and small attention given to its food value. These restrictions on its
greater popularity, while not insurmountable, will take time and patience
to overcome.

In a measure, these objections apply to the recommendations of a further class of food investigators who wish to abolish the use of the superfine
white flour, especially for bread making. This has occupied the attention
of some of our best writers on rational living—persons of high experience and sound judgment. While these deductions are correct, as must be
admitted by the unprejudiced, the objectors to this plan have some basis
for their argument. The whole grain flour, containing the life element,
has inferior keeping qualities to the artificial white flour, which has this
important life principle removed. The necessity for milling in quantities only sufficient for the more immediate demands is better satisfied by
home grinding or by the small mills found in bygone times in almost every
community. Contrast this with the huge establishments of to-day, concen-

trated in a few localities, with their equipment for the manufacture and storage of the present day white flour in undreamed of quantities.

An attempt has been made at solving this problem by mixing white flour and bran; but at best, this is only a half measure. The natural proportions can hardly be present in such a makeshift, and it lacks the Vitamins or Life-containing elements of the kernel, such as proteid, fats, and the organized mineral matter or salts.

To illustrate the serious mistakes made in extracting the ultra-fine white flour from the wheat berry, the following diagram of a section of a wheat kernel, greatly enlarged, is given. These wasteful processes, which eliminate from 50 to 75 per cent. of the organic salts in the kernel, are not only confined to the wheat grains, but barley, rice and other cereals are peeled and polished to "improve" the appearance.

The outer line (1) is the bran coat, which furnished very little nourishment, but is necessary in the digestive process as bulk; layers (2) and (3) contain nitrogenous matter and the indispensable salts of phosphorus and potassium, which build bones and teeth; in (4) and (5) is found a cerealine substance that give color and flavor to the kernel; layer (6) consists mostly of gluten, while (7) contains principally starch. (8) is the germ, containing the easily soluble organic salts that supply vitality and the first nourishment to the embryo-plant. In white flour the parts from (1) to (6) inclusive, also (8), the vitamins are removed, and there is left a product entirely insufficient as food [see page 360].

Another deterrent to the more general use of whole grain bread, is that, when properly made—without yeast—as in the manner of the ancients, first class results are not at all easy to obtain.

That there is great room for improvement will be quite evident after reading the following figures taken from a magazine of a few years ago:

"The average crop of the United States in wheat is 750 million bushels, containing 57 pounds to the bushel. But as the result of our present wasteful milling methods every unit of 8 bushels of wheat will produce only 5 bushels of highly-milled flour, white 3 bushels of the grain kernel's most nourishing parts, indispensable to a rational nutrition, the brown bran, yellow germ, and white or gray middlings are rejected by men and turned over to cattle. These 3 bushels of rejected products are indispensable to a rational nutrition, and without them no flour will support life; with them man and his children can live indefinitely, even though he eats nothing else."

Getting down to the practical part of this food question, it will be seen that the ideal food must be palatable, nutritious, moderate in price, easily obtained and prepared and have keeping qualities. To the question, "Is there such a food?" we gladly answer, "Yes"—in the old-fashioned **Whole-grain Grits**. Whole-grain Grits have all the popular food requirements—wholesomeness, cheapness, tastiness, good keeping qualities, and lend themselves to various ways of preparation. Having full food value, they are alike suitable for the table of the working-man and the well-to-do, the sick and the healthy, the child and the adult. They are equally suitable for the other meals as well as breakfast; and as they do not irritate the intestines, although containing all the parts of the kernel, they fulfill the above mentioned fundamentals of food reform—a seemingly impossible requirement.

They contain all the Organized Mineral Salts, and are neither degerminated nor deprived of the bran, leaving the dietician no grounds for objection.

That their preparation requires less work for the household than either the baking of bread or the cooking of high priced breakfast foods may be mentioned as another advantage.

They are no experiment, as our historical review abundantly proves—a striking contrast to some of our ultramodern prepared foods.

Other advantages, cheapness, and the ease with which they may be obtained, are almost too obvious to repeat.

Summing up what has been said, it is seen that by taking a lesson from our forefathers and reintroducing the daily use of Whole-Grain Grits, we solve not only the social question of food shortage, but also the equally important problems of healing and preventing diseases. Grits are the ideal bone, tooth, and brain builders. The child nourished on this food will be bright in school, and in the grown-up will be efficient in business, provided, of course, the system is not saturated with stimulants and medicines. Being a natural food, the taste for them can soon be acquired and will never be lost, for they can be served in many ways, cooked or uncooked, as porridge, pudding, or fried.

RECIPES

In minor details the preparation of the following dishes will vary, according to locality and season; a uniform condition is, that the grits be well softened by soaking from 12 to 24 hours.

A few lines are necessary to explain why uncooked Grits are so much to be preferred. The light and warmth-giving qualities of the sun are known to be the best healing potencies for body and mind. In this respect the plant is nothing more than a storehouse for these "vital or life principles or sun energy", therefore, our nourishment should be derived from the vegetable kingdom, and as much as possible, in the uncooked state. The enlivening, creating sun has already prepared our food—a food that is filled with the natural vital force is found only in the uncooked food, as it is liberated in cooking. The seeds from a cooked apple, etc., will not reproduce their kind in tree or fruit. Although the chemist can show to a nicety the constituents of a wheat kernel, human wit fails when it tries to produce one that will germinate. Apart from the loss of these vital elements in cooking, the evaporation of water during boiling leaves the earthy residue to be absorbed into the cooking. Very often the water has to be renewed several times to prevent scorching, thus adding to the amount of this body-encumbering inorganic matter.

It is very important that the grain be well cleaned, especially when one is not sure of the source from which it is obtained. The author has had his own experience in this connection. First the grains should be well picked over, to remove such foreign matter as can be eliminated in this way, hulls, pieces of straw, the larger particles of sand and dirt, etc. Some of the less scrupulous dealers are not any too careful to remove these impurities, as they add weight.

After this dry cleaning, the grain is put under the tap to remove such of the finer particles of dirt, sand, etc., as can be separated in this manner. Now, by putting the grain in tepid water the healthy grains will sink to the bottom and the surface will have an ugly looking covering or scum, which must be removed. This mainly consists of a "smut" or fungus that is barely visible on the grain in the dry state. The action of the luke warm water throws it to the surface in the form of thick, black pods. This fungus is very destructive to our organism; the nervous system becomes deranged, the blood circulation is hindered, and a so-called gangrene is the climax.

In all likelihood, pellagra, so prevalent among the Italians, can be explained by the presence of this fungus.

Other impurities in this scum consist of dust, hulls, the feces of mice and rats, etc.

UNFIRED GRITS

1. For each person, soak over night half cupful grits in about one cup-ful cold water, including if desired, some alkaline fruit like unsul-phured figs, prunes, pears, etc. The next morning the mixture will have a pleasant odor and is eaten without cooking or warming.
    Before using any dried fruit it should be soaked for at least 12 hours in an equal amount of cold water. If the fruit has not been sulphur-dried it will have the taste and odor of fresh fruit.

2. Grits like No. 1 are mixed with raisins and fine ground almonds, nuts, dates cut into pieces, canned fruit or fruit juice. Mix and serve cold with raw sauerkraut.

3. Grits like No. 1 may be served with a raw vegetable such as grated carrot or chopped cabbage, etc. Serve cold.

4. Grits as prepared in No. 1, eaten with berries in season such as

loganberries, cranberries, etc., or dried berries cooked with chopped raisins or honey.

COOKED GRITS

5. Gruel, Porridge, Stirabout. Soak grits over night, add in the morning, if necessary, a little more water, bring to a boil and cook for five minutes, stirring occasionally to prevent scorching. A double boiler is used to advantage here.

6. In the morning pour the soaked grits into boiling water, boil as before for about five minutes, and serve warm or cold, with or without milk, brown sugar or honey. While this boils, if rich milk, chopped figs, raisins, dates, or sweet fruit such as apples or berries in season are added, a delicious dish that is a real staff of life is obtained. Cooked grits have the advantage of keeping quite a long time in a cool, dry place. An excess of these may be used up very nicely, as explained in the next recipes, thus giving a pleasant change. Grits that have been placed while warm in round containers, such as the well known one pound baking powder cans, can easily be cut when cold in nice round pieces.

7. Fried Grits. Cook grits and cool in the form mentioned in the above recipes. Cut in half inch thick pieces, dip them in beaten egg and bread crumbs and fry in very hot oil or cocoanut butter; vegetable fats should be about 50 deg. F. hotter than animal fats (about 550 deg.) so that the food does not absorb so much of the fat.

8. Fried Grits. Cooled grits are cut into pieces one half inch thick in the form of cubes, discs, or finger-shaped strips, dipped like fried potatoes into smoking hot fat, nicely browned for a few minutes, and laid on a piece of paper. Serve with or without brown sugar, honey, or raw sauerkraut.

9. For three or four persons use two cups grits; one and a half cups milk, half cup honey; two eggs are to be added later. Grits are to be soaked over night, cooked in the morning for about ten minutes, mixed with the above ingredients, and baked for about thirty minutes or until brown.

10. Take any of the grains to be obtained in a feed store, which are, of course, to be cleaned and washed as previously directed, soak over night; slowly boil for a few hours—a fireless cooker is of good service here. The kernels breaks open, are milky white, and of a nutty flavor.

A practical, fuel-saving way in the winter time of preparing grains is given in the next lines. Place the cleaned grain with sufficient water in a vessel, close with a tight-fitting cover and keep it over night in the ash-pan of the furnace; the steady moderate heat makes the kernels swell and burst.

With the general lack of knowledge regarding the use of medicines can be placed that almost as dangerous and misleading humbug, predigested foods, in which the deluded purchaser imagines he gets nutriment value for the high price he pays. Far too little is this deception realized; even when the buyer knows that he pays for the advertising and fancy containers, he has still paid altogether too much for the food. His ignorance of what to substitute has driven him to accept such conditions.

The remedy is easy. In the following lines is given a recipe that is as healthful as it is inexpensive—and one knows at least what one eats.

11.　Blanched Bran. Purchase for a few cents some bran at a feed store. It should be thoroughly picked over and such foreign matter as particles of straw, etc., removed. Placed in a dish without fat, it is then roasted over a hot fire, similar to the way coffee is roasted, stirring all the while with a spoon. A pinch of brown sugar may be added. The result is a food with a fine nutlike flavor and taste. It is served with sugar, milk, apple, etc. The occasional eating of such a food can be recommended.

12.　Zwieback Grits or Blanched Flour Soup with the characteristic Meat Flavor. For each person take one tablespoonful of fine, ground rye or wheat grits, or so-called low-grade flour, which costs only half as much as the patent flour; brown through and through over a moderate fire, stirring frequently to avoid scorching. Then make a paste by adding cold water, and while stirring, add sufficient boiling water for soup. Allow it to cook evenly for about five minutes. Add a trace of salt, a piece of butter or vegetable fat. Instead of the oil, fried onions, left-over soups or water in which bones have been cooked, may be used.

The enlivening, creating sun has already prepared our food—a food that is filled with the natural vital force is found only in the uncooked food, as it is liberated in cooking.

THE CURATIVE DIET (CONTINUATION)

by William Freeman Havard, N.D.

Herald of Health and Naturopath, XXVI(2) 89-93. (1921)

AN ANSWER

Anticipating the old time worn question of why use acid fruits when the body is already encumbered with acids, we insert here the explanation. Acid fruits are rich in organic salts which become liberated during digestion. The acid character of fruits is destroyed in the stomach and intestines and the salts are absorbed into the blood in the form of feeble alkalis. They are among the most valuable eradicators of the acid wastes which are formed from the proteins, sugars and fats.

Do not make the mistake of confusing an acid condition of the stomach with an acid constitution. Even in acidity of the stomach, acid fruits are not necessarily to be avoided. It will all depend on how the patient's stomach receives these products.

LEMON DIET

This is not an exclusive diet, but may be used in rheumatic conditions or other liver disorders, together with a moderate mixed diet. The best method I have found to carry out such a diet is to begin with the juice of one-half lemon three times a day and to increase by one and a half lemons each day until nine lemons are taken and then reduce by dropping off a lemon and a half a day, until the starting point is reached. If necessary this regimen may be repeated after a period of ten days has elapsed. After taking a quantity of lemon juice, the mouth should be thoroughly rinsed, as an excess of lemon acts on the teeth.

RAW VEGETABLE DIET

In hyperacidity of the stomach and chronic constipation, a raw vegetable diet is to be highly recommended. It provides the necessary bulk for elimination and where such substances as rhubarb, spinach, beet tops, or such other greens as are in season are used, will produce good action on the liver. Watermelons, Cantaloupes and other gourds are valuable eliminators in their season.

STOMACH OR INTESTINAL ULCERS

Moderate fasting for not more than three or four days at a time should be decreed in such cases with the drinking of warm water. High enemas should be given nightly over a sufficient period to assure cleanliness of the alimentary tract. This should be followed by a diet consisting of milk, very thin gruels which have been thoroughly cooked and worked through a sieve and vegetable juices, or, where they can be tolerated without giving distress, finely chopped or grated raw vegetables. Three-day fasts alternated with seven days of dieting carried on over a period of six weeks should be sufficient to cure the stubborn cases.

FOR CONSUMPTIVES

This is one condition that requires careful feeding and also one condition that seems to be an exception to the general rule of feeding largely to produce elimination. The consumptive requires to be fed, but not stuffed. His food must be properly prepared with the aim of giving him the proper nutrition and yet at the same time maintaining the elimination.

To arrest the destruction of tissue, the foods must contain an abundance of lime salts. The diet of the consumptive should consist largely of vegetables both raw and steamed, well cooked cereals, easily digestible proteins, which can be obtained from milk, and olive oil. Goat's milk is preferable and Syrian olive oil is far superior to all other brands for this purpose. Sub-acid and sweet fruits, together with a few almonds and pine nuts make an ideal lunch.

As the fever in the consumptive rises toward evening, it is advisable to arrange the menu in such a manner as to provide the nutritive foods before three o'clock in the afternoon.

GARLIC AND ONIONS

Garlic is an excellent purifier of both the intestines and blood, as well as a wonderful nerve tonic. It is also an excellent remedy for pin worms in children. It is a remedy which the American people would do well to acquaint themselves.

Toast several pieces of whole wheat bread in the oven, butter them and into each rub one piece of garlic. Eat while still warm.

The following is a good tonic for children, in the spring of the year as well as an intestinal renovator. Into one pint of milk drop six pieces of well scored garlic. Place on stove and allow to heat slowly until it reaches the simmering point. This quantity should be taken every morning for one week.

Onions are also splendid purifiers and should be eaten frequently—at least three times a week. Onions are good eliminators in any style except boiled.

PRODUCTS EXCLUDED FROM A CURATIVE DIET

Meats, Fish, Fowl, White Sugar, Animal Fats, Vinegar, Fermented Cheese, Pastry, Pies, Cakes, Boiled Vegetables, Canned Goods (fruits or vegetables), yeast bread.

PRODUCTS TO BE EXCLUDED FROM AN ELIMINATIVE DIET BUT WHICH MAY BE USED SPARINGLY OR AS DIRECTED IN A CONSTRUCTIVE DIET

Peas, Beans, Lentils, Eggs, Corn Meal Products, Buckwheat, Oats, Starch, Fried Foods, Fresh Cheese, Breadstuffs.

VEGETABLE COOKING

Vegetables contain a high percentage of soluble organic salts, which give them their most valuable properties. Leafy or other vegetables which grow above the ground, need no cooking and are better eaten in their raw state.

Vegetables growing below the ground are sometimes improved by cooking, provided they are cooked in such a manner as to preserve the organic salts. Baking, where practical, is the best form of cooking, but otherwise some means must be devised of cooking them without water. In the first place the vegetables must be crisp, not withered. They can be cooked either in casserole dishes in the oven, or if the kitchen is provided with a "waterless cooker" they may be cooked on top of the stove. Waterless cookers are made of agate ware and have a tightly fitting lid which prevents the escape of the steam. Fireless cookers may also be used. Whichever method is employed, the vegetables should be washed in cold water, cut into convenient sizes and placed in the pot with sufficient oil or butter to cover the bottom. This prevents scorching. If cooked in casserole the dish must be tightly covered. If cooked in a waterless cooker on top of the stove, an asbestos pad must be used to protect the cooker from direct contact with the flame and the gas turned very low. The lid must not be removed until the vegetables are thoroughly cooked. A little experimenting will enable the cook to determine the length of time required for each kind of vegetable. After steam begins to form, they require from twenty-five to forty-five minutes.*

Boiled vegetables are almost devoid of organic salts, as well as flavor. The above method of preparation will preserve both. If a richer dish is required, add sweet cream after the vegetables are done, allowing it to heat thoroughly, but not to boil.

Peas, beans, lentils are more akin to cereal than to vegetables and cannot be cooked in the above manner. They require boiling.

---

*Cooking times seem excessive but we must keep in mind that cooking was a precautionary measure at the time when refrigeration was not commonly available. *Ed.*

DIET MENUS GENERAL

DIET NO. 1. ACID FRUIT DIET

Breakfast: Acid fruit—Grape fruit, grapes, orange or pomegranate. Preferably one kind of fruit at the meal.

Lunch: Acid Fruit with cereal.
Almonds and raisins, small dish.

Dinner: Acid fruit with small dish of cereal and cream.

Six to eight grape fruit or their equivalent in other fruit should be eaten each day. Cereal eight ounces, cream four ounces per day.

This diet may be continued for from seven to twenty-one days and is indicated in rheumatism, obesity, recurrent biliousness and all liver complaints, such as congestion, jaundice, gall stones, sclerosis, etc. After twenty-one days a change to either Diet No. 2 or No. 3 is advisable for a week or ten days, going back again to Diet no. 1 and alternating in this manner for a period of three months.

DIET NO. 2. RAW VEGETABLE DIET

Breakfast: Selection—Celery, Watercress, Parsley.

Lunch: Salad: Salad—Lettuce with tomatoes and cucumbers or chopped cabbage, onions and sweet peppers, or other raw vegetable combination.

Dinner: Salad—Large, consisting of lettuce and grated raw vegetables—carrots, beets, turnips, black raddish, horseraddish, oyster plant* or parsnips.

Two triscuits or their equivalent in whole wheat biscuits. A small amount of olive oil and lemon juice may be used on these salads.

This Diet is particularly recommended in chronic constipation, intestinal indigestion, acidity of the stomach, in rheumatic ailments in thin people, and in cases of extreme acidosis. It should be followed for twenty-one days and then Diet No. 3 should be used for a week or ten days, going back to Diet No. 2 for two or three weeks and continue thus until all symptoms disappear.

---

* Oyster plant, sometimes spelled oister plant, refers to the widely known species of the salsify genus, *Tragopogon*. *Ed.*

DIET NO. 3. THE MIXED DIET

Breakfast: One acid and one sub-acid fruit.

Lunch: Vegetable salad; cereal with cream or biscuits and one glass of milk.

Dinner: Vegetable salad, two cooked vegetables (in cold weather a soup), whole wheat bread or biscuits.

If there is difficulty with the bowels, eat a handful of dry prunes before retiring.

This diet is a common diet and an alternate for No. 1 and No. 2.

DIET NO. 4. MILK AND FRUIT

8:00 A.M. One orange or grape fruit, or other acid fruit in season.

9:30, 10 A.M. and **10:30 A.M.** One glass of milk.

11:30 A.M. Seasonable fruit—one acid and one sub-acid.

12:30 A.M. And every hour until 4:30pm, one glass of milk.

5:00 P.M. A meal of sweet dried fruits—figs, dates, raisins or prunes. One glass of fruit juice before retiring.

DIET NO. 5. MILK AND RAW VEGETABLES

8:00 A.M. Salad of grated, raw vegetables or chopped greens. One glass of milk every hour from **9:00 A.M.** until **11:30 A.M.**

12:00 P.M. Vegetable salad. One glass of milk every hour from **1 P.M.** until **5 P.M.**

6:00 P.M. Vegetable salad or large dish of greens.

Diets No. 4 and No. 5 are suitable for almost any condition except acute disorders and can be used to great advantages during convalescence from acute diseases and after fasting. People inclined to obesity will find Diet No. 4 more suitable while those who are inclined to be below normal in weight will receive more benefit from No. 5. Either to be effective should be followed for at least twenty-one days without interruption.

DIET NO. 6. FOR ACUTE DISEASES—FEVERS

*Fruit juice when thirsty or plain vegetable broths, made by
boiling together 4 to 6 different kinds of vegetables for two
or three hours and straining through a sieve.*

Cool fruit juice is better in most cases, except where there is violent irritation or inflammation of the alimentary tract as in typhoid or typhus, fevers, appendicitis, gastritis, ptomaine poisoning, etc., when the vegetable juices will prove of better value. In many such cases however, an absolute fast would be advisable.

It must be remembered that so called acute disease are in themselves nature's method of causing the oxidation and elimination of surplus and waste material. They are the result of the body's reaction to irritating poisons and such a process must not be interfered with. Rest and abstinence from food are two factors which are necessary to complete recovery. In severe reactions rational hydrotherapy may be employed. Nor is "stuffing" essential during convalescence although the constructive diets should be employed.

CONSTRUCTIVE OR REGENERATIVE DIETS

The period required to effect elimination varies with the age, of the person, the character and duration of the disease. The younger the person the more rapidly metabolism regains its balance under dietetic correction. The longer the body has been laboring under the stress of waste encumbrance the longer will be the eliminating process. To determine the exact time to stop the strictly eliminative diet and begin the constructive diet is often a difficult matter. The safest plan is to gradually add building foods to our daily menu or to adopt a milk diet for from three to six weeks.

MILK DIET

As a building food milk affords all the nutritive elements that the body requires, consequently after a fast, after an acute illness or after a period of a strictly eliminating diet, the milk diet is the safest. It is a difficult diet to regulate properly so as to get the maximum nutrition, as an excess invariably produces such a rapid peristalsis that diarrhoea results while an insufficient quantity tends to constipate. In commencing the milk diet (after a fast or a period of elimination) the patient should take two quarts the first day and increase the quantity by the addition of between a pint and a quart a day. For the average person five to six quarts a day will prove sufficient. If constipation develops during the first few days, enemas should be used and the quantity of milk may be increased more rapidly, while if the bowels become too loose the quantity of milk should be cut down to a point where the bowels move normally and then built up again more slowly. The use of a few dates or two or three oranges a day will tend to check diarrhoea while the addition of a few figs or prunes will over come constipation.

Milk should be taken at regular intervals, in the beginning a glass every hour which must be increased to two or more glasses an hour as the daily quantity is increased. It should be sipped very slowly or sucked through a straw in order to become thoroughly mixed with saliva.

Experience has proven that the unpasteurized milk from Holstein Cows is best suited to human digestion.

In cases where violent diarrhoea develops skimmed milk or clabber may be used for a few days in place of fresh milk.

The milk diet should be pursued for three to six weeks in order to achieve the best results.

BUILDING FOODS

In grains, nuts, legumes, eggs, milk and its products, we find all the substances that are required to build tissue and produce heat. From these we may select articles to form the base of our menus. Monotony must be avoided and the menus varied from day to day although too great a variety or mixture must not be attempted at any one meal. If cereal dishes and nuts are used, do not have legumes and eggs at the same time. With sedentary workers experience has proven to me that they thrive best on the following diet.

Breakfast: Two kinds of fruit or one fruit and small dish or cereal with cream.

Lunch: A fruit or vegetables salad, two slices of whole wheat and rye bread, a glass of buttermilk or sweet milk.

Dinner: A large salad, a cereal dish, or an egg dish or legumes, two cooked vegetables, whole wheat bread, milk.

The physical worker may have a large side of cereal for breakfast with the addition of eggs or cereal at lunch and a greater quantity of milk, cheese and legumes in his diet.

> [The Milk Diet] is a difficult diet to regulate properly so as to get the maximum nutrition, as an excess invariably produces such a rapid peristalsis that diarrhoea results while an insufficient quantity tends to constipate.

SOME THOUGHTS ON THE VALUE OF VEGETARIANISM AND RAW FOODS IN HEALTH AND DISEASE

by Louise Lust, N.D.

Herald of Health and Naturopath, XXVI(7), 323-324. (1921)

Those who will adopt as far as possible during the summer months a natural, unfired diet, will find it will supply all the necessary elements for the nutrition of the body and in the right proportions. Cooking, when not properly done, destroys the vital or life principle of the food. Boiling milk, for example, kills it and prevents it from turning sour. Although eating of raw food compels slow mastication and thus aids digestion, there are many who, through a misconception, are prejudiced against it. The dyspeptic fears raw food and must have everything doubly cooked and made into a mushy mess before he will eat it. Some however discover that vegetables cooked in the ordinary way by boiling in salt water, increase their distress, while raw salads and grated vegetables relieve it, stop fermentation and neutralize the acids and toxins. These are wise.

The change from cooked to raw foods should be made gradually in order to permit the stomach and intestines to accustom themselves to it. In this way they will escape the depression, which usually follows the discarding of the stimulating flesh food, pastries, cakes and sugared beverages.

We find a number of dyspeptics among the vegetarians, who have stopped their diet reform after discarding the meat. They try to live, as so many people do, on white bread and butter, predigested cereals, milk, tea, coffee, pastry, milk puddings and sugared stewed fruits. Such vegetarians should remember that the secret of physical health lies just as much in discarding sugared beverages and starchy, devitalized foods as in leaving out the meat. After a would-be vegetarian has been living for some time on a diet composed mainly of nuts, fruits, salads and vegetables he loses all taste for meat. Green and root vegetables are antiseptic. They neutralize poisons and toxins as well as stop gaseous fermentation and eradicate poisons from the walls of the bowels.

We have had patients suffering with ulcerated and cancerous stomachs where cooked foods, even though carefully prepared, could not be retained or digested, while raw spinach mixed with apples, or lettuce or water cress mixed with grated celery, and the gradual addition of raisins, prunes, fresh peaches and a variety or fresh root vegetables could be taken without discomfort. Nature, aided by an appropriate diet and hygienic treatment, has done a great deal to relieve such cases, and even if a cure was not entirely effected, life was made bearable. Any treatment for indigestion must be directed toward cleansing the stomach and bowels

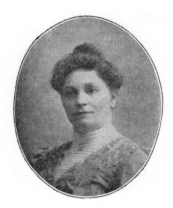

Louisa Lust.

of their poisonous accumulations. This treatment must be deliberately and persistently kept up, sometimes for months, until a complete restoration or digestive health has been established. The meals and habits must be systematized and regulated. The diet is corrected by the free use of natural uncooked foods. Water is used to wash out the sour poisons and toxins from the stomach and bowels. Dyspeptics should avoid milk altogether because, owing to the milk sugar that it contains, it is very often detrimental to the working of the digestive functions. If the digestive organs are enfeebled by dietetic errors and rapid eating, milk will intensify the fermentation that is present. The milk sugar will further break down into lactic acid which, in the bowels, is very astringent and binding. Milk, either hot or cold, used as a beverage with meals is generally bad. If milk is taken at all it should be sipped slowly without any other food. Sour milk or buttermilk exert a less injurious action upon digestion than fresh milk but the merits of sour milk and its germs are much exaggerated. It is better to keep away from milk in any shape or form while there is any tendency to indigestion. Raw food is the safest and best, particularly in the hot weather. This applies to the sick and well alike.

> *Dyspeptics should avoid milk altogether because, owing to the milk sugar that it contains, it is very often detrimental to the working of the digestive functions.*
>
> *The milk sugar will further break down into lactic acid which, in the bowels, is very astringent and binding.*

THE LIFE WORTH WHILE
EDWIN J. ROSS

LIGHT ON DIETETIC PROBLEMS
ALEX EMIL GIBSON

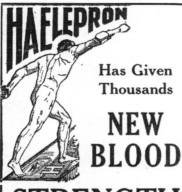

HAELEPRON

Has Given
Thousands

NEW
BLOOD

STRENGTH
and ENERGY

HAELEPRON TABLETS
(Formerly called: Begee-Haematogen Tablets)

**For weak, anaemic women,
men and children**

Contains no medical poison or alcohol

A scientific food preparation,
containing 90% nutritives, including 10% mineral salts (not a patent medicine).

Superior to all other preparations of similar nature, surpassing the world known liquid Haematogen 1:3.

Indicated in the treatment of impaired nutrition, nervous conditions (lack of appetite, general prostration due to fevers, such as typhoid, pneumonia, influenza, or incident to anaemia, severe operation, etc.)

Agents wanted, samples free to physicians

Price per box containing 48 large
tablets $1.00, postpaid

Haelepron Sales Co.
109 BROAD STREET, Dpt. BL.
NEW YORK, N. Y.

Nutriceuticals with their promises.

THE LIFE WORTH WHILE

by Edwin J. Ross

Herald of Health and Naturopath, XXVII(3), 117-118. (1922)

ACID FOODS

There is widely prevalent a fear amounting almost to panic that certain so-called acid foods are dangerous to the health and must be avoided at all costs.

This fear is based on the illusion that an "acid-stomach" is caused by the eating of these "acid-foods."

The very contrary may be said to be true. Fruits such as lemons, limes, oranges, pineapple, etc., most of the varieties of berries, and vegetables such as cucumbers, tomatoes, etc., are often misnamed "acid-foods." While it is true that these foods contain "acids," these acids are nevertheless absolutely harmless to the body. In fact, they are of the very greatest benefit to the health of everyone—and most particularly to those who are afflicted with sour or "acid-stomach." They tend to neutralize the "acid-condition" of the contents of the stomach, and they act as cleansers—purging the stomach of the fermenting and rotting food with which it is loaded.

Furthermore, the "acids" in these foods are not only good and beneficial for all who eat them, but chemically they even cease to be acids, but instead turn alkaline almost as soon as they enter the stomach. In other words, they are "acids" only outside, and before they have entered the stomach. On the other hand, starchy and protein as well as fatty, oily, or hydro-carbon food easily sets up a process of acid-producing fermentation in any but the healthiest of stomachs.

All varieties of "meat" or flesh are greatly productive of uric acid in the process of digestion. Beans, peas, lentils, eggs, butter and cheese, are greatly productive of uric and butyric acids. White-sugar, pastries, bread and cereals of very sort and potatoes as well, are perhaps the chief causes of stomach-fermentation of the wrong sort. These, the starches or carbohydrates, are the greatest trouble-makers in the weakened digestive system.

There is no reason for being frightened, however, "Acid-stomach" is easily cured. Simply refrain from eating too much. Eat sparingly, and not too great a variety of foods.

Avoid pastries, and saucy, gooey, complicated dishes. Eat as little as possible of meats and fish of every sort. Avoid starches as much as possible.

And above all, eat "acid" fruits and vegetables. They will cure you of "acid-stomach," "'acidulous blood," and "acid-mouth," all at the same time.

On following these direction, within the space of a few weeks you will realize the utter, absolute folly and mischievousness of the "acid food" hysteria.

Light On Dietetic Problems

by Alex Emil Gibson

Herald of Health and the Naturopath, XXVII(8), 371-372. (1922)

Should Fruit Be Cooked Or Eaten Raw?

Here again comes up the equation of individuality and idiosyncrasy. In cooking the fruit its vital-electric energies become largely reduced and modified. Hence in cases of constitutionally high-strung and over-wrought subjects—with their nervous system constantly quivering under interior irritation, the cooked fruit would be more agreeable, while to the easy-going well-poised, phlegmatic nature the raw fruit is preferable. As to children, whose digestion is still unaccustomed to acid digestion it is safer to have their fruit cooked—though raw orange juice, taken by the teaspoon, may in case of gastritis caused by undigested milk-curds, be of greatest medicinal value. Furthermore in cases of neuralgia, Bright's disease, gastric ulceration, colitis and general systemic acidity, raw fruit may prove to induce severe physiological reactions for the diseased membranes; while cooked fruit of low sugar and acid percentage, such as apples, blackberries, huckleberries, blueberries—if enjoyed alone or with some pecan nuts, well masticated—may be safe even under these conditions.

It is one of the greatest mistakes in our modern forms of cooking to combine fruit with our meals. Fruit is a creation all by itself—a fairy fabric of sunbeams, electricity, ozone and magnetism, pivoted on a basis of attenuated organic salts—as different in composition to the substances contained in the grain, the meat and the vegetable as silk-texture is different to sole leather, or the wing of a butterfly to the wing of a Dutch windmill; while their admixture in a meal is not more compatible and reasonable than to patch up a child's face with a piece of pigskin. A dessert of fruit at the end of a dinner is practically a physiological dynamite thrown in with the fuel into the body furnace and followed by reactions in terms of vegetable vital explosions in the digestive tract.

The mistake in combining fruit with meat is readily seen when realizing that the former owing to its high oxygen percentage and delicately poised structure only requires seventy minutes for its digestion, while meat, grains and vegetables need a period, varying from three to six hours before it is ready to leave the stomach; and furthermore that the meat is digested both in regard to time of digestion, in the stomach, but the fruit in the duodenum—involving a discrepancy both in regard to time of digestion, place of digestion and secretions of digestion of the stomach contents. The consequences is a handicapped digestion that may delay the process for hours and, if the digestive powers are feeble, may react in fermentation and alcoholization of the entire meal.

The main argument against combining fruit with starches is based on the danger of fermentation and alcoholization, which, unless the digestive system of the individual is powerful, is practically unavoidable. The prevention of fermentation in the face of fruit and starch mixtures has its sole possibility in calling into action the physiological reserve forces, normally intended to maintain the energies of life in undiminished vigor and efficiency even at the high age of one hundred years and more. In our shortsightedness we fail to recognize that in overcoming the consequences of our present errors of living we use up the very energies which were to give a fulcrum career. We readily realize our sufferings, but seldom discover our losses, in most cases only after it is too late for repair.

There is a profound significance between the passing seasons of the year to the products of the earth brought forth at each season in relation to the need of the human body. It should be our effect to adjust our diet to the seasons, especially when it concerns fruit and vegetables. In the long course of evolution nature has established a definite relationship between the living things of earth, and reciprocally adjusted vegetative life to animal life. In the course of the year, each season produces such foods as the animals and humans need at that particular time for the expression of their best efforts. Hence we should not use the fruits in our winter diet which grew in the spring and summer seasons. From a general point of view the rule holds good that fruits should be enjoyed in their fresh uncooked state wherever they are found growing, but only at their respective seasons; while when dried or preserved should be used only in territories where they otherwise could not be obtained. For as a general rule it will be found that in climates too severe for any but a limited cultivation of fruit, the percentage of oxygen in the atmospheric air is considerably higher than in those semi-tropical countries yielding fruit the year round—thus indicating that oxygen is the greatest biological as well as physiological purifier of the earth, either through the medium of fruit, or in the absence of the latter, as in the arid and frigid regions—through its own vitalizing and eliminating element. In other words, fruit is an expediency, introduced in nature as a power of balance by eliminating the excess of impurities accumulating in the body through a mixed and incongruous system of living.

Thus it is readily seen that in the artificial conditions arising from enforced indoors occupation with its limited access to pure air, even the vitally reduced products of conserved or preserved fruit finds a great usefulness in the maintenance of health and endurance of these people. In other words, cooked and canned fruit, though partly devitalized, will yet suffice to combat the accumulated waste products in the tissues and successfully carry on the physiological house-cleaning under these unyielding fields of conditions. Thus is opened a natural channel of co-operation, by which the people of the fruit countries may supply the people of the arid regions where there is found an abundance of oxygen to content and peptonize the acid elements of the fruit. A knowledge of the balancing powers in evolution will assist the individual to adjust his individual life processes to the cosmic process and bring about poise and power between man and his environment.

The mistake in combining fruit with meat is readily seen when realizing that the former owing to its high oxygen percentage and delicately poised structure only requires seventy minutes for its digestion, while meat, grains and vegetables need a period, varying from three to six hours before it is ready to leave the stomach; and furthermore that the meat is digested both in regard to time of digestion, in the stomach, but the fruit in the duodenum—involving a discrepancy both in regard to time of digestion, place of digestion and secretions of digestion of the stomach contents.

Cowless Milk
Alice M. Reinhold, N.D.

Foods And Nutrition
Dr. A. J. Kennedy

GOAT MILK KOUMISS CURE.

And Outdoor Camp for Consumptives.

A camp located in one of the most healthful sections of the United States, for the treatment of catarrhal diseases of the nose, throat and lungs, and all wasting diseases, chronic bronchitis, etc. In addition to camp life, surrounded by lakes of extreme beauty and grandeur, and the finest of fishing and hunting at one's command, we employ the

GOAT'S MILK KOUMISS CURE.

Statistics prove this to be the greatest therapeutic remedy that there is for the treatment of consumption, debility, and all wasting diseases. By taking Goat's Milk Koumiss patients may regain their health without change of climate. Write for literature.

——— Address :———

R. AYERS, Secretary,   **26 Park Gate Building, Chicago.**

Fermented goat milk was advertised as a curative for patients with tuberculosis.

Cowless Milk

by Alice M. Reinhold, N.D.

Herald of Health and Naturopath, XXVIII(1), 31. (1923)

In the March number of *The Vegetarian Magazine* was an interesting story about the rice milk. I am not a bit surprised about it, however, as it is long since we learned to use "milk of the grain," and proved that it is not at all necessary to use any sort of dairy product to keep in good health.

For years before our son was born, neither his father nor I used dairy products of any kind, nor did we use animal flesh in any form. Result—our boy was born (weight 10 pounds) without any pain or trouble, and tasted of nothing except his mother's milk for the first year of his life.

He never tasted of animal or dairy products until over 4 years old, and then only because we went to live in a new colony where there was not much else for a time. Yet he never once had a meal of animal food, and got away from the dairy stuff just as soon as possible.

Now, at 20 years of age, he has never had a sickness in his life, never was vaccinated, does not smoke, swear or have any habits that are called bad. He is over 6 feet tall and quite strong and muscular, weighing over 170 pounds.

I have raised and helped to raise several motherless babies without either cow's or goats' milk. I used "milk of the grain"—wheat, oatmeal, cornmeal, etc., sweetened a little with honey; and never had a sickness among the children. For the benefit of those interested, I give the recipes.

Use a little Dana grinder. Grind up your own hard wheat, yellow cornmeal, oatmeal or barley, raw. Stir a small quantity into distilled water for a few moments. Then strain through cheese cloth. Very slowly warm it in a double boiler, stirring the while, until creamy (use your own judgment about the time, but never allow the heat over 98 degrees F. or you will coagulate the tender albumen). Serve warm in a nippled bottle as with milk. Use a little honey to sweeten. You can vary the grain according to condition of child. A weakly child requires barley as well as wheat.

Just recently there was an epidemic of "septic sore throat" among children in the suburbs of Portland, Ore., and twelve of the babies and small children died as the result. Such an epidemic is likely to appear at any time, and in any place, with like fatal results, as our "health boards" insist on each cow being vaccinated when her raw milk is served in dairy form.

If a baby must have artificial food, why not at least take it first-hand fresh from the grasses and grains as the cow does, and not wait to get it second-hand from the big cow after she has eaten the food fresh from nature from which she has evolved her milk, flesh and blood, and waste materials?

Lazy, ignorant people revert to avatism by eating the cow and her products, with the consequent train of diseases. Wise, educated vegetarians take their food fresh from nature's hand and are not troubled with diseases. They are also able to produce their own milk for their own babies with "human natures" instead of "cow natures."

—*The Vegetarian Magazine*

I have raised and helped to raise several motherless babies without either cow's or goats' milk. I used "milk of the grain"— wheat, oatmeal, cornmeal, etc., sweetened a little with honey; and never had a sickness among the children.

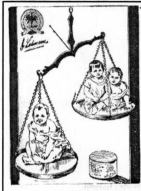

DR. LAHMANN'S

Non-Constipating   Cocoa
Oatmeal-Cocoa, Chocolate
Vegetable   Salt   Extract
Vegetable Milk

To be had in groceries, druggists and
Naturopathic and Kneipp Institutions

Write for booklet and samples

KASTOR & HAASTERS
SOLE LICENSEES AND IMPORTERS
127 FRANKLIN ST.   NEW YORK CITY

When making purchases, please say "I saw your ad. in THE NATUROPATH"

Swiss Oat Cocoa offered a nutritious beverage for the sick.

FOODS AND NUTRITION

by Dr. A. J. Kennedy

Herald of Health and Naturopath, XXVIII(8), 385-386. (1923)

For the maintenance of health, as well as recovery from sickness, there is nothing so fundamental as nutrition. No matter how valuable a remedy may be for the destruction of an invading disease, if the patient cannot be nourished, the remedy is of very little curative value. Naturally, the most important time of life for attention to nutrition is during the growing period, since the extent to which the child develops physically and mentally and the particular development of every organ of the body, is in a great measure influenced by nutrition. Should nutrition, during this period, be interfered with by wrong combination of food, a lifelong injury would be inflicted upon the developing organism.

ESSENTIALS TO PROPER NUTRITION

1. Pure, digestible foods, free from poisons or injurious substances, and capable of supplying all nutritive requirements of the body.

2. Eating at regular intervals and of proper combinations.

3. Following a program between meals that will not detract from thorough digestion of food, or from its normal distribution of all the tissues of the body.

WHAT IS FOOD?

A food is a substance that supplies the elements necessary for nutrition but does not contain harmful elements that will weaken the body. Thus foods should contain, in a pure state and in a proper proportion, sufficient starches, albumin, fats, mineral elements and vitamines. This does not mean that we must measure the several elements in exact amount, or that any scientist has yet acquired knowledge as to the exact quantity of each element required. Such a basis would treat all human beings in a uniform manner, and in doing so we would err in having too much of certain elements and an impoverished diet in other elements.

VARIETY IS IMPORTANT

It is of great importance that all these elements be provided in sufficient quantity; and no harm is done if slightly liberal allowance of all the essential elements is provided. For adequate nutrition it is necessary that all of them be provided in the dietary. A large portion of chronic diseases are, as a matter of fact, diseases from deficient nutrition, and can be corrected largely through proper diet, aided by a general program that will assist digestion and absorption.

Preparation Of Food

Food should be thoroughly prepared. Baked foods, as a rule, are better than boiled foods. Fried foods are generally difficult to digest. The oil surrounds the starchy elements, and as the saliva of the mouth has no effect upon fats, it is thus prevented from acting on the starch granules.

One of the chief causes of faulty nutrition lies in the manner of eating. Food eaten hastily and washed down is, as a rule, poorly digested. Chewing food well insures not only grinding it into such fine particles that the saliva can act upon the individual starch granules, but making more certain the mixing and mingling of the essential digestive fluids, such as saliva, gastric juice in the stomach, bile and pancreatic juice in the intestine. Secretion from the digestive glands is stimulated by the presence of food in the mouth and by the pleasure which comes from the flavors of food, which can be developed only by thorough mastication. To taste food, it is necessary to have it in solution; and it is the action of the saliva that makes the starch soluble. This, therefore, brings out the flavors, which in turn aid all the processes of digestion.

Regularity Of Meals; Food Combinations

There should be regularity in the time of meals, and especial importance should be given to the refraining from food between these regular periods of eating. The order in which foods are eaten is of considerable importance. Soups are best taken at the end of a meal; all acid or sour fruits should be set aside and eaten at the end of the meal. It is better to begin a heavy meal by eating crackers, zwieback, or substances that require thorough chewing.

For the best results in nutrition, one should eat but a small variety at each meal. It would be better if only two or three kinds of food were selected for each meal, variety being obtained by eating different foods at different meals rather than by too large a combination at one meal. It is impossible to gather together a large number of combinations without getting a questionable mixture. Sugar, confections and rich pastries combine poorly with most of the food elements; the less used the better.

Good Cheer And Diversion A Tonic

After food is eaten, one should not be in a state of worry or in a discouraged mood, because depression of any sort casts its influence over every function of the body. It is also unwise to engage in strenuous mental or physical work immediately after meals. A half hour's diversion, recreation, or rest following meals is excellent, though moderate work taken up directly after eating is not harmful to a person having good digestion.

Cold liquids should not be taken sooner than a half hour after meals, and it is desirable to wait an hour. Liquids are better taken between meals than during the meal. We must not lose sight of the value and importance of water in nutrition, for it is an essential in supplying fluids necessary to make up a large part of the secretions of all the digestive glands.

It is better to be unconscious of what has been eaten than to meditate upon some food that might be questioned. So vital is the nutrition of the cells and tissues of the body to the maintenance of life and health that particular attention should be directed to this subject by every one who takes seriously the problems of life, and is interested in his productive value in the world. To a great extent a man is what he makes himself, and nutrition plays a part second only to spiritual influences in making us what we are.

REFERENCES

Ammann, D. (1918). Cocoa bread. *Herald of Health and Naturopath*, XXIII(2), 175-177.

Barclay, E. (2012). A nation of meat eaters: see how it all adds up. NPR, June 27, 2012.

Bilz, F. E. (1900). Diet for patients and convalescents. *The Kneipp Water Cure Monthly*, I(7), 118-119.

Blad, V. (1914). Eugene Christian—the food scientist. *The Naturopath and Herald of Health*, *XIX(9)*, 605-606.

Bloch, S.A. (1906). Adulteration of food. *The Naturopath and Herald of Health*, VII(4), 167.

Buettgenbach, F. J. (1900). Biscuits, light bread, or whole wheat bread? *The Kneipp Water Cure Monthly*, I(12), 228-229.

Campbell, D. (1913). Building brain by diet. *The Naturopath and Herald of Health*, XVIII(11), 727-728.

Carqué, O. (1906). The nutritive value of unpolished rice. *The Naturopath and Herald of Health*, VI(1), 35-36.

Carqué, O. (1911). Care and feeding of infants. *The Naturopath and Herald of Health*, XVI(12), 788-790.

Carqué, O. (1912). California "likefresh" fruit. *The Naturopath and Herald of Health*, XVII(12), 730-735.

Christian, E. (1912). The food we eat and the food we should eat. *The Naturopath and Herald of Health*, XVII(1), 6-7.

Clark, A. (1906). Green salads and vegetables as medicine. *The Naturopath and Herald of Health*, VII(6), 254.

Cristadodo, C. (1909). Unbleached flour. *The Naturopath and Herald of Health*, XIV(5), 308.

Daniel, C. R., Cross, A. J., Koebnick, C., Sinha, R. (2011). Trends in meat consumption in the United States. *Public Health Nutr.* 14(4), 575–583.

Drews, G. J. (1913). The cruciferae. *The Naturopath and Herald of Health*, XVIII(3), 201-204.

Drews, G. J. (1913). Curled dock. *The Naturopath and Herald of Health*, XVIII(4), 266.

Drews, G. J. (1914). Edible thistle. *The Naturopath and Herald of Health*, XIX(12), 832.

Drews, G. J. (1915). How to eat dahlia tubers. *The Naturopath and Herald of Health*, XX(2), 69-70.

Drews, G. J. (1915). The dasheen. *The Naturopath and Herald of Health*, XX(6), 399-400.

Drews, G. J. (1915). Dulse as food. *The Naturopath and Herald of Health*, XX(11), 714.

Drews, G. J. (1916). Milk for apyrtrophers. *Herald of Health and Naturopath*, XXI(2), 119-120.

Drews, G. J. (1916). Spring suggestions. *Herald of Health and Naturopath*, XX(6), 403.

Eales, I. J. (1919). The cause of disease. *Herald of Health and Naturopath,* XXIV(6), 276.

Ehret, A. (1917). My diet of healing. *Herald of Health and Naturopath,* XXII(2), 257-260.

Ehret, A. (1919). Paradise health. *Herald of Health and Naturopath,* XXIV(3), 145-146.

Gibson, A. E. (1915). Life and death in diet. *The Naturopath and Herald of Health,* XX(2), 99-101.

Gibson, A. E. (1922). Light on dietetic problems. *Herald of Health and Naturopath,* XXVII(8), 371-372.

Gray, J. A. R. (1904). Modern systems of healing. *The Naturopath and Herald of Health,* V(8), 184-185.

Hara, O. H. (1906). Fruit and nut diet. *The Naturopath and Herald of Health,* VII(6), 223-225.

Havard, W. F. (1920). Fasting. *Herald of Health and Naturopath,* XXV(6), 277-282.

Havard, W. F. (1920). The curative diet. *Herald of Health and Naturopath,* XXV(10), 504-508.

Havard, W. F. (1921). The curative diet (continued). *Herald of Health and Naturopath,* XXVI(1), 29-33.

Havard, W. F. (1921). The curative diet. *Herald of Health and Naturopath,* XXVI(2), 89-93.

Ives, C. G. (1906). This nation suiciding. *The Naturopath and Herald of Health,* VII(6), 230-231.

Kellogg, J. H. (1908). A remarkable discovery. *The Naturopath and Herald of Health,* IX(10), 319-323.

Kellogg, J. H. (1908). The simple life in a nutshell. *The Naturopath and Herald of Health,* IX(9), 260-270.

Kennedy, A.J. (1923). Foods and nutrition. *Herald of Health and Naturopath,* XXVIII(8), 385-386.

Kneipp, S. (1900). Honey. *The Kneipp Water Cure Monthly,* I(4), 58.

Lahmann, H. (1909). Dr. Lahmann's vegetable milk. *The Naturopath and Herald of Health,* XIV(1), 19-22.

Lahn, H. E. (1921). Grits and bread. *Herald of Health and Naturopath,* XXVI(2), 67-72.

Leppel, S. (1903). Should we drink? *The Naturopath and Herald of Health,* IV(4), 87-89.

Leppel, S. (1918). A nut and fruit dietary for brain workers. *Herald of Health and Naturopath,* XXIII(6), 575-576.

Lindlahr, A. (1910). Suggestions for cooking vegetables. *The Naturopath and Herald of Health,* XV(2), 107-108.

Lindlahr, A. (1910). Raw Food. *The Naturopath and Herald of Health,* XV(4), 239-240.

Lindlahr, H. (1908). Why we favor a vegetarian diet. *The Naturopath and Herald of Health,* IX(10), 302-306.

Lindlahr, H. (1910). The magnetic properties of food. *The Naturopath and Herald of Health,* XV(2), 103-105.

Lindlahr, H. (1910). Standard foods. The Naturopath and Herald of Health, XV(5), 259-263.

Lindlahr, H. (1910). Overeating. *The Naturopath and Herald of Health*, XV(10), 611-612.

Lindlahr, H. (1912). The vegetarian kitchen, to salt or not to salt. *The Naturopath and Herald of Health*, XVII(4), 218-220.

Lust, B. (1900). Kneipp health food. *The Kneipp Water Cure Monthly*, I(1), 14.

Lust, B. (1900). Olive oil as a remedy. *The Kneipp Water Cure Monthly*, I(3), 36.

Lust, B. (1900). Nut foods. *The Kneipp Water Cure Monthly*. I(8), 141-142.

Lust, B. (1900). Milk. *The Kneipp Water Cure Monthly*. I(10), 180.

Lust, B. (1901). Diet treatment. *The Kneipp Water Cure Monthly*, II(1), 27-28.

Lust, B. (1902). Regeneration. *The Naturopath and Herald of Health*, III(3), 107-109.

Lust, B. (1902). In praise of the onion in medicine. *The Naturopath and Herald of Health*, III(11), 468.

Lust, B. (1903). Diet. *The Naturopath and Herald of Health*, IV(8), 226-227.

Lust, B. (1903). A naturopathic silhouette. *The Naturopath and Herald of Health*, IV(8), 247-249.

Lust, B. (1904). Naturopathic kitchen: non-stimulating diet, vegetarian or naturopathic. *The Naturopath and Herald of Health*, V(7), 173-174.

Lust, B. (1905). New theory on eating. *The Naturopath and Herald of Health*, VI(2), 53-56.

Lust, B. (1905). About the value of a good gluten graham bread. *The Naturopath and Herald of Health*, VI(11), 316.

Lust, B. (1905). The new tuber food. *The Naturopath and Herald of Health*, VI(11), 331-333.

Lust, B. (1907). Cause and cure of ailmetns according to natur-therapeutics. *The Naturopath and Herald of Health*, VIII(4), 97-98.

Lust, B. (1908). Diet for the corpulent people. *The Naturopath and Herald of Health*, IX(2), 38.

Lust, B. (1908). Vegetarian method of life. *The Naturopath and Herald of Health*, IX(5), 148-149.

Lust, B. (1908). Why peanuts are hard to digest. *The Naturopath and Herald of Health*, IX(11), 355.

Lust, L. (1909). Cooked and uncooked foods. *The Naturopath and Herald of Health*, XIV(2), 98-99.

Lust, L. (1918). Kitchen and table. *Herald of Health and Naturopath*, XXIII(3), 278.

Lust, L. (1921). Some thoughts on the value of vegetarianism and raw foods in health and disease. *Herald of Health and Naturopath*, XXVI(7), 323-324.

Miller W. H. (1907). Biographical sketches of Chicago's prominent nature cure physicians. *The Naturopath and Herald of Health*, VIII(6), 168-170.

Moershell, R. (1911). Conducting a fast. *The Naturopath and Herald of Health*, X(2), 592-593.

Moershell, R. (1915). Scientific dietetics—fasting. *The Naturopath and Herald of Health*, XX(2), 104-106.

Neff, J. H. (1911). Drink at meals. *The Naturopath and Herald of Health*, XVI(6), 381.

Opland, M. B. (1920). For mothers and children. *Herald of Health and Naturopath*, XXV(9), 449.

Reinhold, A. M. (1923). Cowless milk. *Herald of Health and Naturopath*, XXVIII(1), 31.

Ross, E. J. (1922). The life worth while. *Herald of Health and Naturopath*, XXVII(3), 117-118.

Scholta, A. (1904). Some foods as remedies. *The Naturopath and Herald of Health*, V(6), 139-140.

Sherry, H. (1913). A plea for an Apyrotropher society. *The Naturopath and Herald of Health*, XVIII(1), 50-52.

Sherry, H. (1913). Do you 'troph'? *The Naturopath and Herald of Health*, XVIII(2), 123-125.

Tunison, E. H. (1918). Healthful eating. *Herald of Health and Naturopath*, XXIII(7), 652.

Wilson, E. C. (1909). Substitutes for meat and their values. *The Naturopath and Herald of Health*, XIV(8), 569-572.

INDEX

Name Index

RECIPES INDEX

About the Editor, NCNM, NCNM Press

Sussanna Czeranko, ND, BBE, is a 1994 graduate of CCNM (Toronto). She is a licensed ND in Ontario and in Oregon. In the last twenty years, she has developed an extensive armamentarium of nature-cure tools and techniques for her patients. Especially interested in balneotherapy, botanical medicine, breathing and nutrition, she is a frequent international presenter and workshop leader. She is a monthly Contributing Editor (Nature Cure —Past Pearls) for NDNR and a Contributing Writer for the Foundations of Naturopathic Medicine Project. Dr. Czeranko founded The Breathing Academy, a training institute for naturopaths to incorporate the scientific model of Butyeko breathing therapy into their practice. Her next large project is to complete the development of her new medical spa in Manitou Beach, Saskatchewan, on the shores of a pristine medical waters lake.

NCNM (National College of Natural Medicine, Portland, Oregon) was founded in 1956. It is the longest serving, accredited naturopathic college in North America and home to one of the two U.S. accredited graduate research programs in Integrative Medicine. NCNM is also home to one of North America's most unique classical Chinese medicine programs, embracing lineage and a powerful mentoring model for future practitioners.

NCNM Press, an ancillary venture of NCNM, publishes distinctive titles that enrich the history, clinical practice, and contemporary significance of natural medicine traditions. The rare book collection on natural medicine at NCNM is the largest and most complete of its kind in North America and is the primary source for this landmark series— *In Their Own Words*—which brings to life and timely relevance the very best of early naturopathic literature.

The Hevert Collection: *IN THEIR OWN WORDS*

A Twelve-book Series

ORIGINS of Naturopathic Medicine

PHILOSOPHY of Naturopathic Medicine

DIETETICS of Naturopathic Medicine

PRINCIPLES of Naturopathic Medicine

PRACTICE of Naturopathic Medicine

PHYSICAL CULTURE in Naturopathic Medicine

HERBS in Naturopathic Medicine

WATER CURE in Naturopathic Medicine

MENTAL CULTURE in Naturopathic Medicine

VACCINATION in Naturopathic Medicine

CLINICAL PEARLS of Naturopathic Medicine, Vol. I

CLINICAL PEARLS of Naturopathic Medicine, Vol. II

From the NCNM Rare Book Collection On Natrual Medicine.
Published By NCNM Press, Portland, Oregon.

CPSIA information can be obtained at www.ICGtesting.com
Printed in the USA
BVOW07s1239240914

368095BV00001B/4/P